OPHTHO NOTES

The Essential Guide

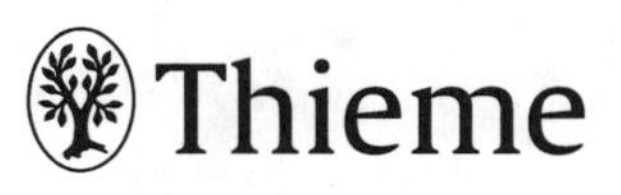

OPHTHO NOTES

The Essential Guide

Randall L. Goodman, M.D.

Chief of Ophthalmology
Mike O'Callaghan Federal Hospital
Las Vegas, Nevada

Thieme

New York · Stuttgart

Thieme New York
333 Seventh Avenue
New York, NY 10001

Consulting Medical Editor: Esther Gumpert
Assistant Editor: Owen Zurhellen
Director, Production and Manufacturing: Anne Vinnicombe
Production Editor: David R. Stewart
Marketing Director: Phyllis Gold
Director of Sales: Ross Lumpkin
Chief Financial Officer: Peter van Woerden
President: Brian D. Scanlan
Compositor: Thomson Press International
Printer: Sheridan Books, Inc.

Library of Congress Cataloging in Publication Data is available from the publisher

Important note: Medical knowledge is ever-changing. As new research and clinical experience broaden our knowledge, changes in treatment and drug therapy may be required. The authors and editors of the material herein have consulted sources believed to be reliable in their efforts to provide information that is complete and in accord with the standards accepted at the time of publication. However, in view of the possibility of human error by the authors, editors, or publisher of the work herein, or changes in medical knowledge, neither the authors, editors, or publisher, nor any other party who has been involved in the preparation of this work, warrants that the information contained herein is in every respect accurate or complete, and they are not responsible for any errors or omissions or for the results obtained from use of such information. Readers are encouraged to confirm the information contained herein with other sources. For example, readers are advised to check the product information sheet included in the package of each drug they plan to administer to be certain that the information contained in this publication is accurate and that changes have not been made in the recommended dose or in the contraindications for administration. This recommendation is of particular importance in connection with new or infrequently used drugs.

Printed in the United States of America

5 4 3 2 1

TNY ISBN 1-58890-171-8
GTV ISBN 3-13-135781-9

Contents

Foreword

Ophtho Notes: The Essential Guide is a compendium of ophthalmology knowledge and review subjects expressed in a concise and factual manner. As such, this work forms a useful clinical review for the resident as well as the practicing ophthalmologist.

From residency into clinical practice, ophthalmologists are deluged with large volumes of well-written basic science materials from experts in their respective fields. New residents in ophthalmology are sometimes overwhelmed with the depth and breadth of material that places them at risk of "missing the forest for the trees." While there is no substitute for mastering the basic sciences, residents may benefit from this pocket review, especially when under less than optimal clinical and time pressures as on morning rounds and during the weeks prior to exams.

This compendium may also serve a different but equally useful purpose in terms of providing a relevant, concise, and quick review for busy professionals in their clinical practice. In addition, medical students interested in a career in ophthalmology would find it a quick overview of basic materials.

While admittedly abbreviated and lacking scientific notations, the author has combined into one book not only his own accumulated notes from years of training and experience, but has attempted to expand it for even more completeness and value. The author also encourages the reader to consult references by leading authorities in the field, thereby having the option to add to or update the material from his or her own study.

With pleasure, I take this opportunity to commend Dr. Goodman for his effort to assist ophthalmologists in-training as well as clinical ophthalmologists through the communication and sharing of his collective ophthalmology notes.

HOWARD V. GIMBEL, M.D., M.P.H., F.R.C.S.C.
Gimbel Eye Centre
Calgary, Alberta, Canada

Preface

Like most medical review books of this type, *Ophtho Notes: The Essential Guide* grew out of years of collected knowledge from various sources. It began as jottings and notes compiled as a "peripheral brain" during residency. As additional material was assembled and collated, the notes began to take on the form of a small book that soon became more complete.

The book is organized into chapters largely based on anatomic areas of the eye. The chapter sequence begins anteriorly and proceeds posteriorly (e.g., orbit, cornea, retina, etc.), much like the succession of a thorough eye examination that begins externally and moves orderly through the eye tissues.

Each anatomic chapter is organized in a similar fashion. The first section of the chapter, Anatomy and Physiology, discusses pertinent basic science material for that area. Next, the Signs and Symptoms section records common differential diagnoses by presenting complaint or exam finding. The third section, Exam and Imaging, contains important exam skills and tests for that anatomic region. This sequence was chosen because this is generally how a patient is clinically approached: a good understanding of the basic sciences is needed first, then patient history is taken, followed by examination, then a diagnosis can be made.

Following the three opening sections, the greater part of each anatomic chapter discusses diseases of that region organized by etiology. Every disease is classified into one of the following sections: Congenital and Genetic Disease, Infectious Disease, Neoplastic Disease, Metabolic and Degenerative Disease, Systemic and Vascular Disease, Physical Disease (trauma, toxic, etc.), and Inflammatory and Immune Disease. Each anatomic chapter then ends with a Surgery section discussing relevant surgical techniques for that ocular area.

Because this organization is consistent throughout the anatomic chapters, ophthalmic diseases can be easily referenced. For example, retinoblastoma is discussed in the Retina and Vitreous chapter under the Neoplastic Disease section. However, the differential diagnosis for corneal edema (not a disease but a physical exam finding) is listed in the Signs and Symptoms section of the cornea chapter. Classifying disease by etiology allows better recollection and hopefully improved understanding of the material.

Several chapters do not lend themselves to anatomic organization. For example, the book begins with a General chapter that covers diverse topics such as genetics, optics, pathology, lasers, etc. Glaucoma is discussed following the cornea chapter because the inaugural pathology is in the anterior chamber angle. Glaucomatous diseases are classified based on whether they are congenital or primary or secondary and open or closed angle. Uveitis and intraocular inflammation precedes the Lens chapter because many uveitides involve the iris. After a brief discussion of the iris, the chapter classifies the uveitic diseases according to their primary presentation as anterior, intermediate, posterior, or panuveitis.

The Pediatrics and Strabismus chapter has an expanded Congenital and Genetic Disease section that chiefly discusses syndromes, phakomatoses, and other pediatric diseases not easily classified under a single anatomic chapter. However, most pediatric diseases are not discussed in this chapter and can be found based on their pathophysiology under the anatomic chapters (for example, as above, retinoblastoma is categorized in the neoplastic section of the retina chapter). Strabismic diseases are then organized into Esotropia, Exotropia, and Vertical Deviation sections. And lastly, the book ends with a chapter detailing common ophthalmic medications.

Because it is designed to be a concise review of ophthalmology, most subjects in *Ophtho Notes* are only briefly covered. Therefore the diagnostic, therapeutic, and practice recommendations contained in this work should be verified prior to use with information provided from an independent source and considered in light of a particular patient's clinical condition. The ultimate arbiter of any diagnostic or therapeutic decision remains the individual clinician who assumes full responsibility for all patient care.

This work comes to you largely without quotes or references, although many such acknowledgments could be made, and a number of sources could be credited. Most of the material in this book was gleaned from reading, lectures, and clinical experience. As such, I owe a particular debt of gratitude to the faculty and residents of the San Antonio Uniformed Services Health Education Consortium (SAUSH-EC) Ophthalmology Residency, San Antonio, Texas. Specifically, I am thankful for the contributions and review of the chapters by the following ophthalmologists: R. Gary Lane, M.D., Charles Reilly, M.D., David E.E. Holck, M.D. (oculoplastics); Daniel A. Johnson, M.D. (cornea); Erin Doe, M.D. (glaucoma and lens); J. Brian Reed, M.D. (uveitis and retina); Martha Schatz, M.D. (neuro-ophthalmology); and Mary O'Hara, M.D. (pediatrics and strabismus).

In addition, I thank Emil Sauer, a talented Las Vegas artist, who illustrated most of the figures. Lastly, the grace of God and the love and patient support of my wife, Karen, receive the lion's share of credit for making this work possible. I hope that you enjoy this book, and I welcome your comments or suggestions.

RANDALL L. GOODMAN, M.D.

List of Abbreviations

The following list contains the most common abbreviations used in this book.

Ab: antibody
ABK: aphakic bullous keratopathy
AC: anterior chamber
AC/A: accommodative convergence/accommodation (ratio)
ACAID: anterior chamber associated immune deviation
ACG: angle-closure glaucoma
ACh: acetylcholine
ACT: alternate cover test
Ag: antigen
AIC: adult inclusion conjunctivitis
AIDS: acquired immunodeficiency syndrome
AION: anterior ischemic optic neuropathy
AK: astigmatic keratotomy
AKC: atopic keratoconjunctivitis
ALK: automated lamellar keratoplasty
ALT: argon laser trabeculoplasty
AMD: age-related macular degeneration
AMPPE: acute multifocal placoid pigment epitheliopathy
ANA: antinuclear antibodies
ANCA: antineutrophil cytoplasmic antibodies
APD: afferent pupillary defect
ARC: anomalous retinal correspondence
ARN: acute retinal necrosis
ARPE: acute retinal pigment epitheliitis
ATR: against-the-rule (astigmatism)
AV: arteriovenous
AVM: arteriovenous malformation
BARN: bilateral acute retinal necrosis
BCC: basal cell carcinoma
BCVA: best corrected visual acuity

BI: base-in (prism)
BLRR: bilateral lateral rectus recession
BM: basement membrane
BMRR: bilateral medial rectus recession
BO: base-out (prism)
BRAO: branch retinal artery occlusion
BRVO: branch retinal vein occlusion
BSCL: bandage soft contact lens
BSS: balanced salt solution
CA: cancer
CACG: chronic angle-closure glaucoma
CAMP: cyclic adenosine monophosphate
CAR: cancer-associated retinopathy
CB: ciliary body
C:D: cup to disk (ratio)
CDCR: canaliculodacryocystorhinostomy
CE: cataract extraction
CHRPE: congenital hypertrophy of the retinal pigment epithelium
CIN: conjunctival intraepithelial neoplasia
CIS: carcinoma in situ
CJDCR: conjunctivodacryocystorhinostomy
CL: contact lens
CLW: contact lens wear
CME: cystoid macular edema
CMV: cytomegalovirus
CN: cranial nerve
CNVM: choroidal neovascular membrane
CPEO: chronic progressive external ophthalmoplegia
CPF: capsulopalpebral fascia
CRA: central retinal artery
CRAO: central retinal artery occlusion
CRVO: central retinal vein occlusion
CSM: central, steady, and maintained (visual acuity)
CSME: clinically significant macular edema
CSNB: congenital stationary night blindness
CT: cover test; computed tomography
CVOS: Central Vein Occlusion Study
CWS: cotton wool spot
CXR: chest x-ray
D: diopter
DCG: dacryocystography
DCR: dacryocystorhinostomy
DD: disk diameters

DDT: dye disappearance test
DFE: dilated fundus exam
DLK: diffuse lamellar keratitis
DME: diabetic macular edema
DR: diabetic retinopathy
DUSN: diffuse unilateral subacute neuroretinitis
DVD: dissociated vertical deviation
E: esophoria
EBMD: epithelial basement membrane dystrophy
ECCE: extracapsular cataract extraction
EIC: epidermal inclusion cyst
EKC: epidemic keratoconjunctivitis
ELISA: enzyme-linked immunosorbent assay
EOG: electro-oculogram
EOM: extraocular muscles
ERG: electroretinogram
ERM: epiretinal membrane
ESR: erythrocyte sedimentation rate
ET: esotropia
E(T): intermittent esotropia
EVP: episcleral venous pressure
FA: fluorescein angiogram
FAZ: foveal avascular zone
FBS: foreign body sensation
FEVR: familial exudative vitreoretinopathy
F/F: fix-and-follow (visual acuity)
FGX: fluid–gas exchange
FMG: focal macular grid
FTA-Abs: fluorescent treponemal antibody absorption test
FTWS: full-thickness wedge resection
5-FU: 5-fluorouracil
Fuchs' HIC: Fuchs' heterochromic iridocyclitis
GAG: glycosaminoglycans
GARPE: geographic atrophy of the retinal pigment epithelium
GCA: giant cell arteritis or temporal arteritis
GPC: giant papillary conjunctivitis
gtt: drop
GVHD: graft versus host disease
H: hyperphoria
H & E: hematoxylin and eosin (stain)
HAART: highly active antiretroviral therapy
HE: hard exudate
Hgb: hemoglobin

HIV: human immunodeficiency virus
HLA: human leukocyte antigen
HOF: herniated orbital fat
HPMG: hard palate mucosal graft
HPV: human papilloma virus
HST: horseshoe tear
HSV: herpes simplex virus
HT: hypertropia
HVF: Humphrey visual field
HZV: herpes zoster virus
ICCE: intracapsular cataract extraction
ICE: iridocorneal endothelial (syndrome)
ICG: indocyanine green
ICSR: idiopathic central serous retinopathy
Ig: immunoglobulin
IK: interstitial keratitis
ILM: internal limiting membrane
INO: intranuclear ophthalmoplegia
IO: inferior oblique (muscle)
IOF: inferior orbital fissure
IOFB: intraocular foreign body
IOL: intraocular lens
ION: ischemic optic neuropathy
IOO: inferior oblique overaction
IOP: intraocular pressure
IPD: interpupillary distance
IPE: iris pigment epithelium
IR: inferior rectus (muscle)
IRMA: intraretinal microvascular abnormality
ISS: inferior scleral show
JOAG: juvenile open-angle glaucoma
JPA: juvenile pilocytic astrocytoma
JRA: juvenile rheumatoid arthritis
JXG: juvenile xanthogranuloma
K: keratometry
KC: keratoconjunctivitis
KCS: keratoconjunctivitis sicca
KP: keratic precipitates
LASEK: laser-assisted in situ epithelial keratomileusis
LASIK: laser-assisted in situ keratomileusis
LF: levator function
LGN: lateral geniculate nucleus
LK: lamellar keratectomy

LN: latent nystagmus
LP: light perception (visual acuity)
LPI: laser peripheral iridotomy
LR: lateral rectus (muscle)
LTS: lateral tarsal strip (procedure)
Ma: microaneurysm
MCT: medial canthal tendon
MEN: multiple endocrine neoplasia
MEWDS: multiple evanescent white-dot syndrome
MG: myasthenia gravis
MGD: meibomian gland dysfunction
MHA-TP: microhemagglutination—*Treponema pallidum*
MLF: medial longitudinal fasciculus
MMC: mitomycin C
MMP: matrix metalloproteinase
MP: membrane peel
MPS: mucopolysaccharides
MR: medial rectus (muscle)
MRA: magnetic resonance angiography
MRI: magnetic resonance imaging
MS: multiple sclerosis
MTMT: maximal tolerated medical therapy
MVR: microvitreoretinal
NAION: nonarteritic anterior ischemic optic neuropathy
NAT: nonaccidental trauma
NBS: nystagmus blocking syndrome
NF: neurofibromatosis
NFL: nerve fiber layer
NLD: nasolacrimal duct
NLDO: nasolacrimal duct obstruction
NLP: no light perception (visual acuity)
NPC: near point of convergence
NPDR: nonproliferative diabetic retinopathy
NRC: normal retinal correspondence
NTG: normal tension glaucoma
NV: neovascularization
NVA: neovascularization of the angle
NVD: neovascularization of the disk
NVE: neovascularization elsewhere
NVG: neovascular glaucoma
NVI: neovascularization of the iris
OA: ocular albinism
OAG: open-angle glaucoma

OCP: ocular cicatricial pemphigoid
OCT: optical coherence tomography
OD: right eye (L. *oculus dexter*)
OHS: ocular histoplasmosis syndrome
OHT: ocular hypertension
OKN: optokinetic nystagmus
OIS: ocular ischemic syndrome
ON: optic nerve
ONH: optic nerve hypoplasia
ONSD: optic nerve sheath decompression
OPL: outer plexiform layer
OS: left eye (L. *oculus sinister*)
OU: both eyes
PACG: primary angle-closure glaucoma
PAM: primary acquired melanosis
PAS: peripheral anterior synechiae
PBK: pseudophakic bullous keratopathy
PC: posterior chamber
PCA: posterior communicating artery
PCO: posterior capsule opacification
pD: prism diopters
PD: pupillary distance
PDG: pigment dispersion glaucoma
PDR: proliferative diabetic retinopathy
PDS: pigment dispersion syndrome
PDT: photodynamic therapy
PED: pigment epithelial detachment
PEE: punctate epithelial erosions
PEK: punctate epithelial keratitis
PF: palpebral fissure
PFV: persistent fetal vasculature
PHPV: persistent hyperplastic primary vitreous
PI: peripheral iridectomy
PIC: punctate inner choroidopathy
PION: posterior ischemic optic neuropathy
PIP: pseudoisochromatic plates
PK: penetrating keratoplasty
PMB: papulomacular bundle
PMMA: polymethylmethacrylate
PO: by mouth, orally (L. *per os*)
POAG: primary open-angle glaucoma
PPA: peripapillary atrophy
PPMD: posterior polymorphous membrane dystrophy

PPRF: paramedian pontine reticular formation
PRK: photorefractive keratectomy
prn: as circumstances may require (L. *pro re nata*)
PRP: panretinal photocoagulation
PSC: posterior subcapsular (cataract)
PTC: pseudotumor cerebri
PTK: phototherapeutic keratectomy
PUK: peripheral ulcerative keratitis
PVD: posterior vitreous detachment
PVR: proliferative vitreoretinopathy
PXG: pseudoexfoliative glaucoma
PXS: pseudoexfoliation syndrome
qd: every day
qid: four times a day
RA: rheumatoid arthritis
RB: retinoblastoma
RCE: recurrent corneal erosion
RD: retinal detachment
RF: rheumatoid factor; radio frequency
RGP: rigid gas-permeable contact lens
RK: radial keratotomy
ROP: retinopathy of prematurity
RP: retinitis pigmentosa
RPB: relative pupillary block
RPE: retinal pigment epithelium
R & R: resect and recess (strabismus surgery)
RRD: rhegmatogenous retinal detachment
SAC: seasonal allergic conjunctivitis
SBP: scleral buckle procedure
SC: sickle cell (disease)
SCC: squamous cell carcinoma
SCL: soft contact lens
SEI: subepithelial infiltrate
SiO: silicone oil
SJS: Stevens-Johnson syndrome
SLD: staphylococcal lid disease
SLK: superior limbal keratoconjunctivitis
SMAS: superficial musculoaponeurotic system
SO: superior oblique (muscle)
SOAG: secondary open-angle glaucoma
SOF: superior orbital fissure
SOO: superior oblique overaction
SOOF: suborbicularis oculi fascia

SPCT: simultaneous prism cover test
SPK: superficial punctate keratitis
SR: superior rectus (muscle)
SRF: subretinal fluid
SS: scleral spur
STK: sub-Tenon's Kenalog
SVP: spontaneous venous pulsation
TAB: temporal artery biopsy
TBUT: tear break-up time
TIA: transient ischemic attack
tid: three times a day
TID: transillumination defect
TM: trabecular meshwork
TON: traumatic optic neuropathy
TRD: tractional retinal detachment
TRIO: thyroid-related immune orbitopathy
TSH: thyroid-stimulating hormone
TTT: transpupillary thermotherapy
TVO: transient visual obscurations
UGH: uveitis-glaucoma-hyphema (syndrome)
UV: ultraviolet (light)
VA: visual acuity
VDRL: Venereal Disease Research laboratory test
VEGF: vascular endothelial cell growth factor
VEP: visual evoked potential
VF: visual field
VH: vitreous hemorrhage
VKC: vernal keratoconjunctivitis
VKH: Vogt-Koyanagi-Harada disease
VMT: vitreomacular traction
VOR: vestibulo-ocular reflex
W4D: Worth four-dot test
WEBINO: wall-eyed bilateral intranuclear ophthalmoplegia
WTR: with-the-rule (astigmatism)
WWP: white without pressure
X: exophoria
XLD: X-linked dominant
XLR: X-linked recessive
XT: exotropia
X(T): intermittent exotropia

CHAPTER 1

General Topics in Ophthalmology

Approach to the Patient: Exam and History

- History: demographics, referring doctor, chief complaint, history of present illness, past ocular history, ocular medications, past medical and surgical history, medications and allergies, family history
- External and orbit: inspection, palpation, lymph nodes, skin, interpupillary distance, exophthalmometry, globe displacement, eyelid position, lid eversion, Schirmer's testing
- Visual acuity (VA): distance with and without correction, pinhole, near acuity, stereopsis, color, contrast, retinoscopy, cycloplegia, refraction, lensometry, prescription
- Visual fields: confrontation, Amsler's grid, Goldmann or Humphrey automated perimetry
- Motility: ductions, versions, Hirschberg's test, cover tests
- Pupils: shape, size and reactivity, swinging flashlight testing for APD
- Slit lamp examination: lids/lacrimal/lashes, conjunctiva/sclera, cornea, anterior chamber (AC), iris, lens, gonioscopy, fundus biomicroscopy
- Tonometry: applanation, time of day
- Dilated fundus examination: disk/macula/vessels/periphery, direct and indirect ophthalmoscopy, scleral depression, color drawings, photos, fluorescein angiography, ultrasound
- Assessment, plan, counseling: in general, all ophthalmology problems are problems with either optics or anatomy. Attempt to stratify disease into typical versus atypical: if typical, then treat typically or observe; if atypical, then do full work-up.

Embryology and Development

NEURAL ECTODERM Derived from the folds of the neural plate and forms the optic vesicle and cup. Gives rise to the retinal pigment epithelium (RPE), iris sphincter and dilator muscles, iris pigment epithelium (IPE), the pigmented and nonpigmented ciliary epithelium, and the optic nerve (ON).

SURFACE ECTODERM Forms lens, corneal epithelium, lacrimal gland, epidermis of the lids, and epithelium of the adnexal glands and conjunctiva.

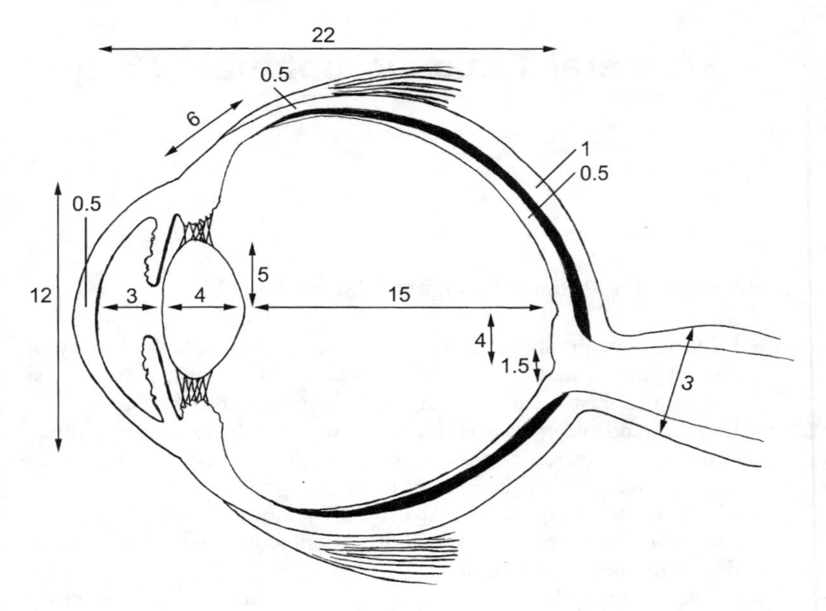

Figure 1–1 Average eye measurements in millimeters.

NEURAL CREST Forms most connective tissues of the eye and its adnexal structures. Gives rise to the corneal keratocytes and endothelium of the cornea and trabecular meshwork (TM), the iris and choroidal stroma (pigmented and nonpigmented cells), the ciliary smooth muscle, the fibroblasts of the sclera, and the ON meninges. Also forms orbital fibroadipose tissues, the satellite cells of the extraocular striated muscles, the pericytes of the vascular channels of the orbit, the orbital nerves (including the trigeminal ganglion) and associated Schwann's cells, and the orbital cartilage and bone.

MESODERM Contributes very little to the head and neck mesenchyme through the somites. Forms the striated extraocular muscles, vascular endothelia, and circulating blood elements.

EYE MEASUREMENTS See Figure 1–1.

Emergencies

IMMEDIATE INTERVENTION Chemical burns, central retinal artery occlusion, orbital hemorrhage.

URGENT ATTENTION Endophthalmitis, orbital cellulitis, globe laceration or intraocular foreign body (IOFB), macula-on RD, acute glaucoma.

Epidemiology/Statistics

LEADING CAUSES OF BLINDNESS Cataract, glaucoma, and trachoma account for more than 70% of cases of blindness throughout the world. The leading cause of pediatric blindness is xerophthalmia from vitamin A deficiency. Other leading causes include onchocerciasis, ocular trauma, bacterial and fungal keratitis, leprosy, diabetes mellitus, and age-related maculopathy.

POPULATION STATISTICS For a normal bell curve, one standard deviation above and below the mean includes 66% of the observed population; two standard deviations above and below the mean encompass 95%; three standard deviations above and below the mean include 99% of the population.

STATISTICAL TESTING The *p* value is the probability that the null hypothesis, if true, will be rejected.

- Posttest probability: Bayes' theorem
- Sensitivity = true positives ÷ total with disease. Describes how good the test is to find disease; thus, a good screening test has high sensitivity.
- Specificity = true negatives ÷ total without disease. Describes how good the test is to rule out disease; thus, a good confirmatory test has high specificity.
- Type 1 error: rejecting a null hypothesis that is in fact true; the probability of commiting a type 1 error is designated as α, which is conventionally 0.05 for most studies.
- Type 2 error: failing to reject a false null hypothesis or chance effect cannot be ruled out (often from inadequate sample size). The chance of a type 2 error, or missing a specified difference should it exist, is designated as β and is often 0.10. The power of a study is the complement of β or 1 − type 2 error.

Genetics

See Table 1–1 for a list of selected heritable ocular disorders with known genetic mutations.

TABLE 1–1
Selected Heritable Ocular Disorders with Known Genetic Mutations

Condition	Gene	Locus
Anterior Segment Conditions		
Aniridia	*PAX6*	11p13
Avellino dystrophy	β*ig-h3*	5q31
Axenfeld-Rieger anomaly	FKHL7	6p25
Corneal dystrophy, granular (CDGG1)	β*ig-h3*	5q31
Corneal dystrophy, Meesmann	K3	12q12–q13
	K12	17q12–q21
Cornea plana congenita (CNA1 and CNA2)		12q21
Iridogoniodysgenesis anomaly (IRID1)		6p25
Iridogoniodysgenesis syndrome (iris hypoplasia)	*RIEG1*	4q25
Lattice corneal dystrophy (LCD1)	β*ig-h3*	5q31
Macular corneal dystrophy		16q22
Megalocornea (X-linked)		Xq12–q26
Microcoria		13q31–q32
Peters' anomaly	*PAX6*	11p13
	PITX2	4q25
Posterior polymorphous dystrophy		20q11
Reis-Buckler (CDRB)	β*ig-h3*	5q31
Rieger syndrome, type 1	*RIEG1*	4q25
Rieger syndrome, type 2		13q14
Schnyder's crystalline corneal dystrophy		1p36–p34.1
Lens Disorders		
Cataract, anterior polar 1 (CTAA1)		14q24–qter
Cataract, anterior polar 2 (CTAA2)		17p13
Cataract, cerulean type I (CCA1)		17q24
Cataract, cerulean type II (CCA2)	*CRYBB2*	22q11.2–q12.2
Cataract, congenital total		Xp
Cataract, dominant, congenital	*CRYGA*	21q22.3
Cataract, Coppock-like (CCL)	*CRYGA*	2q33–q35
Cataract, Marner type (CAM)		16q22.1
Cataract, posterior polar (CPP)		Lpter–p36.1
Cataract, Volkmann type		1p36
Cataract, dominant, zonular pulverulant (CZP)	GJA3	13q11–q12

TABLE 1–1 (*Continued*)

Selected Heritable Ocular Disorders with Known Genetic Mutations

Condition	Gene	Locus
Cataract, lamellar, zonular pulverulant, Coppock	GJA8	1q21.1
Cataract, zonular with sutural opacity (CCZS)		17q11–q12
Ectopia lentis, simple	Fibrillin	15q21.1
Primary Glaucomas		
Glaucoma, adult onset POAG (GLC1B)		2cen–q13
Glaucoma, adult onset POAG (GLC1C)		3q21–q24
Glaucoma, adult onset POAG (GLC1D)		8q23
Glaucoma, adult onset POAG (GLC1E)		10p15–p14
Glaucoma, open angle, juvenile onset (GLC1A)	Myocillin	1q23–q25
Glaucoma, primary infantile (GLC3A)	CYP1B1	2p21
Glaucoma, primary infantile (GLC3B)		1p36
Glaucoma, pigment dispersion type		7q35–q36
Vitreoretinopathies		
Familial exudative vitreoretinopathy (EVR1)	Norrin	11q13–q23
FEVR X-linked (EVR2)		Xp11.4–p11.23
Myopia, Bornholm eye disease, X-linked		Xq28
Neovascular inflammatory vitreoretinopathy		11q13
Norrie disease	Norrin	Xp11.4–p11.23
Primary retinal dysplasia, X-linked (PRD)	Norrin	Xp11.4–p11.23
Retinoschisis (RS)	XLRS1	Xp22.2–p22.1
Stickler's syndrome, type I (STL1)	COL2A1	12q13.1–p13.3
Stickler's syndrome, type II (STL2)	COL11A2	6p22–p21.3
Wagner syndrome type 1 (WGN1)		5p14.3
Wagner syndrome type 2 (WGN2)	COL2A1	12q13.11
Retinal Disorders		
Achromatopsia 1	CNGA3	14
Achromatopsia 2		2q11
Achromatopsia 3		8q21–q22
Albinism		
Oculocutaneous, OCA1-A (tyrosinase −)	Tyrosinase	11q14–q21
Oculocutaneous, OCA1-B (yellow)	Tyrosinase	11q14–q21
Oculocutaneous, OCA2 (tyrosinase +)	P	15q11.2–q12

(*Continued*)

TABLE 1–1 (*Continued*)

Selected Heritable Ocular Disorders with Known Genetic Mutations

Condition	Gene	Locus
Oculocutaneous, OCA3 (brown)	TYRP-1	9p23–p22
Chédiak-Higashi syndrome (CHS1)	LYST	1q42.1–q42.2
Hermansky-Pudlak syndrome (HPS)	Transmembrane protein	10q23.1–q23.3
Ocular albinism, OA1 (Nettleship-Falls)	OA1	Xp22.3
Ocular albinism, OA2 (Åland eye dis.)		Xp11.4–p11.23
Ocular albinism with sensorineural deafness		Xp22.3
Atrophia areata (helicoid chorioretinal degen.)		11p15
Bardet-Biedl syndrome, BBS 1		11q13
Bardet-Biedl syndrome, BBS 2		16q21
Bardet-Biedl syndrome, BBS 3		3p13–p12
Bardet-Biedl syndrome, BBS 4		15q22.2–q23
Bardet-Biedl syndrome, BBS 5		2q31
Central areolar choroidal dystrophy		17p
Choroideremia	REP1	Xq21.1–q21.3
Color vision defects		
Blue cone monochromacy (CBBM)	Red, green genes	Xq28
Deuteranopia	Green genes	Xq28
Dominant tritanopia	Blue genes	7q31.3–q32
Protanopia	Red genes	Xq28
Cone dystrophies		
Cone dystrophy, dominant (COD3)	GUCA1A	6p21.1
Retinal cone dystrophy 1 (RCD1)		6q25-q26
Retinal cone dystrophy 2 (RCD2)	Recoverin	17p13.1
XL progressive cone dystrophy (COD1)		Xp11.4
XL progressive cone dystrophy (COD2)		Xq27
Cone rod dystrophy, CORD 1		18q21.1–q21.3
Cone rod dystrophy, CORD 2	CRX	19q13.1–q13.4
Cone rod dystrophy, CORD 3	ABCR	1p21–p13
Cone rod dystrophy, CORD 5		17p13–p12
Cone rod dystrophy, CORD 6	GUC2D	17p13
Cone rod dystrophy, CORD 7		6cen–q14
Congenital stationary night blindness		
Oguchi's disease, RHOK-related	RHOK	13q34
Oguchi's disease, SAG-related	Arrestin (SAG)	2q37.1
CSNB 1		Xp11

TABLE 1–1 (*Continued*)

Selected Heritable Ocular Disorders with Known Genetic Mutations

Condition	Gene	Locus
CSNB 2	CACNA1F	Xp11.23
CSNB 3, PDE6B-related	PDE6B	4p16.3
CSNB 4, RHO-related	RHO	3q21–q24
CSNB, Nougaret	GNATI	3p21
Doyne's honeycombed retinal dystrophy	EFEMP1	2p16
Gyrate atrophy	OAT	10q26
Leber's congenital amaurosis, LCA 1	GUC2D	17p13
Leber's congenital amaurosis, LCA 2	RPE65	1p31
Leber's congenital amaurosis, LCA 3	CRX	19q13.3
Macular dystrophies		
Macular dystrophy, age-related (ARMD1)	ABCR	1q25–q31
Macular dystrophy, age-related (ARMD2)	RDS/peripherin	1p21–p13
Macular dystrophy, peripherin-related		6p21.2–p11.2
Macular dystrophy, dominant cystoid		7p21–p15
North Carolina macular dystrophy (MCDR1)		6q14–q16.2
Progressive bifocal chorioretinal atrophy	TIMP3	6q14–q16.2
Sorsby's fundus dystrophy	*ABCR*	22q13–qter
Stargardt's disease, STGD 1		1p21–p13
Stargardt's disease, STGD 2		13q34
Stargardt's disease, STGD 3		6cen–q14
Stargardt's disease, STGD 4		4p–1q13
Vitelliform macular dystrophy (Best's)	VMD21	11q13
Retinoblastoma	p100	13q14
Retinitis pigmentosa		
Digenic RP (ROM/RDS)	RDS/peripherin	6p21.2–p11.2
Over 10 autosomal recessive genes	Arrestin, ROM1, etc.	2q37, 11q13, etc.
Over 10 autosomal dominant genes		1p21–p13, etc.
At least 5 X-linked genes identified	ABCR, etc.	Xp21, etc.
Mitochondrial RP	RPGR, etc.	mtDNA
Usher's syndrome, USH 1A	MTTS2	14q32
Usher's syndrome, USH 1B		11q13.5
Usher's syndrome, USH 1C	Myosin 7A	11p15.1
Usher's syndrome, USH 1D		10q
Usher's syndrome, USH 1E		21q21

(*Continued*)

TABLE 1–1 (*Continued*)

Selected Heritable Ocular Disorders with Known Genetic Mutations

Condition	Gene	Locus
Usher's syndrome, USH 1F		10
Usher's syndrome, USH 2A		1q41
Usher's syndrome, USH 2B		not 1q
Usher's syndrome, USH 3		3q21–q25
Retinitis punctata albescens	RDS / peripherin	6p21.2–p11.2
	RHO	3q21–q24
	RDH5	12q13–q14
	RLBP1	15q26
Optic Nerve Disorders		
Coloboma of ON with renal disease (ONCR)	*PAX2*	10q24.3–q25.1
Dominant optic atrophy, Kjer type (OPA1)		3q27–q28
Leber's hereditary optic neuropathy		MtDNA
X-linked optic atrophy (OPA2)		Xp11.4–Xp11.2
Lid Disorders		
Blepharophimosis syndrome, BPES1		3q22–q23
Blepharophimosis syndrome, BPES2		7p21–p13
Congenital ptosis, dominant		1p34.1–p32
Eye Movement Disorders		
Congenital fibrosis of extraocular muscles 1		12p11.2–q12
Congenital fibrosis of extraocular muscles 2		11q13.2
Congenital fibrosis of extraocular muscles 3		16q24.2–q24.3
Kearns-Sayre syndrome		MtDNA
Progressive external ophthalmoplegia 1 (PEO1)		10q23.3–q24.3
Progressive external ophthalmoplegia 2 (PEO2)		3p21.2–p14.1
Progressive external ophthalmoplegia 3		4q
Nystagmus, dominant congenital		6p12
Nystagmus, X-linked congenital		Xq26–q27
Ocular Development Disorders		
Anophthalmos, X-linked		Xq27–q28
Holoprosencephaly	SIX3	2q21
Microphthalmia		14q32
Microphthalmia with linear skin defects (NILS)		Xp22

TABLE 1–1 (*Continued*)
Selected Heritable Ocular Disorders with Known Genetic Mutations

Condition	Gene	Locus
Myopia 2 (MYP2)		18p11.31
Myopia 3 (MYP3)		12q21–q23
Nanophthalmos		11p
Selected Systemic Disorders with Ocular Findings		
Abetalipoproteinemia	MTP	4q22–q24
Alagille syndrome	JAG1	20p12
Alport's syndrome (autosomal recessive)	COL4A4	2q35–q37
Alport's syndrome (X-linked)	COL4A5	Xq22–q24
Ataxia-telangiectasia	ATM	11q22–q23
Gardner's syndrome	APC	5q21–q22
Incontinentia pigmenti (type I)		Xp11.21
Incontinentia pigmenti (type II)		Xq28
Lowe's oculocerebrorenal syndrome	InsP-ase	Xq24–q26
Marfan syndrome	Fibrillin	15q21.1
Multiple endocrine neoplasia (type II A and B)	RET	10q11.2
Myotonic dystrophy	Myotonin	19q13.2–q13.2
	DM2	3q
Neurofibromatosis (NF1)	Neurofibromin	17q11.2
Neurofibromatosis (NF2)	Schwannomin	22q12.2
Neuronal ceroid lipofuscinosis		
Infantile (CLN1)	Palmitoyl-thioesterase	5p32
Classic late infantile (CLN2)		11p15.5
Juvenile, Batten disease (CLN3)	CLN2	16p12.1
Variant late infantile (CLN5)	CLN3	13q21.1–q32
Variant late infantile (CLN6)	CLN5	15q21–q23
Oculodentodigital dysplasia (ODDD)		6q22–q23
Oculopharyngeal muscular dystrophy	PAPB2	14q11.2–q13
Osteoporosis-pseudoglioma syndrome (OPS)		11q12–q13
Refsum's disease with increased pipecolic acid		10p
Renal-coloboma syndrome	PAX2	10q24.3–q25.1
Spinocerebellar ataxia with muscular dystrophy	SCA7	3p21.1–p12
Tuberous sclerosis 1	TSC1	9q34
Tuberous sclerosis 2	TSC2 (tuberin)	16p13.3

(*Continued*)

TABLE 1–1 (*Continued*)
Selected Heritable Ocular Disorders with Known Genetic Mutations

Condition	Gene	Locus
von Hippel-Lindau disease (VHL)	Transmembrane protein	3p24-p25
Waardenburg's syndrome, WS1	PAX3	2q35
Waardenburg's syndrome, WS2A	MITF	3p14.1–p12.3
Waardenburg's syndrome, WS2B		1p21–p13.3
Waardenburg-Klein syndrome, WS3	PAX3	2q35
Waardenburg-Shaw syndrome, WS4	SOX10, etc.	22q13, etc.
Wilson's disease	P-type ATPase	13q14.3
Wolfram syndrome	WFS1	4p16 or mtDNA
Zellweger syndrome	PEX2, etc.	7p11.23

Imaging: Computed Tomography (CT)

MECHANISM OF ACTION X-ray beams are attenuated according to the tissue density; gives excellent bony detail. Array of thin collimated x-ray beams in rows and columns (voxel = volume where beams intersect). Hounsfield unit is value assigned to each voxel from exiting attenuated beams from rows/columns (+1000 to −1000). 'Window' stipulates narrow range of Hounsfield unit to enhance resolution of specific tissue (bone, soft tissue, etc.).

INDICATIONS

- Orbital trauma (suspected fractures or foreign bodies)
- Infectious or noninfectious orbital inflammation
- Ocular trauma to rule out foreign body (severe ruptured globe in which clinical exam or B-scan may cause additional disruption)
- Bone lesions (osteoma, fibrous dysplasia, suspected metastatic disease, etc.)
- Preoperative imaging for orbital decompression (TRIO)
- Lesions that may contain calcium (retinoblastoma, orbital varices, ON drusen, etc.)
- Lacrimal gland lesions

ALWAYS ORDER

- CT of orbits and sinuses, including cavernous sinus

- Axial and direct coronal views (if direct coronal views are not available, then order coronal reconstructions)
- Soft tissue and bone windows

ADDITIONAL CONSIDERATIONS

- For routine studies, 3 mm cuts are usually adequate (order 1.5 mm axial cuts if coronal reconstructions are needed).
- For suspected foreign body or traumatic optic neuropathy, order 1.0 to 1.5 mm cuts.
- For loss of consciousness or suspected intracranial trauma, also order CT of brain. Remember to clear the cervical spine.
- For suspected vascular lesions, infections, or inflammations (orbital pseudotumor, etc.), also order intravenous (IV) contrast (always will see contrast in sinus mucosa in CT and magnetic resonance imaging [MRI]).

Imaging: Magnetic Resonance Imaging (MRI)

MECHANISM OF ACTION A signal is generated with a particular frequency when protons in a magnetic field are exposed to a radio frequency pulse, usually 1.5 tesla coils (1 tesla = 10,000 gauss, or 1 in 1 million protons are aligned). Protons are spinning with a "north" and "south" pole and are randomly aligned (net vector force = 0). In a magnetic field, the hydrogen atoms mostly align with the axis of the magnetic field. Each proton has spin and precess, or "wobble," like a spinning top, with a relationship between the spin and the magnet (Larmor's equation: precess frequency = gyro mag ratio × field strength).

- Radio frequency (RF) is applied 90 degrees away from the magnetic axis, and hydrogen protons that are precessing (1 in 1 million) change orientation to resonate at that frequency. When the RF signal is turned off, the protons graduallly reorient to the magnet, emitting a signal. Signals deteriorate at different times for different tissues. Transverse relaxation time (T2) is the time to loss of phase coherence (decay), and longitudinal relaxation time (T1) is the time to reorient (recovery). Tissues with a shorter T1 time constant (e.g., fat) give off more energy and appear brighter. Tissues with a longer T2 time constant (e.g., vitreous) give off more energy and appear brighter; T2 is always shorter than T1.
- Signals of T1 and T2 have same frequency, but the spin (RF signal) to echo (listen) varies and is termed TE. TR is the time to RF. T1 has short TR and TE and causes pulses to repeat prior to tissue returning to equilibrium to maximum T1 signals. T2 has long TR and TE and allows time for water signals to show up. Proton density: T2 with long TR and short TE.

- Fluid-attenuated inversion recovery (FLAIR) and fast spin echo (FSE) optimization allow a faster study. Slice generated by gradient magnetic field to select specific precessional frequency.

INDICATIONS

- Optic neuritis (obtain MRI of brain)
- Central nervous system (CNS) pathology (pituitary lesions, occipital lobe lesions, aneurysms)
- Cavernous sinus/orbital apex pathology
- ON glioma or sheath meningioma (parasagittal views and gadolinium are especially important)
- Suspected lymphangioma (no gadolinium)
- Suspected ON sheath hemorrhage
- Wooden foreign bodies
- Suspected fungal sinusitis

ALWAYS ORDER

- MRI of orbits and sinuses, including cavernous sinus
- Axial, coronal, and parasagittal views
- Fat suppression (ask for specific techniques available)
- Gadolinium: paramagnetic agent, shortens T1 relaxation time (do not order gadolinium if short-tau inversion recovery [STIR], an older type of fat suppression, is used)

ADDITIONAL CONSIDERATIONS

- Vitreous is dark in T1 and bright in T2, and orbital fat is bright in T1 and dark in T2.
- With fat suppression (T1), vitreous and orbital fat will appear dark, but the muscles will be bright.
- The majority of orbital tumors will be dark in T1, but most orbital tumors will be bright in T1 once gadolinium is injected.
- To see the ON on the films, find the clinoids, as they are at level of the ON.

LESIONS THAT MAY APPEAR BRIGHT IN T1 WITHOUT GADOLINIUM

- Lesions containing fat (dermoids, liposarcoma, etc.)
- Subacute hemorrhage: lymphangioma, varix, orbital hemorrhage, hematic cyst, hemorrhagic choroidal detachments (acute blood < 3 days is dark in T1)
- Lesions containing mucus: mucocele, mucinous adenocarcinoma, dacryocystocele, dermoids
- Tumors containing melanin (e.g., melanoma), certain types of fungal sinusitis, mascara on the lids

Immune System/Inflammation

INFLAMMATION The eye is an immunoprivileged site with special relationship to the immune system (no lymphatics as in the CNS, but with residual ocular cells, such as Müller's, RPE, and Langerhans' cells, which have immunofunction).

- Acute reactions are mediated by neutrophils (exudative response); chronic reactions are mediated by lymphocytes (proliferative response) or plasma cells (B cells). Three stages of acute reactions:
    - Vascular dilation, change in flow, and increased permeability
    - Cellular margination, emigration, attachment, and ingestion
    - Humoral responses, especially interleukin-1 and interleukin-6, increase vascular permeability
- Chronic inflammation may be granulomatous (T lymphocytes, histiocytes, epithelioid cells) or nongranulomatous (B cell mediated).
    - Granulomatous reactions may be diffuse (e.g., sympathetic ophthalmia and Vogt-Koyanagi-Harada syndrome [VKH]), focal (sarcoid, tuberculosis), or zonal (foreign body reactions, phacoanaphylaxis).

HYPERSENSITIVITY REACTIONS The Greek word *atopy*, meaning "out of place," is used to define an inappropriate response to allergen. Five types (mnemonic ACIDS):

- **A**naphylaxis: type 1 hypersensitivity with immediate IgE-mediated response to allergen. Common allergic reactions to pollens, dust, and danders. Upon the initial exposure, the allergen binds to IgE on the mast cell and "cocks the pistol" awaiting the next exposure. The subsequent exposure to the allergen causes a dramatic release of cyclic adenosine monophosphate (cAMP) in the cell membrane, stimulating membrane arachidonic acid metabolism to mediators such as kinins, leukotrienes, and prostaglandins. Also causes increased tubulin production for microtubules to guide the degranulation of vasoactive amines (i.e., histamines). Treatment of this type of allergy is often aimed at treating the mast cell.
- **C**ytotoxic: type 2 allergic reaction from cell-to-cell interaction.
- **I**mmune-complex: type 3 hypersensitivity from B cell antibody production. Treat the B cells (Cytoxan, etc.).
- **D**elayed hypersensitivity: type 4 reaction.
- **S**timulating antibodies: type 5 reaction (e.g., antibodies that stimulate interleukin-12 production).

Optics

ABERRATIONS Lower order aberrations (sphere and cylinder) are the most common; when corrected, they usually give the patient excellent vision.

Higher order optic aberrations are pupil size dependent: the smaller the pupil size, the more the vision is diffraction limited. Wavefront sensors such as the Hartmann-Shack identify higher order aberrations of the eye.

- Astigmatism of oblique incidence: tilting a spherical lens produces astigmatism. An undercorrected myope may tilt spectacles by raising the temples to gain increased minus sphere and minus cylinder in the axis of tilt.
- Chromatic aberration: blue/green rays are refracted more than red (about 1.5 D difference in the eye).
- Spherical aberration: peripheral rays passing through a lens are refracted more (thus larger pupil size may induce myopia).
- Stiles-Crawford effect: the retina is most sensitive to light rays striking it directly perpendicular (thus one reason that a pinhole provides a sharper image as it collimates light rays). As the pupil size increases, the number of tangential rays, and thus visual distortion, also increases.

ACQUIRED HYPEROPIA

- Decreased refractive power
  - Lenticular: aphakia, posterior lens dislocation
  - Weak accommodation: Adie's tonic pupil, trauma, chloroquine, phenothiazines, antihistamines, benzodiazepines, marijuana
- Decreased axial length (retina pushed forward): central serous retinopathy, tumor (choroidal melanoma or hemangioma), retrobulbar orbital mass

ACQUIRED MYOPIA

- Increased refractive power
  - Lenticular changes: cataract, diabetes, and retinopathy of prematurity
  - Anterior lens displacement: ciliary muscle pushed forward (toxemia of pregnancy, chlorthalidone, miotics, sulfonamides, tetracycline, carbonic anhydrase inhibitors) or anterior lens dislocation
  - Increased ciliary muscle tone: antihistamines, excessive accommodation, inadequate fogging with refraction
  - Increased cornea power: keratoconus, infantile glaucoma
- Increased axial length: infantile glaucoma, posterior staphyloma

ANISOMETROPIA Patients may have reading complaints or feel as if eyes are crossing, usually after cataract extraction with anisometropia. Patients usually can tolerate up to 1.5 D difference, but if they have more anisometropia, then the minus lens may induce base-down prism in reading position. Thus, check vision with a base-up prism to correct the induced phoria, and consider prescribing "slab off" for that amount.

CONTACT LENSES Write prescription as base curve/diameter/power. Base curve stated in millimeters (use 0.3375/radius of cornea curvature in meters to get diopters of cornea power). Bifocal contact lens: push −0.50 far and +0.25 near, only 1 base curve and diameter.

DECREASED VA EVEN AFTER REFRACTION Try to pinhole over manifest refraction, refine with high-power Jackson cross-cylinder, and improve eye chart contrast. Many causes (cataract, dry eye, retinal disorders, etc.).

GLASSES COMPLAINTS

- Check glasses: axis/power/compare base curve (Geneva lens clock); look for prism (ground in or unintentional shift in optical center); check glasses frame, astigmatic grinding front versus back surface, coating/tints.
- Bifocals: check segment height (best if level with lower lid), design (progressive; Varilux is different), power.
- Refraction: sphere; consider cycloplegic refraction, any change in cylinder, and refractive change such as cataract.

HEADACHE AND ASTHENOPIA Cover test to rule out phoria; check for prism, cycloplegic refraction (latent hyperopia, etc.), accommodation (early presbyopia, etc.).

OPHTHALMIC INSTRUMENTS

- Direct ophthalmoscope: uses the optics of the eye as a simple magnifier (14×) but has limited field of view (5–7 degrees).
- Geneva lens clock: measures the radius of curvature of spectacle lenses (most are calibrated for crown glass). May use for patient dissatisfied with new spectacles to measure the base curvature and determine front versus back surface cylinder.
- Gonioscopy: mirrored contact lens designed to overcome the total internal reflection of the anterior chamber at the tear-air interface. Total internal reflection occurs when the incidence angle of light rays exceeds the critical angle, and all light is reflected inward (e.g., light leaving the AC angle). Governed by Snell's law, which says that from a lower to higher index of refraction, light bends toward the normal, giving a tear-air critical angle = 48.6 degrees.
- Indirect ophthalmoscope: the illumination system uses mirrors to place the light source close to the examiner's pupils (nearly coaxial) and passes through a handheld condensing lens that forms an inverted aerial image between the examiner and the lens.
- Keratometer: determines corneal curvature by measuring the size of a reflected mire. Diopter scale is derived from the radius scale: $D = (n - 1)/r$, where $n = 1.3373$.

TABLE 1–2
Characteristics of Selected Diagnostic Lenses

Lens and Power	Magnification	Field	Image	Comment
Hruby (−55 D)	12×	10 degrees	Upright, virtual	
Goldmann contact lens (−64 D)	10×	20 degrees	Upright, virtual	Mirrors to view angle and retinal periphery
20 D	3×	45 degrees	Inverted	12 mm view, 400 μm spot
30 D	2×	50 degrees	Inverted	400 μm spot
78 D	10×	30 degrees	Inverted	
90 D	7.5×	40 degrees	Inverted	High plus

- Lensometer: measures the power of a lens. Based on the optometer principle, which allows the dial to be linear (i.e., dial moves the same amount whether from 1 to 2 D or from 8 to 9 D, etc.). This works by placing the unknown lens at the primary focal point of a "standard" plus lens, then moving the illuminated target to the secondary focal point.
- Retinoscope: detects the far point of the eye. The neutralized meridian is perpendicular (and axis is parallel) to the streak orientation. When the light reflection is neutralized, the far point of the eye is at the retinoscope peephole; "with" movement indicates the far point is beyond the peephole (behind the examiner), and "against" movement indicates the far point is between the patient and the peephole.
- Slit lamp: optical cross section can be seen using a narrow slit beam. Both the illumination system and the binocular stereo microscope (a reversible Galilean telescope) are imaged at a common pivot point.
- Characteristics of diagnostic lenses (Table 1–2).

OPTICS FORMULAS See Table 1–3.

REFRACTIVE ERRORS The emmetropic eye has a far point at infinity (the point on the line of sight that is conjugate to the retina when accommodation is completely relaxed).

- Astigmatism: has a far line instead of a far point.
- Hyperopia (farsighted): far point is located behind the eye; the refractive power of the eye is too weak or the eye is too short; the eye is naturally focused farther than infinity.
- Myopia (nearsighted): far point is located anterior to the retina; the refractive power of the eye is too strong or the eye is too long; the eye is naturally focused closer than infinity.

TABLE 1–3
Optics Formulas

Basic Formulas

Vergence formula: $U + D = V$; where U = object vergence, V = image vergence

Index of refraction: $\dfrac{\text{speed of light in air}}{\text{speed of light in substance}}$

air $n = 1.00$, water $n = 1.33$, cornea $n = 1.37$, lens $n = 1.42$

Retinal image size: $\dfrac{\text{object height}}{\text{retinal image height}} = \dfrac{\text{mm from nodal point}}{17\text{ mm}}$

Snell's law: $n_1 \sin\Phi_1 = n_2 \sin\Phi_2$, where n_1 = index of refraction of the incident medium, Φ_1 = angle of incidence, n_2 = index of refraction of the refractive medium, and Φ_2 = angle of refraction

Power Formulas

Fluid changing lens power: $\dfrac{D_{air}}{D_{fluid}} = \dfrac{n_{lens} - n_{air}}{D_{lens} - n_{fluid}}$

Effectivity of lens: $D_2 = \dfrac{D_1}{1 - s \times D_1}$

D_1 = old lens, D_2 new lens, s = meters lens is moved toward eye (negative if moved forward, positive if moved backward)

Lens effectivity alternate method: locate focal point of old lens ($1/D$, which is far point of the emmetropic eye), then measure from the far point to the new lens, and take a reciprocal for the new lens power. Moving lens away from eye increases its effective plus power (hyperope CL is stronger plus, myope in CL needs more accommodation to read).

Spherical refracting surface power: $D = \dfrac{n_2 - n_1}{r}$

n_1, n_2 = refractive indices, r = radius of curvature (m)

r is (+) for convex surfaces and (−) for concave surfaces

Power of lens calculation: $D = \dfrac{100\text{ cm}}{f} = \dfrac{1\text{ m}}{f}$

D = lens power (diopters), f = focal length (cm)

Corrective Lenses

Power cross: write prescription in both (+) and (−) cylinder forms. Put the sphere of the (−) prescription on the minus meridian and the sphere of the (+) prescription on the plus meridian. Or place sphere of prescription on axis, then add sphere (+) cylinder and place at other meridian. Do not confuse with axis cross.

AC/A ratio:

1. Gradient (lenses) $= \dfrac{\text{deviation with lens - deviation without lens}}{D\text{ of lens}}$

2. Heterophoria (PD) $= \dfrac{\text{deviation at near - deviation at distance}}{D\text{ of accommodation}} + \text{PD (cm)}$

(Continued)

TABLE 1–3 (*Continued*)

Optics Formulas

IOL POWER CALCULATION: $D = A - 2.5$ (axial length) – 0.9 (average K)

D = IOL power, A = IOL constant, axial length (cm)

RGP PRESCRIBING: if too steep, add minus (SAM) or too flat, add plus (FAP). To steepen or tighten a lens (if apical bearing on fluorescein exam), decrease base curve or radius or increase diameter.

1. Choose base curve 0.5 *D* larger than lower *K* to account for the minus tear lens.
2. Convert prescription to minus cylinder, and drop the cylinder.
3. Convert to zero vertex distance (if >4 *D*).
4. Subtract 0.50 *D* tear lens.

ADD PRESCRIBING: average accommodative amplitude at age 40 is ~6 *D*, age 44 ~4 *D*, age 60 ~1 *D*.

1. Take reciprocal of working distance to find how much near power is required.
2. Subtract $\frac{1}{2}$ of expected or measured accommodative amplitude (keep in reserve).
3. Prescribe the rest as the prescription add.

- Kestenbaum's rule: estimate the near add needed for low vision patients to read newsprint by taking the reciprocal of best distance Snellen acuity (divide the denominator by the numerator).
- Bifocal distortion: image jump is worse with round top segments for all lenses; image displacement (which is more bothersome) is worse with flat top segments for plus lenses and round top segments with minus lenses. Thus, give a flat top bifocal segment for minus lenses (less image jump and displacement) and round top with plus lenses (more image jump but less displacement).

PRENTICE'S RULE: $pD = h \times D$

pD = prism diopters, h = distance from optical center (cm), D = diopter of lens power

Real image is displaced toward base, virtual image toward apex.

RAY TRACING: three rays used to locate objects and images in an optical system.

1. Central ray drawn from tip of object through the center of an ideal thin lens and continues in a straight line.
2. Ray that emerges from the tip of the object traveling parallel to the principal axis is refracted through the primary focal point (F).
3. Ray passing through or heading toward the secondary focal point (F') is refracted parallel to the principal axis.

By convention, light rays always travel from left to right. A converging or plus lens has the focal point to the right of the lens. A diverging or minus lens has the focal point to the left of the lens, and the image is always virtual, erect, smaller than the object, and located between the object and the lens.

TABLE 1–3 (*Continued*)

Optics Formulas

Magnification Formulas

Transverse magnification: $M = \frac{\text{image height}}{\text{object height}} = \frac{\text{image distance}}{\text{object distance}} = \frac{U}{V}$

M = magnification, U = object vergence, V = image vergence

Also known as linear or lateral magnification.

Axial magnification (depth): M^2, where M = transverse magnification

Mirror reflecting power (spherical): $D = \frac{100}{f} = \frac{200}{r\ (\text{cm})} = \frac{2}{r\ (\text{m})}$

f = focal length (cm), r = radius of curvature; central ray goes through center of curvature

- Convex mirror: has minus power, image is virtual, erect, minified (e.g., rear view mirror, cornea)
- Concave mirror: has plus power (e.g., shaving mirror). If object is closer than 1/2 of radius of curvature, then image is virtual, magnified, and upright. If object is between 1/2 of the radius and the center of curvature, then the image is real, minified, and inverted.

Angular magnification: $M = \frac{D}{4}$

M = magnification, reference distance = 25 cm

Telescope magnification (angular): $M = \frac{D_{eyepiece}}{D_{objective}}$

Telescope accommodation: = normal accommodation × (telescope magnification)^2

1. Astronomical: 2 plus lenses; length is $1/D_{\text{eyepiece}} + 1/D_{\text{objective}}$ (longer length; gives inverted image; e.g., lensometer)
2. Galilean: minus eyepiece with plus objective; length is $1/D_{\text{eyepiece}} - 1/D_{\text{objective}}$ (shorter length; gives an upright image; e.g., microscope, loupes, or a corrected aphakic patient whose −12.5 *D* error lens is the eyepiece ÷ 10 *D* spectacles objective lens = 1.25 or 25% magnification)

VISUAL ACUITY 20/20 vision is equivalent to 1 minute of arc or 30 cycles per degree of contrast.

- Snellen's optotypes: standard visual angle of 1 minute of arc; numerator corresponds to the testing distance; denominator corresponds to the distance at which the test letters subtend an angle of 5 minutes of arc.

Pathology

FIXATION Use alcohol for tissues containing water-soluble crystals and formalin for protein.

GROSS PATHOLOGY OF GLOBES Orient posteriorly to see the ON and four vortex veins with superior oblique muscle (SO) insertion superotemporally and inferior oblique muscle (IO) inferotemporally. Dissect in the meridian of interest: vertical through surgical wounds, horizontal through macula, or in the meridian of a tumor. Start the cut 2 mm lateral to ON, and exit 2 mm inside limbus.

HISTOLOGIC STAINS AND CLINICAL USES See Table 1–4.

IMMUNOLOGIC STAINS See Table 1–5.

INTERMEDIATE FILAMENTS See Table 1–6.

TABLE 1–4
Selected Histologic Stains and Clinical Uses

Alcian blue	MPS (faint blue), macular dystrophy
Calcofluor white	Binds to cell walls of fungi and *Acanthamoeba*, see with fluorescent scope
Colloidal iron	Acid mucopolysaccharides, macular dystrophy, vitreous
Congo red	Amyloid
Dieterle and Warthin-Starry	Spirochetes, *Bartonella*, melanin
Fite	Acid fast
Giemsa	Intracytoplasmic organisms or inclusions as in chlamydia, also fungi
H&E	Hematoxylin stains nuclei blue; eosin stains cytoplasm pink (pink = protein)
Potassium hydroxide (KOH)	Fungi; base disrupts epithelial cell membranes
Luxol fast blue	Myelin, granular dystrophy
Masson trichrome	Collagen, smooth muscle, hyaline (granular dystrophy)
Oil-red O	Lipid, sebaceous CA (need fresh tissue)
Periodic acid Schiff (PAS)	Glycogen, BM, fungi, *Propionibacterium acnes*
Prussian blue	Iron (old hemorrhage, siderosis)
Silver stains (e.g., GMS)	Fungi (organisms are always black)
Sudan black	Lipid
Verhoeff van Gieson	Elastin, solar elastosis
von Kossa	Calcium (looks black, blocks transmitted light)
Ziehl-Neelsen	Acid fast

GMS, Gomori methenamine silver.

TABLE 1–5

Selected Immunologic Stains

Immunologic Stain	Target Tissue
Chromogranin	Neuroendocrine tumors like carcinoid
Cytokeratins	Epithelial cells, carcinomas
Desmin	Skeletal, smooth, and cardiac muscle
Epithelium membrane antigen (EMA)	Epithelial cells (cell membrane glycoprotein)
Factor 8	Vascular endothelium, Kaposi's sarcoma
Glial fibrillary acidic protein (GFAP)	Astrocytes, gliomas, ganglia, Schwann's cells

INTRACELLULAR BODIES Russell's bodies—represent stored Ig in plasma cells that are antibody (Ab) factories seen with chronic inflammation. Dutcher bodies—represent Ig in lymphocytes.

INTRACELLULAR INCLUSIONS (Mnemonic: Give your HEN a CBC). **H**erpes viruses have **e**osinophlic intra**n**uclear inclusions versus **c**hlamydia, which has **b**asophilic **c**ytoplasmic inclusions.

TABLE 1–6

Intermediate Filaments

Filament	Cellular Association
KP1	Histiocytes
L26	B lymphocytes
Leukocyte common antigen (LCA)	Lymphocytes, granulocytes, monocytes, dendritic cells
Melanoma specific antigen, HMB-45	Melanoma, nevi
Muscle specific actin (MSA)	Skeletal, smooth, and cardiac muscle
Neurofilaments	Neurons
Neuron specific enolase (NSE)	Neurons, myoepithelia, neuroendocrine
S100	Neural ectoderm, neural crest, neurons, adipose, melanocytes, cartilage
Smooth muscle actin (SMA)	Smooth muscle
UCHL-1	T lymphocytes
Vimentin	Cytoplasmic intermediate filaments in all mesenchymal tissue, sarcoma

TABLE 1–7
Selected Culture Mediums

Culture Medium	Organisms
Blood agar	Aerobic organisms; bacteria, fungi, amoebae
Chocolate agar	Aerobic organisms; contains hemolyzed blood, which will support the growth of fastidious organisms such as *Hemophilus* (requires NAD and hemin) and *Neisseria*
Löffler's serum	*Moraxella* and *Listeria*
Lowenstein-Jensen	*Mycobacterium tuberculosis*; atypicals will grow on blood agar
Sabouraud's	Fungi; culture is a dextrose agar without cycloheximide, which would inhibit saprophytic fungi
Thayer-Martin agar plate	*Neisseria*
Thioglycollate broth	Anaerobes

NAD, nicotinamide adenine dinucleotide.

SIGNS OF MALIGNANCY Atypia (single-cell abnormality), dysplasia (abnormal structure among cells), faulty maturation, loss of polarity

SKIN PATHOLOGY TERMINOLOGY

- Acantholysis: separation of epidermal cells; rapid growth, as in inverted follicular keratosis (IFK)
- Acanthosis: thickening of squamous, prickle cell layer
- Dyskeratosis: intraepithelial keratinization (mnemonic: "dys don't belong here").
- Hyperkeratosis: thickening of keratin layer; denotes rapid tissue growth
- Parakeratosis: absence of granular layer with nuclei in keratin; immature tissue; rapid growth
- Pseudoepitheliomatous hyperplasia (PEH): reactive process; invasive acanthosis

CULTURE MEDIUMS See Table 1–7.

Pregnancy

NORMAL OCULAR CHANGES Decreased IOP from enhanced uveoscleral outflow and lowered episcleral venous pressure (EVP); minimal corneal edema may lead to refractive changes and contact lens intolerance.

TABLE 1–8
Tissue Effects of Lasers (Mnemonic: ABCD)

Action	Chromophore	Mechanism	Example	Uses
Ablative and sublimation	Nucleic acid and protein	Bond-breaking	Excimer ArF (193 nm)	Refractive surgery
Coagulation	Uveal and RPE melanin	Thermal	Argon green (514 nm), dye	Retinal laser
Disruption	Plasma	Acoustomechanical	YAG (1064 nm)	Capsulotomy, LPI

PREGNANCY MAY INCREASE THE RISK OF, EXACERBATE, OR PRECIPITATE Cortical blindness; idiopathic central serous retinopathy (ICSR); ischemic optic neuropathy (ION); toxemia of pregnancy with potential serous choroidal or retinal detachments (frequently bilateral); progression of diabetic retinopathy (DR) (5% risk of proliferative diabetic retinopathy in patients with moderate nonproliferative disease); Graves' disease; pituitary adenoma; and meningioma.

Radiation/Laser

LASER PRINCIPLES Amplification of narrow wavelength (monochromatic) light, emitting intense and coherent (synchronous with respect to time and space) radiation. Power × time = energy. See Table 1–8 for tissue effects of lasers.

- Chromophores: substances that absorb laser energy; in the retina mainly RPE melanin, but also xanthophyll (intraretinal, peak with blue light), hemoglobin (peak with yellow light), lipofuscin, and visual pigments.
- Parameters for retinal treatments
  - Exposure time: 0.1 seconds for most treatments. A shorter time increases the blast effect with increased risk of tissue rupture, hemorrhage, and increased temperature. A longer time increases the "cooking" of tissue and increases overflow with less defined burn.
  - Power: start low and increase.
  - Size: for panretinal photocoagulation (PRP) and to close tears, use 250–500 μm or larger spot (must increase power if the size increases to maintain the same energy density); use smaller 50–100 μm in macula to limit scotoma size.
- Argon and krypton lasers are generated from a high voltage passed across gas-filled tubes and emit continuously.
  - Blue (488 nm): not used often, as it is absorbed by xanthophylls in the macula.

TABLE 1–9
The Electromagnetic Spectrum

Shorter wavelengths
Gamma rays 10^{-14} m, x-rays 10^{-10} m, ultraviolet 10^{-6} m, UVA 150–200 nm
Visual spectrum
Violet ~400 nm, blue 450–500 nm, green 500–550 nm, yellow ~600 nm, red ~650 nm
Ophthalmic lasers
Excimer 193 nm, argon green 514 nm, HeNe 633 nm, diode 800 nm, YAG 1064 nm
Longer wavelengths
Radar 10^{-2} m, FM radio, TV, shortwave radio 10^{2} m, AM radio 10^{4} m

- Green (514 nm): superficial RPE; good for most conditions, highly absorbed by hemoglobin; may cause more direct closure of choroidal neovascular membrane (CNVM) vessels.
- Krypton red (647 nm): deeper RPE; choriocapillaris; hurts more; use red or diode to treat through hemorrhage or nuclear sclerotic cataract; low scatter.
- Dye yellow (577 nm): minimal xanthophyll absorption; low scatter, high hemoglobin absorption; useful in vascular lesions.

- Diode (800 nm): solid-state continuous-wave laser (do not need a large cooling bath as with argon lasers); portable and highly efficient. Treats deeper RPE and choriocapillaris (can always see the lesion; hurts more, spares inner retina more).

ULTRAVIOLET RADIATION (MNEMONIC: ABC):
- Ultraviolet **A** (UVA); longest wavelength; **a**ges skin, blocked by lens
- Ultraviolet **B** (UVB); 150–200 nm; **b**urns skin and responsible for most skin cancer
- Ultraviolet **C** (UVC); < 150 nm; most powerful and **c**arcinogenic, but largely blocked by ozone

ELECTROMAGNETIC SPECTRUM See Table 1–9.

Surgery

PREOPERATIVE EVALUATION Overall perioperative mortality of eye surgery is 0.06 to 0.18%.
- Anticoagulants: for most surgeries, except topical clear-corneal cataract surgery, have patient stop aspirin 7 to 10 days prior, stop other nonsteriodal anti-inflammatory drugs (NSAIDs) 1 or 2 days prior, and stop warfarin (Coumadin) 3 to 5 days before surgery.

  - Patients at high risk for thromboembolic disease (prosthetic heart valves, prior embolic stroke, recent deep venous thrombosis, or pulomary embolus) may need to discontinue warfarin and be hospitalized for 24 to 48 hours prior to surgery for heparin, which can then be stopped 4 to 6 hours prior to surgery. For emergent surgery, reverse warfarin with 2 to 4 units fresh frozen plasma or vitamin K 10 mg intramuscularly (IM) or subcutaneous (SQ) every 12 hours.
  - One month after deep venous thrombosis (DVT) there is a 1% risk of a DVT-related event without warfarin. The risk decreases even further with time; thus, can usually stop anticoagulation 3 months after a DVT for outpatient surgery unless the patient is hospitalized or otherwise immoblized.
- Cardiac disease: accounts for half of postoperative complications; avoid elective surgery within 6 months of a myocardial infarction. In general, patients are okay to proceed with elective surgery without further testing if they have mild and stable angina, have had a heart attack more than 6 months prior, have stable congestive heart failure (CHF) and can climb one flight of stairs without stopping. Otherwise refer for patient evaluation and clearance.
- Cerebrovascular disease: avoid elective surgery within 3 months of a transient ischemic attack or stroke.
- Chronic obstructive pulmonary disease (COPD): aggressive preoperative treatment to prevent coughing; patient may not be able to lie flat for surgery.
- Diabetes: ask about prior history of ketoacidosis; oral hypoglycemics should be stopped the morning of surgery; insulin patients should receive 1/2 dose before surgery and be maintained on intravenous fluids containing glucose until they are taking orals.
- Hepatic disease: avoid elective surgery until 1 month after liver function tests have normalized.
- Hypertension: in general, avoid surgery if blood pressure is > 200/110 mmHg; patients may take their usual antihypertensive dose on the morning of surgery.
- Platelets: transfuse for < 30,000; each unit adds 10,000.
- Renal failure: dialyze the day before surgery to optimize fluid and electrolyte balance and to eliminate anticoagulants used in dialysis; beware of associated qualitative platelet defects (assess with bleeding time; greater risk with blood urea nitrogen [BUN] > 60).
- Steroids: patients taking more than 7.5 mg of prednisone × 3 months or 40 mg of prednisone × 1 week are at risk for adrenal suppression and may need a "stress" steroid dose (for most ophthalmic surgeries, 25 mg hydrocortisone on the day of surgery is sufficient).
- Valvular heart disease: clean ophthalmologic procedures pose little risk for endocarditis; thus, no antibiotic prophylaxis is typically necessary.

TABLE 1–10

Comparison of Suture Materials

Type	Material	Tensile Strength	Tissue Reactivity	Knot Security	Absorption
Absorbable (< 60 days tensile strength)					
Plain gut	Beef or sheep intestine	7–10 days	High	Poor	60–90 days
Chromic gut	Beef or sheep intestine	10–20 days	High, but less than plain gut	Poor	90 days
Fast-absorbing gut	Beef or sheep intestine	5–7 days	High	Poor	2–4 weeks
Dexon	Polyglycolic acid	30 days	Low, braided	Good	90 days
Vicryl	Polyglactin 910	32 days	Low, tightly braided	Good	70 days
PDS	Polydioxanone	28 days	Low, stiff monofilament	Poor	180 days
Maxon	Polytrimethylene carbonate	High	Low	Good	210 days
Monocryl	Polyglecaprone	High	Low	Good	120 days
Nonabsorbable (> 60 days tensile strength)					
Silk	Silk (silkworm)	1 year (variable)	High	Good	2 years (variable)
Nylon	Polyamide	6 months to 2 years	Low, monofilament, braided	Poor–fair	15–20%/year
Prolene	Polypropylene	High, indefinite	Low, monofilament, smooth	Poor	Indefinite
Polydek, Mersilene	Polyester	High, indefinite	Low, braided synthetic	Good	Indefinite
Novafil	Polybutester	High	Low	Good	Indefinite

PRINCIPLES OF SURGERY Understand that surgery is iatrogenic trauma and that most eye tissues can only repair themselves and not regenerate.

- Determine goal; have a clear knowledge of surgery purpose.
- Develop a well-defined plan.
- Be adaptable and flexible.
- Maintain good visualization of surgical field.
- Minimize trauma.
- Restore tissues to normal states.
- Practice economy and control.
- Continue with development and improvement.

SUTURE MATERIALS See Table 1–10.

CHAPTER 2

Orbit, Eyelids, and Ocular Adnexa

Anatomy and Physiology

BONY ORBIT (Fig. 2–1) Average 30 cc volume (about that of a shot glass with a 6 cc globe inside), 35 mm height, 40 mm depth (22 mm globe and 18 mm from posterior globe to the orbital apex; thus, the 25 mm intraorbital optic nerve (ON) has ~7 mm redundancy), and 45 mm width. Average interpupillary distance (IPD) = 60 mm. Optic axis is 23 degrees lateral to anteroposterior axis. Maximum circumference is ~1 cm behind rim (at the globe equator). All bones are of neural crest origin except superotemporal orbit (ectodermal); orbital growth completed by 7–9 years. Seven bones comprise the bony socket: frontal, zygomatic, greater and lesser wings of the sphenoid, maxillary, lacrimal, ethmoid, and palatine.

- Two bones in the roof: frontal and lesser wing of the sphenoid. Bordered by anterior cranial fossa and frontal sinus. Trochlea is 4 mm behind rim. Houses the lacrimal gland fossa (postseptal). Optic canal travels through lesser sphenoid, 37 degrees off optic axis.
- Two bones in the lateral wall: zygomatic and greater sphenoid wing. Bordered by temporal and pterygopalatine fossa. Lateral walls are perpendicular to each other, thickest (1.0–1.5 mm) and strongest orbital bones but least protective of globe.
    - Lateral orbital tubercle ~4 mm posterior to the rim on the medial aspect of zygoma; also called Whitnall's tubercle. The "4 L's" attach here: **l**ateral canthal (palpebral) tendon, **L**ateral rectus (LR) check ligament, **l**ateral horn (aponeurosis) of the levator muscle, **L**ockwood's suspensory ligament of eye (equivalent to Whitnall's in upper lid).
- Three bones in the floor: maxillary, palatine, and zygomatic bones. Bordered by infraorbital canal and maxillary sinus. The floor slopes upward from the inferior orbital rim toward the apex but does not reach the apex and ends at pterygopalatine fossa. It is the only wall without a sphenoid bone contribution.
- Four bones in the medial wall (mnemonic: SMEL): **s**phenoid, **m**axillary, **e**thmoid, and **l**acrimal bones. Bordered by ethmoid and sphenoid sinuses, cribriform plate at frontoethmoidal suture (therefore stay below the ethmoidal neurovascular foramina during decompression surgery). Medial walls are parallel to each other and ~25 mm apart

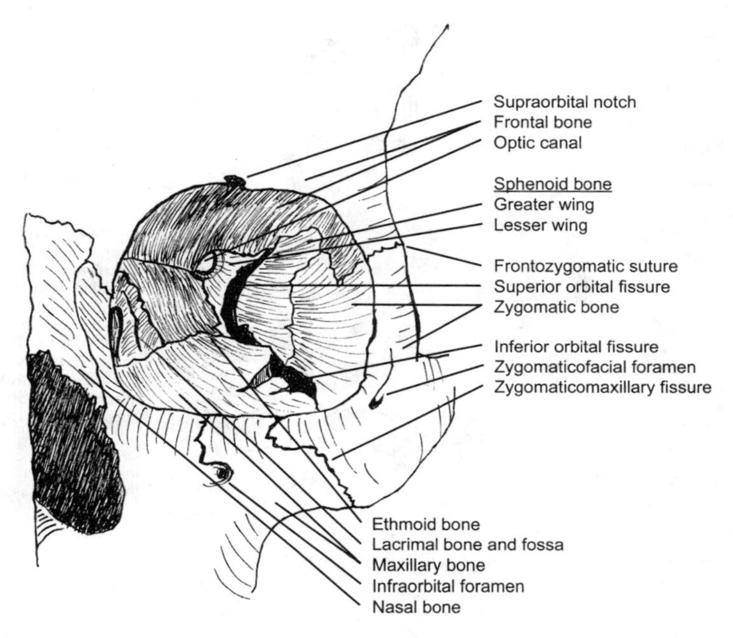

Figure 2–1 Frontal view of the left orbit, showing the bones that contribute to the bony socket (palatine bone not shown).

between the medial canthi and are the thinnest walls (~0.3 mm; called lamina papyracea because they are "paper thin"). Houses the lacrimal sac fossa (preseptal).

- Rule of halves (mnemonic: 24-12-6): anterior ethmoidal aperture (AEA) is 24 mm posterior to the anterior lacrimal crest, posterior ethmoidal aperture (PEA) is 12 mm posterior to the AEA, and the optic canal is 6 mm posterior to the PEA. Thus, total medial wall length is ~42 mm long; remember this during medial orbitotomy.

FISSURES Two main fissures (Fig. 2–2 shows orbital apex anatomy and contents of the orbital fissures):

- Inferior orbital fissure (IOF): "lower tier" of the apex opens into pterygopalatine fossa (behind maxillary fossa). Twice as long as the superior orbital fissure. Contents (mnemonic: PIMP): **p**terygoid nerve of cranial nerve (CN) V_2, **i**nferior orbital vein, **m**axillary nerve (from CN V_2), and the **p**terygopalatine ganglion nerve (postganglionic secretory innervation for the lacrimal gland).
- Superior orbital fissure (SOF): "middle tier" of the apex opens into cavernous sinus. A pencil stuck through the middle of the globe would

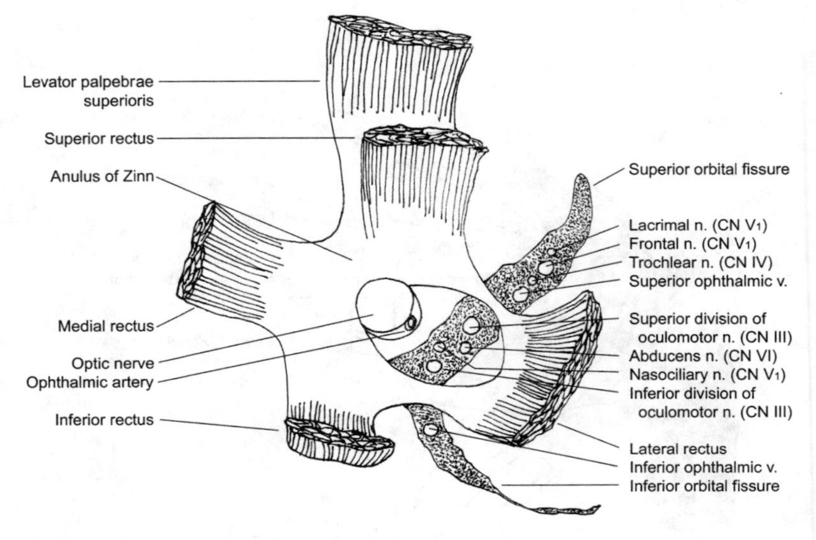

Figure 2–2 The left orbital apex and associated structures.

go through the SOF into the cavernous sinus. The SOF is 22 mm long and separated by LR origin (and thus anulus of Zinn) into:

- Superior division (mnemonic: "Look: Michigan State football team"): **l**acrimal nerve of CN V_1 (most lateral structure at apex), **m**iddle meningeal artery recurrent branch, **s**ympathetic nerves, **f**rontal nerve of CN V_1, and **t**rochlear nerve (CN IV, the least affected muscle from a retrobulbar block because it is outside the muscle cone)
- Inferior division (mnemonic: $NASO_2$): **n**asociliary branch of CN V_1, **a**bducens nerve (CN VI), **s**ympathetic nerves, **o**culomotor nerve (CN III), and the superior **o**rbital vein

FORAMINA Eight main orbital foramina (Fig. 2–3 shows skull base anatomy and openings):

- Optic: the "upper tier" of the apex, located at the level of the anterior clinoid and opens into the middle cranial fossa (MCF). Contains the ON, ophthalmic artery, sympathetic nerves (also enter orbit with nasociliary nerve through SOF). It is ~6.5 mm wide and ~10 mm long. At the apex, the optic foramen is superior and nasal and points up and in toward the MCF.
- Supraorbital: is a foramen in ~20% of the population and a notch in ~80%. Protects the supraorbital vessels and nerve (branch of the frontal branch of CN V_1, transmits sensation from forehead).

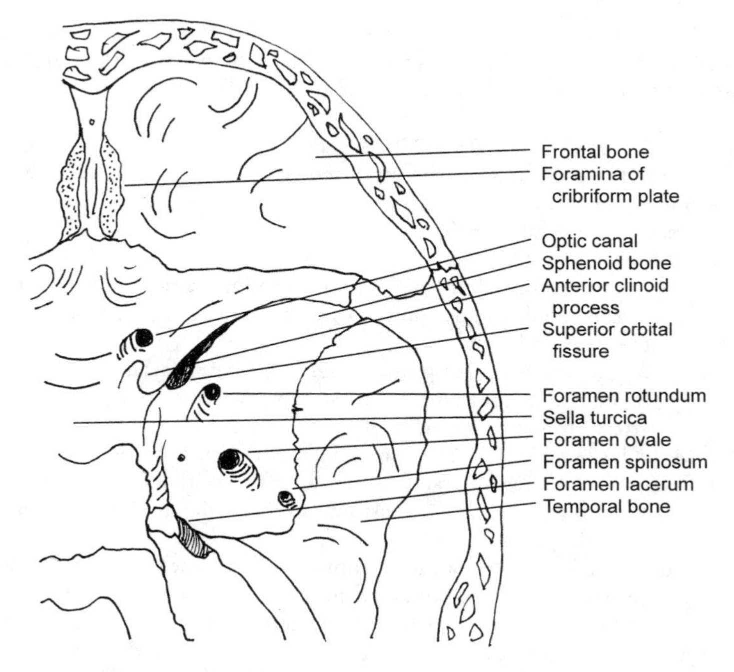

Figure 2–3 Internal view of the right anterior skull base, showing the orbital roof and openings into the orbit.

- Infraorbital: located 5–10 mm below rim and transmits the infraorbital nerve (from CN V_2) that provides sensation from midface, superior gums, and canine teeth.
- Anterior and posterior ethmoidal: transmit vessels and nerves (from CN V_1) at the junction of ethmoid and frontal bones.
- Zygomatic: zygomaticofacial and zygomaticotemporal foramina house their respective arteries and nerves (branches of CN V_2, transmit sensation from the lateral face and temple).
- Nasolacrimal fossa and duct: responsible for lacrimal drainage into the inferior meatus.

BLOOD SUPPLY TO THE ORBIT AND GLOBE First branch of the internal carotid artery is the ophthalmic artery, followed by the middle cerebral, posterior communicating, and anterior communicating arteries. The first branch of the ophthalmic artery is the central retinal artery (CRA). The CRA begins inferior and lateral to the ON, then sweeps over, crossing nasally (is also nasal to the medial rectus muscle. Its branches can be grouped into three circles: posterior (supplying globe: CRA, short and long ciliaries); middle (supplying extraocular muscles and orbit: muscular, anterior ciliary, lacrimal); and anterior (terminal branches to skin: anterior and posterior ethmoidals, supraorbital, supra- and infratrochlear, dorsal nasal).

BRANCHES OF THE OPHTHALMIC ARTERY

- Central retinal: supplies the inner retina
- Small meningeal/pial branch
- Central collateral branch
- Lacrimal
  - Lateral palpebral artery passes into the upper and lower eyelids, runs medially to anastomose with medial palpebral artery to form the palpebral arcades.
  - Zygomatic branches pass through zygomaticofacial and zygomaticotemporal foramina to anastomose with superficial temporal artery (from the ECA).
- Muscular branch to LR (or variably from lacrimal artery)
- Recurrent meningeal branch (may arise from the lacrimal artery): passes through the SOF, anastomoses with the middle meningeal artery (from the ECA)
- Muscular branches to four rectus muscles: two branches to each muscle (except one to the LR). Gives rise to seven anterior ciliary arteries that supply the sclera and conjunctiva and terminate in the major arterial circle of iris, providing 50% of anterior segment blood (remainder is from the long posterior ciliary arteries). Vertical muscles contribute more to the anterior segment circulation than horizontal muscles.
- Ciliary
  - Long posterior ciliary: two vessels pass through the suprachoroid space forward to supply the choroid anterior to the equator, ciliary body, and anastomose with the anterior ciliaries to form the major circle of the iris
  - Short posterior ciliary: usually about seven vessels that then divide into 10 to 20 branches; supply choroid posterior to the equator and form anastomotic ring of Zinn around the optic nerve head, and in 20% of the population give rise to a cilioretinal artery
- Supraorbital: along medial aspect of the levator and superior rectus muscles through supraorbital foramen to the scalp, lying deep to the frontalis muscle, supplying the levator palpebrae muscle, frontal sinus, upper eyelid, and skin of forehead, and anastomoses with the superficial temporal artery (ECA)
- Posterior ethmoid: through posterior ethmoid canal to posterior ethmoid air cells, anterior cranial dura, and upper nasal mucosa
- Anterior ethmoid: through anterior ethmoid canal to anterior cranial fossa through cribriform plate into nose under nasal bone to face, supplying anterior and middle ethmoidal air cells, frontal sinus, meninges, anterior nasal mucous membranes, and skin of nose

- Meningeal: supplies meninges of middle cranial fossa
- Medial palpebral (may also branch from dorsal nasal artery): usually two branches that travel below the trochlea, behind the lacrimal sac, through the septum, above and below the medial palpebral ligament, to pass laterally and enter the upper and lower eyelid and divide into the peripheral and marginal arcades between the orbicularis and tarsus, supplying eyelids and conjunctiva. Marginal arcade is 2 mm from the margin, and peripheral arcade in upper eyelid is 1 mm above the tarsus; both covered by levator (should not see during a blepharoplasty).
- Supratrochlear: above trochlea through septum, supplying skin of forehead and scalp
- Dorsal nasal: terminal branch of ophthalmic artery; lies within upper medial fat pad (beware during surgery) through septum above medial palpebral ligament, supplying lacrimal sac and anastomosing with facial artery (from the ECA) at the medial canthus

BRANCHES OF THE EXTERNAL CAROTID ARTERY

- Superior thyroid
- Ascending pharyngeal
- Lingual
- Occipital
- Facial: becomes the angular artery, which anastomoses with the dorsal nasal artery (from the ICA)
- Posterior auricular
- Maxillary: gives rise to the infraorbital artery in the pterygopalatine fossa, through the IOF, down the infraorbital groove and canal, giving branches to the IR, IO, and lacrimal sac, then courses through the infraorbital foramen to supply the skin of the face, maxillary sinus, and upper teeth (upper superior alveolar artery)
- Anterior tympanic
- Middle meningeal: anastomoses with the recurrent meningeal (from the ICA)
- Superficial temporal: anastomoses with the zygomaticotemporal (from the ICA). The artery lies on the superficial temporal fascia; thus, for a temporal artery biopsy, trace the vessel up from just anterior to the ear. If the cut is too deep, you will see the white glistening temporalis (temporal parietal) fascia that splits about 1 cm above the zygomatic arch into a deep and superficial layer.

ARTERIAL ANASTOMOSES BETWEEN THE ICA AND ECA (MNEMONIC: ZEBRAS RARELY SIP DOUBLE LATTES)

- **Z**ygomaticotemporal and superficial temporal
- **R**ecurrent meningeal and middle meningeal
- **S**upraorbital and frontal (branch of superficial temporal)

- **D**orsal nasal and angular
- **L**acrimal and palpebral

VENOUS SYSTEM Superior ophthalmic vein drains the orbit, travels beneath SR, and runs diagonally across the superior orbit from medial posterolaterally to the SOF. It is lateral to and larger than the ophthalmic artery. Because it is valveless and drains into the cavernous sinus, there is a risk of intracranial spread of infection from orbital cellulitis. The inferior orbital vein drains into the superior orbital vein and smaller branches into the pterygoid plexus. The angular vein of the facial plexus also contributes to venous drainage.

LYMPHATIC SYSTEM There are no orbital lymphatics (debatable but classic teaching; there are likely some lymph vessels present). The upper eyelid drains to the preauricular lymph nodes and the lower to submental nodes. The lateral lids drain into the preauricular nodes, and the medial lids drain into the submandibular nodes.

MUSCLES See Chapter 9 for EOM details.

- Eyelid retractors
  - Capsulopalpebral fascia: retractor of the lower eyelid, analogous to the levator muscle, and arises from the IR sheath. After it splits around the IO muscle, it extends to Lockwood's ligament, then takes a vertical course to the anterior tarsus. Thus, movement of the lower eyelid parallels the globe in downgaze.
  - Levator palpebrae superioris: originates superior to the SR at the orbital apex from the lesser wing of the sphenoid. Its 40 mm muscle belly extends to Whitnall's ligament and is responsible for horizontal pull. Then the 12 mm tendon (aponeurosis) attaches to the lower half of tarsus and provides vertical pull. Gives attachments to the overlying orbicularis and skin (forms the eyelid crease). CN III innervation.
  - Müller's (superior tarsal) muscle: originates from the undersurface of the levator muscle (is "posterior lamella" of the levator) and advances 10–12 mm to the superior tarsus. Gives 2–4 mm lift by sympathetic innervation (thus affected in Horner's syndrome).
- Select muscles of facial expression: CN VII (facial nerve) innervation.
  - Frontalis: part of the anterior scalp, elevates the forehead and brow.
  - Nasalis: lateral aspect of nose, to dilate or compress the nares.
  - Orbicularis oculi: primary protractor of eyelids; innervated by the temporal, zygomatic, and buccal (to a lesser extent) branches of the facial nerve. Its medial attachments contribute to lacrimal pump (thus, epiphora occurs with CN VII palsy from poor pump function in addition to corneal exposure and reflex tearing).

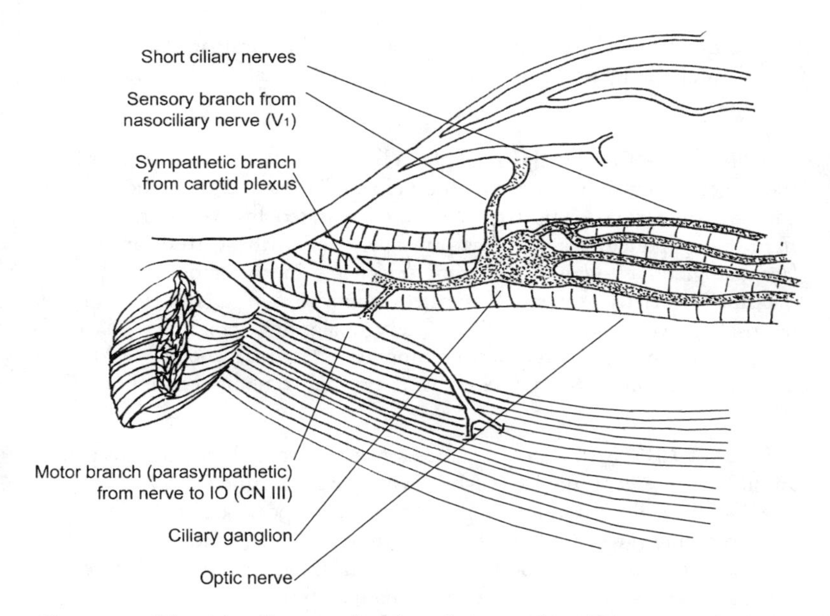

Figure 2–4 The right ciliary ganglion, lateral view, and its tripartite contributions.

Involuntary lid closure (blink) is mostly from the pretarsal orbicularis and voluntary (wink) from the orbital fibers, with preseptal fibers contributing to both.

- Procerus: attaches to frontalis muscle and inserts on the nasal bone; causes horizontal brow wrinkles.
- Superciliary corrugator muscle: originates from the frontal bone, coursing laterally to insert in subcutaneous tissue; responsible for vertical brow wrinkles and rhytids (like a corrugated tin roof).

NERVES See Chapter 8 for cranial nerve details.

- Ciliary ganglion (Fig. 2–4): three roots enter the ganglion, and fibers exit as the short ciliary nerves.
  - The motor root (parasympathetic fibers) arises from CN III branch to the IO muscle and synapse in the ganglion.
  - Sympathetic nerves from the carotid plexus pass through the ganglion without synapsing.
  - Sensory root derives from the nasociliary nerve (CN V_1) and pass through the ciliary ganglion without synapse.
- CN V_1 (trigeminal nerve, ophthalmic division): lacrimal and frontal branches enter the orbit through the superior division of the SOF. The

lacrimal branch supplies the area around the lacrimal gland, and the frontal branch divides into the supraorbital and infratrochlear branches.

LACRIMAL GLAND The lacrimal gland has two lobes; excretory ducts from the larger orbital lobe pass into the palpebral lobe and continue into the conjunctival fornix. The two lobes are separated by the lateral horn of the levator aponeurosis. A salivatory-type gland with no true capsule, the lacrimal gland efferent innervation originates in the superior salivatory (lacrimal) nucleus → nervus intermedius portion of CN VII → greater petrosal nerve → sphenopalatine (pterygopalatine) ganglion → CN V_2 infraorbital nerve → zygomaticotemporal → lacrimal nerve. (Afferent innervation is provided by CN V_1 to the spinal trigeminal ganglion.)

EYELID GLANDS All aqueous glands are eccrine; all oil and mucous glands are holocrine except glands of Moll, which are apocrine.

- Goblet cells: conjunctival glands that are apocrine for a time, then holocrine (gives "wholly" of itself, ruptures and extrudes contents)
- Lacrimal: eccrine (modified sweat gland) and two types of accessory lacrimal glands are present in the conjunctiva:
  - Glands of Krause: present in the conjunctival fornices (glands of Krause are in the "crotch" of the lid); 20–42 in the upper fornix and 6–8 glands in the lower.
  - Glands of Wolfring: present in the "wall" of the palpebral conjunctiva, about three glands near the upper border of the upper tarsus and two near the lower border of the lower tarsus.
- Meibomian: holocrine glands that are hypertrophied sebaceous glands (unique because they are not associated with hairs) and lie within the tarsus
- Zeis: holocrine glands that are rudimentary sebaceous glands connected to a lash follicle
- Moll: apocrine glands that are atypical large sweat glands; loses cytoplasm with secretion and thus produces a thicker solution than sweat; empties into a lash follicle.

EYELID Functions primarily to protect the globe; also important in facial expression. The mucocutaneous junction is a critical eyelid structure because it functions to spread the tears and provides oxygen to the cornea. The mucocutaneous junction is posterior to the eyelashes near the meibomian gland openings; the gray line is anterior lamella and is the edge of the pretarsal orbicularis.

- Eyelid layers (four basic layers near the eyelid margin):
  - Skin: thinnest skin in the body

    - Epidermis has four layers: stratum corneum, granulosum, spinosum, and basale (germinativum). Melanocytes are present in about a 1:10 ratio with epidermal cells, and occasional Langerhans' cells from monocyte precursors express immune antigen (contain Bierbeck granules).
    - Dermis contains hair, sebaceous, Zeis and meibomian glands, eccrine sweat glands, and apocrine glands of Moll. Subcutaneous areolar tissue is present beneath the dermis.
  - Orbicularis muscle: submuscular areolar tissue divides the anterior lamella of skin and orbicularis muscle with the posterior lamella of tarsus and conjunctiva.
  - Septum or tarsus: no cartilage in tarsus and is nonrenewable.
  - Conjunctiva
- Layers of the eyelid that a penetrating wound would pass through:
  - Lower eyelid (Fig. 2–5) (mnemonic: 4-7 rule):

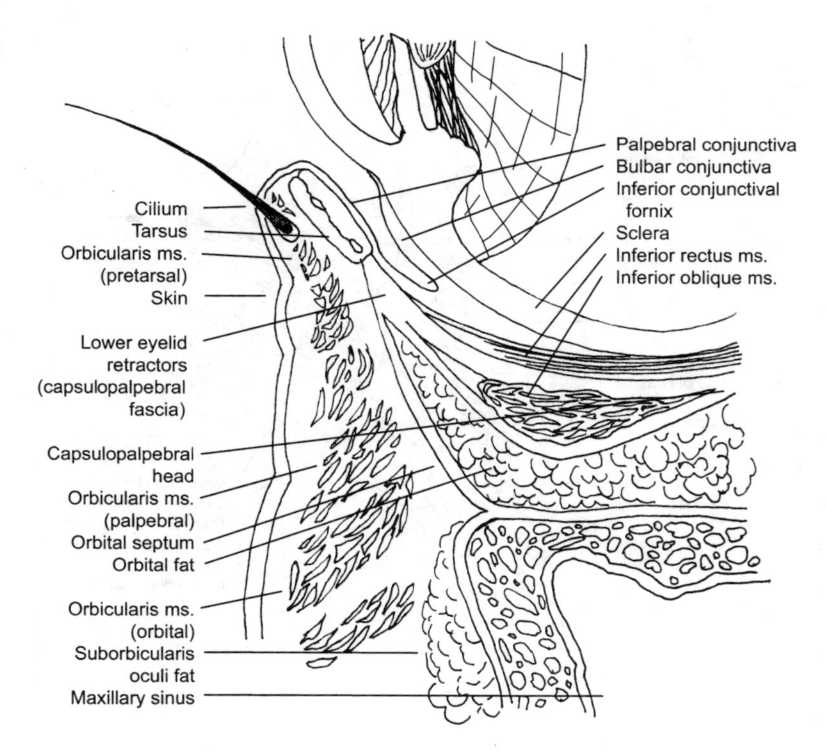

Figure 2–5 The lower eyelid and anterior orbit anatomy, sagittal section.

- The upper 5 mm has 4 layers: skin, orbicularis, tarsus, and conjunctiva.
- The lower 5 mm has 7 layers: skin, orbicularis, septum, pre-CPF (capsulopalpebral fascia) fat, inferior sympathetic muscle (equivalent to Müller's in the upper lid), CPF (equivalent to levator aponeurosis in upper lid), and conjunctiva.

◦ Upper eyelid (Fig. 2–6) (mnemonic: 4-5-7 rule):
  - The lower 5 mm has 4 layers: skin, orbicularis, tarsus, and conjunctiva.
  - The middle 5 mm has 5 layers: skin, orbicularis, levator aponeurosis, tarsus, and conjunctiva.
  - Above 10 mm, the upper eyelid has 7 layers: skin, orbicularis, septum, preaponeurotic fat, levator aponeurosis, Müller's muscle, and conjunctiva.

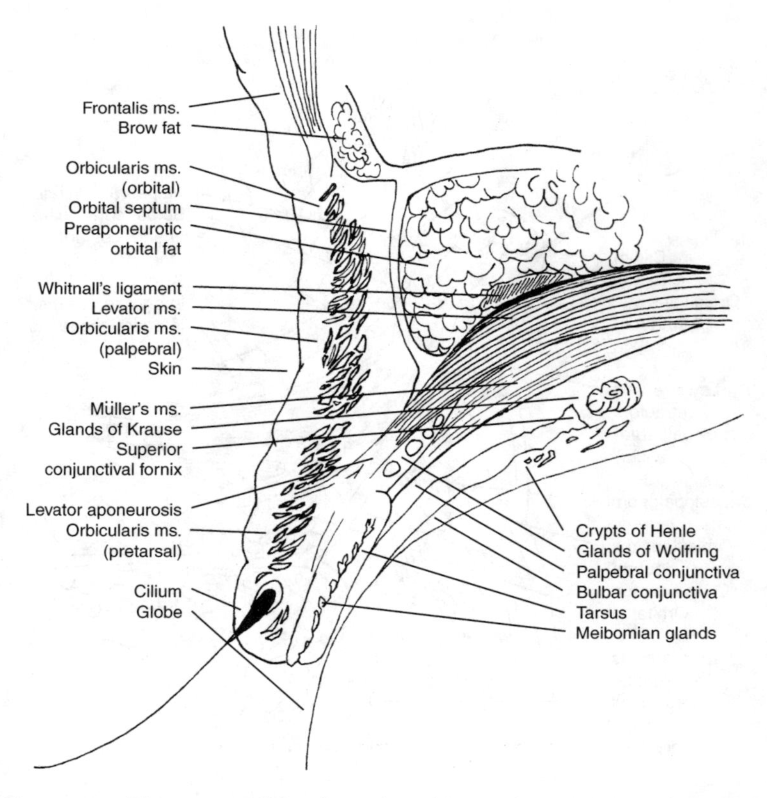

Figure 2–6 The upper eyelid and anterior orbit seen in cross-sectional anatomy.

- Vasculature: upper lid supplied by the marginal and peripheral vascular arcades. The lower lid usually has only a peripheral arcade. The peripheral vascular arcade lies along the peripheral border of the tarsus between the lid retractors and Müller's (inferior tarsal) muscle. The marginal arcade lies anterior to the tarsus 2 mm above the eyelid margin. In eyelid surgery, visualizing these horizontally running vessels indicates that you are below the level of the aponeurosis.

ORBITAL CONNECTIVE AND SUPPORTING TISSUES Most of the orbit is filled with fat.

- Fat pads: removal of too much fat during surgery may result in sunken orbits, EOM restriction, and cicatricial eyelid changes.
    - Upper lid: two fat pads. The large, central, more yellow (higher lutein concentration) preaponeurotic fat pad protects the levator aponeurosis directly beneath it; it is contiguous with deep fat and is less vascular. The smaller, paler medial fat is more vascular and often migrates anteriorly with aging. There is no lateral fat pad in the upper lid because of the presence of the lacrimal gland in that position.
    - Lower lid: three fat pads. The medial and central pads are separated by the IO (essential to avoid the muscle in blepharoplasty) and communicate with deeper orbital fat; thus, excessive traction may lead to orbital hemorrhage. The smaller lateral fat pad is contiguous with the central pad and separated by the arcuate expansion of the IO.
- Orbital septum: an extension of orbital bone periosteum (originates at the arcus marginalis); attaches to the levator aponeurosis 2–5 mm above the superior tarsus in upper lid (attaches lower in the Asian eyelid and thus creates a lower to absent lid crease). Fuses with the lower lid retractors in the lower eyelid within 1–2 mm from the inferior border of tarsus. Is immediately deep to orbicularis muscle and superficial to preaponeurotic orbital fat.
- Suspensory "ligamentous" system
    - Whitnall's ligament (superior transverse ligament): condensation of levator aponeurosis suspended high in orbit, attached medially to the trochlea and laterally to the orbital lobe of the lacrimal gland and also attaches laterally to the orbital wall near the frontozygomatic suture (above but not at Whitnall's tubercle). Acts to change the direction of pull of the levator muscle from horizontal to vertical and limits the extent of lid elevation.
    - Lockwood's ligament: present in the lower lid and is analogous to Whitnall's in the upper lid. Arises from inferior side of IR and continues anteriorly as the CPF (lower lid retractors) with contributions from intramuscular septae and Tenon's capsule. It has medial and lateral horns that attach to the retinaculum, which

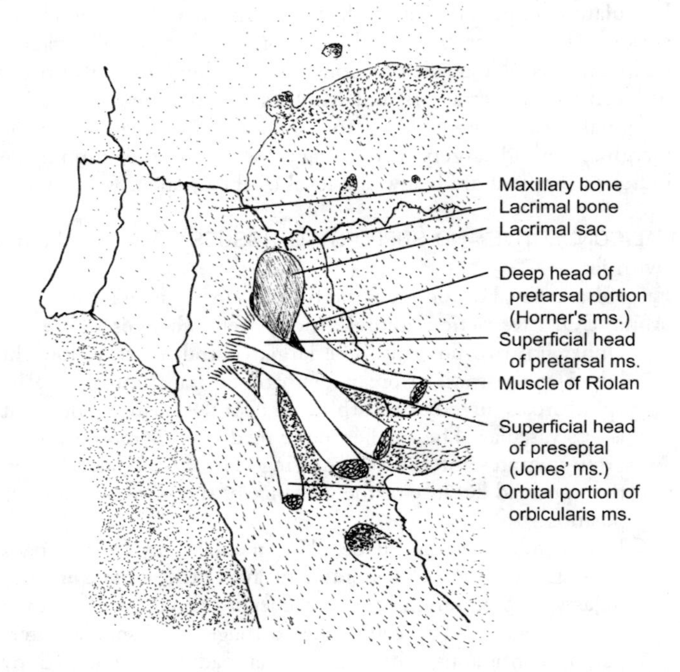

Figure 2–7 The left medial canthus anatomy and tendinous insertions of the orbicularis muscle.

attaches medially to the posterior lacrimal crest and laterally to the lateral orbital tubercle (Whitnall's tubercle), forming a suspensory hammock for the globe.

- Canthal ligaments (also known as tendons) (Fig. 2–7): lateral ligament has a superior and inferior crux. The anterior limb of the medial canthal tendon attaches to the frontal (nasal) process of the maxillary bone; the posterior portion (deep head of the pretarsal and preseptal orbicularis muscle) inserts onto the posterior lacrimal crest and fossa and is important in maintaining apposition of lids to the globe. The tarsus is like a knight's visor that pivots at the canthal tendons.

CARUNCLE Modified lower lid margin composed of nonkeratinized stratified epithelium, with 15 to 20 fine hairs, sebaceous glands, lacrimal glands similar to Krause, and goblet cells. Blood is supplied from the superior medial palpebral artery, innervated from the infratrochlear nerve, and lymph drainage is into the submaxillary nodes.

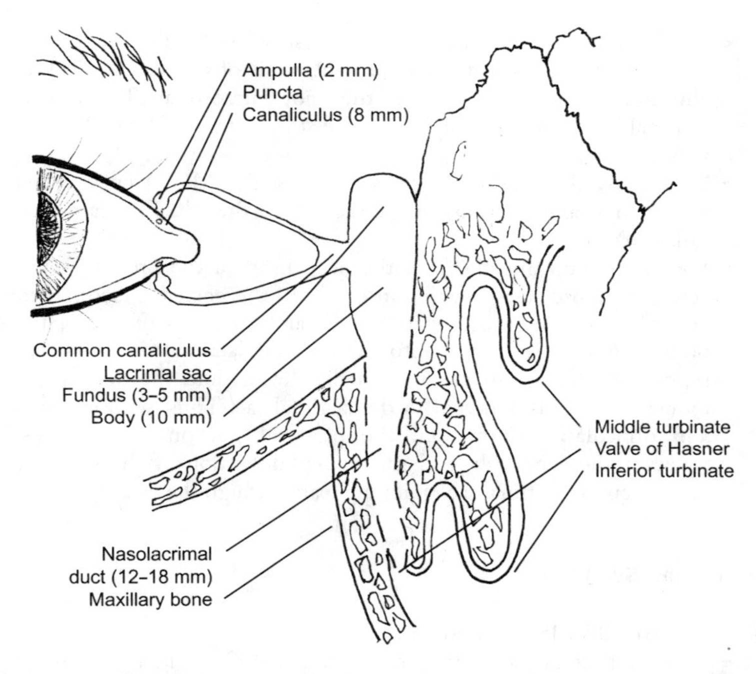

Figure 2–8 The right lacrimal drainage system, showing the soft tissue and bony components.

LACRIMAL DRAINAGE SYSTEM (Fig. 2–8) Begins at the punctum, which extends 2 mm to the ampulla (largest diameter of canalicular system), and into the canaliculus. Nearly 90% of the population has a common canaliculus (1 mm in diameter), which travels 8 mm through the valve of Rosenmüller (Maier's sinus) into the lacrimal sac. Drainage then proceeds through the valve of Krause and Arlt's sinus that open from the sac to the nasolacrimal duct. The spiral valves of Hyrtl and Taillefer are present within the duct that opens through the valve of Hasner into the inferior meatus (1.5 cm up and in from the nasal opening).

- Lacrimal drainage system forms at the 12 mm embryo stage from surface ectoderm (lacrimal gland forms at 25 mm). Nasolacrimal sac forms first, then canalization begins at 4 months (50 mm stage) and precedes bidirectionally (thus valve of Hasner opens last).
- Amniocele and lacrimal sac mucocele are misnomers: they are really imperforate puncta and valve of Hasner with accumulation of lacrimal sac secretions (from goblet cells in the nonciliated pseudostratified columnar epithelium of the sac).

- Lacrimal sac lies between the anterior (strongest) and posterior (most functionally and structurally important) arms of the MCT. The sac is anterior to the septum and is thus not intraorbital. The posterior lacrimal crest is lacrimal bone, and the anterior lacrimal crest is maxillary bone.
- Classically, the fundus of the sac (above the MCT) enlarges with malignancy, and the body of the sac (below the MCT) enlarges with inflammation.
- Lacrimal pump: mostly from the deep head of the pretarsal muscle (Horner's tensor tarsi), which inserts onto the posterior lacrimal crest and also encircles the canaliculi. The anterior head of the pretarsal orbicularis muscle inserts onto the anterior lacrimal crest. The preseptal orbicularis also has two medial heads, and the deep portion (Jones' muscle) is adherent to the lacrimal sac. Thus, with each blink and orbicularis contraction, the pretarsal portion of the muscle squeezes the canaliculi, and the preseptal portion of the orbicularis pulls open the lacrimal sac, pumping tears through the drainage system.

Signs and Symptoms

ABAXIAL GLOBE DISPLACEMENT

- Upward: maxillary sinus tumor, lymphoma, capillary hemangioma, and rhabdomyosarcoma
- Nasal: sphenoid wing meningioma
- Downward: dermoid, encephalocele, arteriovenous shunt, varix, and mucocele
- Temporal: lacrimal sac mass and ethmoid mucocele

AIDS-ASSOCIATED EYELID LESIONS Keratoacanthoma, molluscum contagiosum, and Kaposi's sarcoma. All often have multiple lesions.

"BIG, RED" EYELID LESIONS Capillary hemangioma, Kaposi's sarcoma, hemangiopericytoma, Merkel cell CA (golf ball size), and pilomatricoma (hair cell tumor)

CALCIFIED LESIONS Phlebolith, varix, lymphangioma, chronic inflammation, pleomorphic adenoma, old hemangioma, meningioma, and dermoid. Calcification usually indicates chronicity.

CANALICULAR STENOSIS Infection (herpes simplex virus, trachoma, mononucleosis), inflammation (SJS, OCP), trauma (lacerations, chemical or thermal injury, probings), allergy, radiation therapy, tumors (rare), canaliculitis, and eyedrops (antivirals, strong miotics, epinephrine-containing)

CHORISTOMA Normal tissue (albeit disorganized) in abnormal location (chorista if single-cell type), such as dermoid and lymphangioma (although some believe that there are lymphatics in the orbit)

CLASSIC MASS LOCATIONS
- Central/intraconal orbit: ON glioma, meningioma, hemangioma, and neurolemmoma
- Peripheral orbit: dermoid cysts, neurofibroma, pseudotumor, lymphoma, rhabdomyosarcoma, lacrimal gland tumors, and metastatic cancer
- Subperiosteal: hematoma, mucocele, abscess, and eosinophilic granuloma

CYSTIC LESIONS Dermoid cyst (most common cause), lacrimal cysts, degenerated neoplasms, lymphangioma ("chocolate cysts"), and benign mixed cell tumor (cystic changes helps to differentiate from adenomatous neoplasm)

DEEP SUPERIOR SULCUS Anophthalmos, levator dehiscence, and fat atrophy

DEGENERATIVE DISEASES OF THE ORBIT Fat atrophy (50% of degenerative disease), fat prolapse (27%), myopia (11%), and others

DESTRUCTIVE BONE LESIONS Metastatic cancer (in children usually metastatic neuroblastoma), reparative granuloma, aneurysmal bone cysts, Ewing's and osteogenic sarcoma, fibrosarcoma, histiocytosis X, (Langerhans' cells histiocytoses, especially eosinophilic granuloma), leukemia, lymphoma, and sarcoidosis.

DISTICHIASIS Extra row of short, soft lashes posterior to normal lashes usually in meibomian orifices. May be congenital (autosomal dominant) or secondary to inflammatory conditions (SJS, OCP, chronic blepharitis, etc.).

DYSMOTILITY EOM palsy, myasthenia, CPEO, CN III (rule out aneurysm or tumor) or CN IV or VI palsies

ECTROPION Outward rotation of lid margin, typically lower lid. Signs and symptoms: tearing (no punctal apposition), ocular irritation, canthal dehiscence, inferior scleral show, punctal eversion, lid margin keratinization, and possible keratopathy.
- Involutional: most common, age-related lid laxity with defect of lateral canthal tendon/medial canthal tendon, not tarsus. Treat with horizontal lid tightening or shortening (lateral tarsal strip procedure, full-thickness wedge resection), medial spindle, or two-snip procedure.

- Cicatricial: relative deficit of anterior lamella, often from UV-damaged tight skin, chemical/thermal injury, skin tumors, or inflammatory disease. Treat with skin graft, Z-plasty (changes vertical tension to horizontal), transposition flap, mid-face-lift, or lid shortening if mild.
- Paralytic: CN VII palsy, botulinum toxin. Treat with lower lid recession and LTS with spacer to stiffen the lower lid and gold weight upper lid, lateral tarsorrhaphy, or Arion sling (silicone ocular cerclage).
- Mechanical: tumor, edema. Treat underlying cause.
- Congenital: rare; associated with blepharophimosis.

ENTROPION Inward rotation of lid margin, usually lower lid. Signs and symptoms: foreign body sensation, entropion worse in downgaze or with forcible closure. Check snap back, lateral commissure position, distraction, punctal position, fat atrophy, and orbicularis override (thickening), and evert the lid (scarring, fornix shortening, trachoma).

- Involutional: may have several contributing factors, including CPF dehiscence (inferior cul-de-sac deepened or visible white line), retractor disinsertion or redundancy, horizontal laxity, overriding of preseptal orbicularis, fat atrophy enophthalmos. Involutional entropion of the lower lid is much like involutional ptosis of the upper lid. Often has a spastic component clinically from sustained squeezing or overriding orbicularis. Treat by reattaching the CPF (suture to inferior border of tarsus), lid shortening (LTS), tape applied to the skin, Quickert-Rathbun rotational sutures, and Bick or Wies procedure.
- Cicatricial: deficient posterior lamella (conjunctiva or tarsus) as from chemical injury, OCP, SJS, or trauma. Treat underlying problem, then consider conjunctiva graft (hard palate gives stiffer graft; may also harvest from mouth, vagina, or nasal mucosa, or use amniotic membrane, alloderm, or Gortex).
- Congenital, developmental: usually posterior lamella shortening and anterior lamellar excess, with overriding of preseptal orbicularis onto pretarsus orbicularis. Tarsal kink is rare; more often from epiblepharon.
  - Epiblepharon: extra skinfold, usually in Asians, and usually worse in downgaze. Pulling eyelid down manually helps break spasm. Patients often grow out of it; otherwise, may reform eyelid crease.
- Mechanical: treat underlying cause.

ENLARGING ORBITAL MASS Capillary or cavernous hemangioma, lymphangioma, hemangiopericytoma, varix, and rhabdomyosarcoma

ENOPHTHALMOS Scirrhous breast CA, trauma, floor fracture, congenital absence of sphenoid wing, postradiation therapy and postinflammatory orbital cicatrization

EPICANTHUS Fold of skin covering medial canthus. Classified based on position of the fold:

- Tarsalis: upper lid fold larger (Down syndrome)
- Inversus: lower lid larger (blepharophimosis)
- Palpebralis: equal, upper and lower
- Supraciliaris: from brow to medial canthus

EPIPHORA NLDO, poor punctal position, reflex lacrimation from external disease or CN V irritation, pseudodeficiency of basic secretions, "crocodile tears" (tearing when hungry or eating) from aberrant regeneration of CN VII

EYELID EDEMA (MNEMONIC: CRAB HAD FISH) **C**halazion, **r**enal disease, **a**ngioneurotic edema, **b**lepharochalasis, **h**eart disease, **a**llergy, **d**acryoadenitis, **f**at herniation, **i**nfection (conjunctivitis), **s**uperior vena cava syndrome, **h**ypothyroidism

EYELID RETRACTION Thyroid eye disease is most common cause of unilateral and bilateral retraction (from stimulation of Müller's muscle); may also be caused by Parinaud's dorsal midbrain syndrome (Collier's sign), recession of SR or IR, congenital retraction, surgical overcorrection of ptosis, Marcus Gunn jaw wink, hydrocephalus (such as convergence-retraction nystagmus in periaqueductal stenosis), sympathomimetic drugs, aberrant regeneration, cirrhosis, basal ganglia disease (Parkinson's), or pseudoretraction from ptosis of other lid.

FACIAL ASYMMETRY Fibrous dysplasia, NF, osteosarcoma, congenital hypoplasia, craniofacial dysostoses, and silent sinus syndrome

FIVE ORBITAL COMPARTMENTS Subperiosteal, extraconal, intraconal, subtenons, and subarachnoid spaces

FOUR ORBITAL TUMORS TO EXCISE COMPLETELY (BECAUSE OF RISK OF RECURRENCE WITH MALIGNANT POTENTIAL) Benign mixed tumor (pleomorphic adenoma), hemangiopericytoma, fibrous histiocytoma, and schwannoma

FROZEN GLOBE Metastatic cancer, orbital phycomycosis, and sclerosing pseudotumor

HAMARTOMA Abnormal tissue "at home" in normal location (called hamartia if from single-cell line), such as cavernous hemangioma.

HYPEROSTOSIS OF BONE Prostate CA, orbital osteoma (associated with familial adenomatous polyposis and CHRPE lesions; refer for colonoscopy), meningioma (sphenoid wing 10x more common than ON sheath meningiomas), and fibrous dysplasia

INFILTRATIVE LESIONS Plexiform neurofibroma, lymphangioma, capillary hemangioma, metastatic cancer, malignant fibrous histiocytoma, lymphoma, leukemia, and amyloid

INFLAMMATORY LESIONS OF THE ORBIT 85% are thyroid orbitopathy; of the remaining nonthyroid lesions, most are pseudotumor (46%), infectious (36%), vasculitic (7%), ocular inflammation (5%), Tolosa-Hunt (2.6%), sarcoid (1.3%), or others.

MARCUS GUNN JAW WINKING Eye opens with jaw movement to the contralateral side; associated with aberrant regeneration, congenital ptosis, Duane's syndrome, double-elevator palsy.

MULTIPLE ERUPTIVE SKIN OR EYELID LESIONS Such as seborrheic keratosis, fibroepithelial polyps or acanthoma; consider occult visceral cancer (such as Muir-Torre syndrome).

MUSCLE LESIONS, ENLARGED MUSCLES (MNEMONIC: MASSIVE MUSCLES ARE LIKELY TO CAUSE GIANT TROUBLE) **M**yositis, **m**etastatic cancer, **a**myloid/acromegaly, **l**ymphoma/lymphangioma, **t**hyroid, **c**arotid-cavernous sinus fistula (arteriovenous shunts), **g**ranulomatosis lesions (such as Wegener's granulomatosis), and **t**richinosis/trauma

NEUROGENIC TUMORS Wing meningiomas (30%), glioma (20%), neurofibroma (17%), schwannoma (12%), optic nerve sheath meningioma (9%), and others

ON MASS LESIONS Glioma, meningioma, neurofibroma, metastatic cancer, leukemia

ORBITAL HEMORRHAGE Trauma is primary cause; also varix, lymphangioma, bleeding diathesis, rickets or scurvy, barotrauma, or idiopathic.

ORBITAL LESIONS IN CHILDHOOD (0–20 YEARS OLD) Structural/dermoid (11%), inflammatory (14%), thyroid (10%), and capillary hemangioma (9%), and others

ORBITAL LESIONS IN MIDDLE-AGED PATIENTS (20–60 YEARS OLD) Thyroid (61%), neoplastic (12%), and others

ORBITAL LESIONS IN OLDER ADULTS (>60 YEARS OLD) Thyroid (40%), neoplastic (27%), inflammatory (12%), and lymphoproliferative (11%), and others

PARASELLAR OR SPHENOCAVERNOUS SYNDROME Constellation of cranio-orbital signs from many etiologies encompassing:

- Superior orbital fissure syndrome: CN III, IV, V_1, VI palsies with spared CN II and CN V_2 function. Etiology is similar to orbital apex syndrome.
- Orbital apex syndrome: SOF syndrome plus ON involved. Causes include tumors (most commonly sphenoid wing meningioma or pituitary adenoma, also glioma), trauma, infection, Tolosa-Hunt (name is commonly used as pseudotumor of the apex but is actually a specific granulomatous inflammation around the carotid siphon), sarcoid, sphenoid mucocele, or posterior dermoid.
- Cavernous sinus syndrome: variable signs of SOF or apex syndrome, especially if a Horner's syndrome is present with CN III or VI dysfunction. If CN V_2 is involved, then lesion is in posterior cavernous sinus. Caused by carotid-cavernous sinus or dural fistula, carotid artery aneurysm, infection, or inflammation. Imitators include botulinum and Miller Fisher syndrome.

PRIMARY ORBITAL TUMORS PRESENTING BY AGE Childhood (51%), middle age (41%), older age (8%)

PROPTOSIS Graves' disease (leading cause in adults), cellulitis (leading cause in children); also pseudotumor, tumors, and carotid–cavernous sinus fistulas. Bilateral: Graves' disease (leading cause of bilateral proptosis), pseudotumor, Wegener's granulomatosis, and neoplasm

PROPTOSIS, RAPID Orbital cellulitis, rhabdomyosarcoma, hemorrhage, and lymphangioma with hemorrhage

PSEUDOPROPTOSIS Ptosis of other lid, lid retraction, buphthalmos, myopia, familial, EOM palsy, contralateral enophthalmos

PSEUDOPTOSIS Dermatochalasis, brow ptosis, eyelid edema, chalazion or other tumor, contralateral lid retraction, hypotropia (e.g., double-elevator palsy), enophthalmos (e.g., blow-out fracture), phthisis bulbi, and microphthalmos

PTOSIS DIFFERENTIAL DIAGNOSIS Congenital (myogenic), CPEO, levator dehiscence, Horner's syndrome, botulinum toxin, CN III palsy, trauma

PTOSIS, BLEPHAROPTOSIS Drooping eyelids, which may interfere with superior visual field. Surgical options depend on levator function. If unilateral, remember that surgery on one side may cause the contralateral lid to become more ptotic due to Herring's law because the levator is innervated bilaterally by the caudate CN III nucleus.

- Aponeurotic, involutional: acquired dehiscence of levator aponeurosis with age or from postoperative or other trauma, chronic edema, or blepharochalasis. Signs and symptoms include high lid crease, excellent levator function, thinning of lid superior to the upper tarsal plate. Treat with levator advancement.
- Neurogenic: CN III palsy with levator paresis may be acquired (vascular, aneurysm, trauma, tumors, botulinum toxin) or present congenitally (ptosis is stationary; consider surgery after age 5; monitor for amblyopia). Horner's syndrome affecting Müller's muscle causes a minimal ptosis.
  - Aberrant regeneration of CN III: inferior division of CN III abnormally innervates superior division, and lid may be ptotic in primary gaze but retracts in medial or inferior gaze as the levator is stimulated with the MR or IR (pseudo-Graefe's sign: the lid goes up when eye looks down).
  - Marcus Gunn jaw winking: aberrant levator muscle innervation with the ipsilateral lateral pterygoid muscle (CN V) causes a synkinetic ptosis.
- Myogenic: usually congenital (from poor levator development with a fatty infiltration and fibrosed levator muscle) but rarely acquired in CPEO, oropharyngeal dystrophy, muscular dystrophy, or myasthenia gravis (worse after prolonged upgaze). Poor muscle contraction and relaxation. Do surgery (usually frontalis sling) before school age.
- Mechanical: levator hematoma, trauma to the levator, aponeurosis, or Müller's muscle.
- Others: anterior segment disease (e.g., corneal abrasion) or prolonged topical or subcutaneous steroid, pseudoptosis (contralateral retraction, etc.)

PULSATILE PROPTOSIS Carotid–cavernous sinus fistula or arteriovenous malformations (abnormal vascular flow), mucocele or encephalocele (transmission of normal intracranial pulsations), surgical removal of bone or neurofibromatosis (NF) 1 (absence of sphenoid wing)

PUNCTAL STENOSIS Many causes including infection, trauma, congenital, and secondary to drug reaction such as with chemotherapy (Taxol) and miotics (especially phospholine iodide). Consider two-snip procedure or silicone stent intubation.

SECONDARY ORBITAL LESIONS Extension of nasopharyngeal carcinoma (43%), conjunctival cancer (20%), eyelid cancer (18%), and lacrimal sac tumors (9%)

"S"-SHAPED EYELID Plexiform neurofibroma, dacroadenitis, and sarcoid

SUPERONASAL ORBITAL MASSES Rhabdomyosarcoma, myocele, mucopyocele, encephalocele, neurofibroma

TOUTON GIANT CELL-CONTAINING LESIONS Erdheim-Chester, necrobiotic xanthogranuloma, juvenile xanthogranuloma. Tissue granulomas with a ring of nuclei around the periphery of the giant cell.

UMBILICATED SKIN LESIONS Keratoacanthoma, BCC, and molluscum

UNILATERAL PERIORBITAL INFLAMMATION IN A CHILD Ruptured dermoid cyst, rhabdomyosarcoma (rubor without calor), pseudotumor, leukemia, eosinophilic granuloma, and infantile cortical hyperostosis

VASCULAR NEOPLASMS Capillary hemangioma (41%), lymphangiomas (33%), and cavernous hemangioma (21%)

WELL-DIFFERENTIATED LESIONS Cavernous hemangioma, hemangiopericytoma, peripheral nerve sheath tumors, and fibrous histiocytoma

Exam and Imaging

EXAM, EYELID Record lid measurements; assess corneal protective mechanisms (ensure good blink reflex and CN V function; rule out inferior keratopathy or lagophthalmos; look for Bell's phenomenon; check tear production with TBUT or basal secretion test or Schirmer's). Evaluate brow, lid laxity, canthal tendons, and presence of steatoblepharon. In ptosis evaluation, check for Herring's effect (lift the ptotic lid to see if the contralateral lid lowers), look for jaw wink, and, if new onset, rule out myasthenia and check EOM function. Document with photos, and get superior visual field (VF) evaluation for ptosis or dermatochalasis.

- Brow to upper lid (BUL): measure temporally, centrally, and nasally.
- Excess skin (XS): grade 1–4 for upper and lower lids.
- Herniated orbital fat (HOF): grade 1–4 (two fat pads upper and three lower lid).
- Horizontal palpebral fissure (25–30 mm) interpupillary distance (60 mm). Distance between medial canthal angles (25–30 mm), telecanthus is increased soft tissue distance, and hypertelorism is widened bony distance. Exorbitism is lateral bony orbital walls >90 degrees.

- Levator function (12–14 mm): most important measurement in ptosis evaluation. Perform by eliminating frontalis muscle function, then measure lid excursion as patient looks down, then up. If >10 mm, then good function; fair function: 4–8 mm, poor function: <4 mm.
- Lid laxity: evaluate canthal tendons, snap back (0 normal to 3+ lax), and distraction (<6 mm of lower lid laxity is normal).
- Margin to crease distance (MCD): upper lid crease height normally 7–8 mm (males), 9–10 mm (females); increases with levator dehiscence because the crease is from the insertion of aponeurosis fibers into skin. May also measure margin to fold distance (MFD).
- Vertical palpebral fissure: if >9 mm, then probably has inferior scleral show.
- Margin to reflex distance 1 (MRD_1): distance from upper eyelid margin to the corneal light reflection; normal 3.5–4.0 mm; if >5, suspect superior scleral show.
- Margin to reflex distance 2 (MRD_2): distance from lower eyelid margin to the corneal light reflection; normal 5 mm.
- Inferior scleral show (0 mm)

EXAM, ORBIT Do full eyelid work-up, plus evaluate ON function (BCVA, look for APD, color plates or red top test or D-15), check stereo vision to screen for early strabismus, exophthalmometry, IOP in primary and upgaze, current DFE, and obtain VF for baseline or any visual changes.

- "6 P's" of orbital disease:
    - Pain: inflammation, infection, malignancy, ischemia
    - Proptosis: Graves', pseudotumor, tumor, fistula
    - Progression: hours—trauma, infection, hemorrhage; days—previous plus inflammation, metastatic cancer; weeks—all previous plus neoplasia, vascular, cystic lesions
    - Palpation: masses may cause resistance to retropulsion
    - Pulsation: arteriovenous fistulas or cerebrospinal fluid pulsations
    - Periorbital changes: salmon patch in lymphoma, erythema with inflammation, etc.
- Blowout fractures: do ptosis work-up, plus evaluate motility, hypophthalmos, diplopic VF, forced ductions and generations.
- Thyroid: do ptosis work-up, plus evaluate motility, diplopic VF, Humphrey visual field (HVF), color plates, pupils, manifest refraction if patient is not 20/20, tonometry in primary and upgaze, and exophthalmometry.

EXAM, TEARING Look at lids, anterior segment, and secretory tests such as TBUT (if no anesthetic >15 seconds is normal, determined by goblet cell and oil function) and basal secretion test or Schirmer's I (with anesthetic, >10 mm of wetting at 5 minutes is normal). Lacrimal drainage tests include:

- Dye disappearance test (DDT): excretory test; test is positive if there is significant dye present in the tear film 5 minutes after fluorescein was instilled.
- Jones I (primary dye test): excretory test to determine if tears are passing into nose under normal physiological conditions. Use 2% fluorescein drop in eye and a topical decongestant/anesthetic in nose; place cotton fluff in inferior meatus. If after 5 minutes no fluorescein is recovered, there may be a functional block (but also negative result in 20–30% of normals). Test is positive if dye is recovered in nose. May also use light to look in nose after 10 minutes, or use Calgy swab or have patient blow nose. Gives same information as DDT.
- Jones II (secondary dye test): nonphysiologic test to determine if dye has entered the lacrimal sac. After DDT or Jones I, irrigate through the punctum with saline; recovery of dye in nose indicates lower lacrimal system obstruction. If clear fluid is recovered, obstruction is before the lacrimal sac.
- Jones III: assesses functioning of surgical osteotomy; test is positive if dye is recovered in nose of a post-dacryocystorhinostomy (DCR) or conjunctivodacryocystorhinostomy (CJDCR) patient.
- Probe to evaluate upper system, not the nasolacrimal duct (NLD), except in children.
- Irrigation: 3 cc of saline injected with blunt canula; have patient lean forward, feel sac, and look in nose or have patient report swallowing of fluid.
- Dacryocystography (DCG): nonphysiologic Jones II test using radiopaque dye, then x-ray; can show size and filling defects within sac.
- Dacryoscintigraphy: physiologic test imaging the flow of technetium dye placed in the inferior fornix.

EXOPHTHALMOMETRY Hertel exophthalmometry (upper limits of normal: black males 25 mm, black females 24 mm, white males 22 mm, and white females 21 mm); Naugel exophthalmometry measures from superior and inferior rim (useful after decompression surgery or zygomatic complex fracture), and Luedde exophthalmometry uses ruler (useful with children).

FINE NEEDLE ASPIRATION Limited usefulness and never use for cystic orbital masses or lacrimal gland tumors.

ORBITAL TRAUMA (MNEMONIC: TICS) **T**etanus, **i**ntravenous antibiotics (e.g., Ancef), **c**omputed tomography (CT) thin cuts (3 mm) axial and coronal, and **s**hield for suspected open globe are usually appropriate interventions by emergency personnel while awaiting eye evaluation.

RADIOLOGICAL IMAGING (Fig. 2–9 shows basic orbital structures of the right orbit seen with axial CT images)

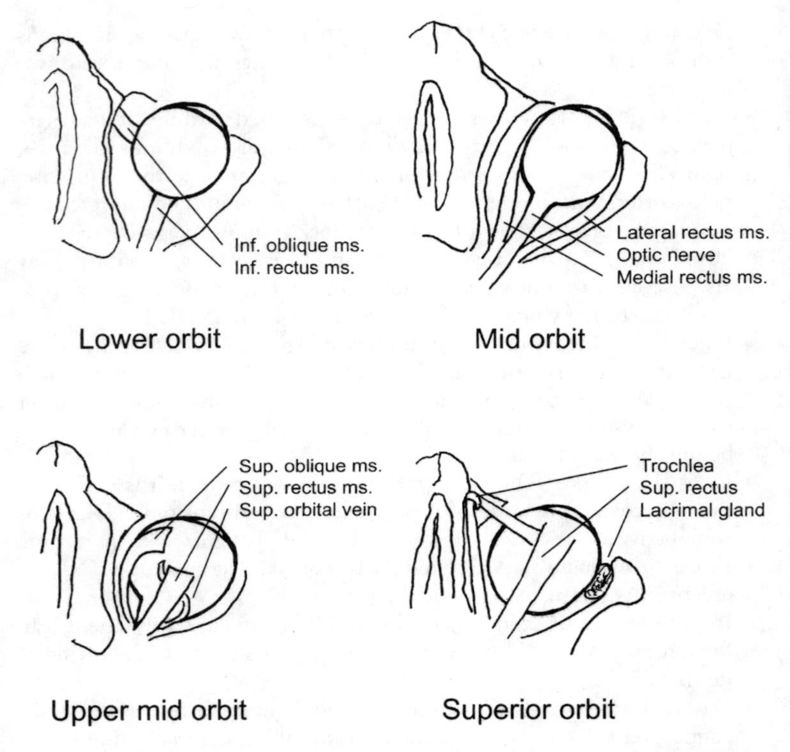

Figure 2–9 Serial diagrams of the right orbit, superior view, showing the basic orbital structures that may be seen on axial CT images.

- CT is the imaging of choice in orbital trauma and gives excellent bony detail.
- Magnetic resonance imaging (MRI) is never the initial imaging modality in trauma or in unconscious patients without adequate history. On MRI, vitreous is dark in T1 and bright in T2 (mnemonic: water is white); orbital fat is bright in T1 and dark in T2.
- Plane x-ray films, especially Waters views, give limited views of the bony orbit and may help localize metallic foreign bodies when CT is not available.

ULTRASOUND A-scan = amplitude mode, 8 MHz. B-scan = brightness mode, 10 MHz (can only see about 25 mm into the anterior orbit). Standardized A-scan is an acoustic biopsy (99% sensitive for melanoma, 90% for metastatic cancer).

- Doppler principle: fluid moving toward probe returns at higher frequency signal and vice versa.
- Intraocular mass ultrasound procedure: in B-scan mode have patient look in direction of lesion, place probe on lid, and measure anteroposterior view straight on (measure lesion distance from ON). Then place probe on sclera with probe 90 degrees away from lesion for a transverse measurement. With probe tip pointing in the meridian of the lesion, take longitudinal measurement. Note the lesion meridian, clock hour, and whether it is anterior or posterior to the equator. Then perform A-scan to evaluate mass characteristics.
  - Melanoma usually has a dome shape, regular surface, collar-button or mushroom, and orange pigment; ultrasound shows orbital shadowing, internal hollowing, choroidal excavation, angle-kappa, and low reflectivity. Metastatic cancer shows irregular surface, often subretinal fluid (SRF).
- Orbital mass ultrasound: useful to evaluate mass topography and quantitative characteristics (internal structure, regularity, reflectivity, sound attenuation posterior to lesion). Kinetic examination is useful to evaluate consistency and vascularity. Use transocular or periocular views to see orbital lesions, muscle or ON lesions. Increased ON thickness may be from tumor or from subarachnoid fluid if the ON thickness decreases by 10% when patient looks from primary gaze to 30-degree abduction.
  - Most tumors, neurofibromas, lymphangiomas, and pseudotumors have high internal reflectivity; however, melanomas, sinus mucoceles, and small cell tumors such as lymphoma and lung and cervical CA have low internal reflectivity.

Congenital and Genetic Disease

ANKYLOBLEPHARON Failure of lids to separate; filiforme variant has strands of tissue connecting lids. Associated with visceral and spinal abnormalities.

BLEPHAROCHALASIS Rare familial disorder with recurrent bouts of lid edema and inflammation in young females. Eventually leads to thickened skin, ptosis from levator dehiscence, or orbital fat prolapse.

BLEPHAROPHIMOSIS SYNDROME (MNEMONIC: PET PEEVE) **P**tosis, **e**picanthus inversus (lower lid), **t**elecanthus, and **p**himosis (horizontal palpebral fissure shortening). Also flattened nasal bridge, lop ears, midfacial hypoplasia, hypertelorism, euryblepharon, lower lid ectropion, but with normal intelligence quotient (IQ). Associated with dysmenorrhea and ovarian failure; thus, greater inheritance in males, as females are often infertile. Most are autosomal dominant, chromosome 3q22, but also sporadic. Treat telecanthus first, then ptosis.

BLEPHAROPTOSIS, MYOGENIC CONGENITAL PTOSIS Also known as simple isolated congenital ptosis. May be sporadic or autosomal dominant, characterized by dysgenesis of the levator muscle, which is atrophic and replaced by fibrous or fatty tissue. Patients may use CN VII to elevate the brow and thus lids. Check for Marcus Gunn jaw wink (synkinesis of CN III and CN V not aberrant regeneration), which may cause surgical overcorrection if not recognized. Other blepharoptosis syndromes include:

- Congenital fibrosis of the EOM: rare, autosomal dominant, bilateral ptosis and external ophthalmoplegia; chromosome 12
- Chronic progressive external ophthalmoplegia (CPEO): manifestation of many disorders (most commonly mitochondrial myopathies), characterized by bilateral, symmetrical, progressive ptosis, and ophthalmoparesis; eyes do not move with head motion.
- Kearns-Sayre syndrome: mitochondrial inheritance with CPEO before 20 years old, plus retinal pigmentary degeneration and heart block.
- Oculopharyngeal muscular dystrophy: late onset progressive dysphagia and bilateral and symmetrical moderate ptosis with good levator function (LF). Ask about swallowing difficulty. Autosomal dominant, chromosome 14q11; usually in French-Canadians.

CLEFTING DISORDERS, EYELID COLOBOMA Usually upper eyelid full-thickness colobomatous defect; rule out other clefting (e.g., Tessier clefts of lip and palate). Lubricate cornea; surgical repair with direct closure or Tenzel flap (no lid sharing techniques in children).

- Goldenhar's syndrome: asymmetric first and second branchial arch disorder (like Treacher Collins syndrome) associated with upper lid colobomatous defect, epibulbar dermoid, Duane's syndrome, preauricular appendages, and bony defects. Also microphthalmia, anophthalmia, ON hypoplasia, ocular colobomas, palatal and facial clefts.
- Pierre Robin syndrome: is a symptoms complex characterized by small jaw and often have clefting; most patients have defined syndromes, most commonly Stickler's.
- Treacher Collins–Franceschetti syndrome (mandibulofacial dysostosis): rare autosomal dominant, first and second branchial arch developmental disorder of mesodermal migration. Patients have "hound dog" faces with bilateral and symmetrical downward slant of palpebral fissures, pseudocolobomas of the lids, midface hypoplasia, and dental and ear abnormalities. Mandibular and laryngeal hypoplasia may be life threatening.

CONGENITAL EYELID EVERSION May be from infection such as chlamydia or associated with Down syndrome. Lubricate; often resolves.

CRANIOSYNOSTOSES Premature closure of cranial sutures (plagiocephaly if one suture); often have hypertelorism and small orbits. All are autosomal dominant except Carpenter's. Common features: midface hypoplasia, proptosis, telecanthus, V-pattern exotropia, and oral, dental, and respiratory problems.

- Crouzon syndrome: autosomal dominant, proptosis, malar hypoplasia, prominent lower lip and base of skull is hypoplastic
- Apert syndrome: autosomal dominant with digital involvement, proptosis
- Pfeiffer syndrome: Apert's with short, broad thumb and big toe, syndactyly, shallow orbits
- Carpenter syndrome: autosomal recessive, polysyndactyly

CRYPTOPHTHALMOS Autosomal recessive failure of eyelids and anterior segment to develop. Has absence of lacrimal gland, hairline grows over eyes, clefting, and usually normal hands.

- Fraser syndrome: cryptophthalmos with genitourinary abnormalities and syndactyly (as in Apert's with "mitten" hands)

DACRYOCYSTOCELE Enlarged lacrimal sac at birth from blocked Hasner's valve. Not a true cyst. Differential diagnosis includes hemangioma, encephalocele, and dermoid. Often resolves but may need massage or patient may become septic if infected and then need IV antibiotics and probing.

DISTICHIASIS Lashes from meibomian glands, usually fine hairs without consequence; autosomal dominant.

EPIBLEPHARON Autosomal dominant altered lower lid retractor attachments allowing override of pretarsal orbicularis muscle above lid margin, causing a congenital entropion (watch for keratopathy from lashes against globe), usually in Asian patients. Also associated with lymphedema (hypoplastic lymphatics that develop at about 10 years of age and persist lifelong even though lid changes improve) and odd malignancies (sarcomas, pheochromocytomas). Lubricate; patients usually outgrow.

EURYBLEPHARON Horizontal PF widening from hereditary descent of lateral canthus (lateral ectropion, antimongoloid slant) with widening of medial canthus. Treat with full-thickness skin graft; may have to address malar hypoplasia with implants and midface lift.

LACRIMAL FISTULA Epithelial-lined communication between common canaliculus or lacrimal sac and skin. If associated with NLDO with reflux through fistula, then treat with antibiotics, probing, and excision of fistulae.

NASOLACRIMAL DUCT OBSTRUCTION, CONGENITAL Present in up to 6% of neonates; 90% resolve without surgery by 12 months old. Tearing differential diagnosis includes congenital glaucoma. NLDO is usually from blocked Hasner's valve as it opens into the inferior turbinate and may have congenital dacryocystocele. Treat with Crigler massage, erythromycin ointment, then probing under general anesthesia with possible inferior turbinate infracture if not resolved by age 12 months. After age 18 to 24 months or several failed probings, consider silicone stent intubation. May also attempt balloon dilation of nasolacrimal duct (e.g., Lacricath), or consider DCR.

PHAKOMATOSES See Chapter 9 for complete description.

- Neurofibromatosis 1: café au lait spots, cutaneous neurofibromas, plexiform neurofibroma ("S"-shaped eyelid), ON glioma, absence of sphenoid wing (pulsatile proptosis), other osseous deformities
- Neurofibromatosis 2: bilateral acoustic neuroma, meningioma, glioma, schwannoma, sphenoid bone dysplasia, orbital, cutaneous, and plexiform neurofibromas
- Tuberous sclerosis: ash leaf spots, fine facial acne (adenoma sebaceum), retinal and CNS astrocytic hamartomas, defect on chromosome 9 (mnemonic: *sclerosis* has nine letters)
- Sturge-Weber syndrome (encephalotrigeminal angiomatosis): unilateral facial, choroidal, or meningeal cavernous angioma
- Louis-Bar's syndrome (ataxia-telangiectasia): telangiectasias on face, neck, or conjunctiva with cerebellar ataxia
- Wyburn-Mason's syndrome (racemose hemangioma): arteriovenous malformations of face, orbit, retina, and brain.
- von Hippel-Lindau disease (angiomatosis retinae): capillary hemangiomas of retina, cerebellar hemangioblastoma, 25% renal cell CA, renal, pancreatic, or other solid organ cysts, meningiomas, pheochromocytomas. Autosomal dominant defect on chromosome 3 (mnemonic: *VHL* is three letters).

Infectious Disease

CANALICULITIS Usually inferior canaliculus with focal swelling, and gritty sensation and resistance with probing. Usually from *Actinomyces israelii* with yellow concretions; may have a dacryolith. Also caused by *Streptomyces*, *Arachnia propionica* (*Streptothrix*), *Nocardia*, *Candida*, and *Aspergillus niger*. Treat with penicillin irrigation, external massage, and curettage.

CAVERNOUS SINUS THROMBOSIS An intracranial infection from infectious thrombosis in cavernous venous plexus. Rare today, but *Mucor* is most common cause, often in a obtunded toxic patient; high mortality.

DACRYOADENITIS Usually noninfectious (pseudotumor), but if infectious, usually viral (Epstein-Barr virus); higher rate in alcoholics.

DACRYOCYSTITIS Swelling and tenderness over lacrimal sac with mucopurulent reflux on palpation. Usually elderly women with NLDO and tear stasis from pneumococci or *Haemophilus influenzae*, *Pseudomonas*, mixed causes, *Actinomyces*, or *Candida*. Acutely treat with systemic (IV or PO and topical antibiotics), warm compresses, and pain control. Incise and drain a pointing abscess. Do not probe; will usually need DCR later.

ECHINOCOCCOSIS, HYDATID CYST DISEASE From dog tapeworm; rupture of cyst may cause severe inflammation. Diagnose with intradermal antigen (Casoni's reaction), and treat with excision of cyst.

HIV AND AIDS ORBITAL LESIONS Higher rate of sinusitis; also consider *Mycobacterium* avium intracellulare (MAI), pneumocystis, aspergillosis, cryptococcus, microsporidia, and rule out syphilis. Masquerades: Hodgkin's and non-Hodgkin's lymphoma are more aggressive, and may invade sinuses and orbit.

HORDEOLUM Acute infection of meibomian gland (internal stye or acute chalazion) or Zeis' or Moll's gland (external or common stye); may become chalazia (chronic). Treat with antibiotics, warm compresses; may excise chalazia if persistent.

MOLLUSCUM CONTAGIOSUM DNA poxvirus that causes a waxy umbilicated nodule; usually affects children and immunosuppressed patients (often multiple lesions) and is contagious. On pathology, Henderson-Paterson corpuscles are filled with poxvirus, and the expulsed virus may cause follicular conjunctivitis and ipsilateral preauricular lymphadenopathy. Resolves spontaneously, but if not, incise and central curettage (make it bleed), excision or Retin-A (tretinoin) treatment.

ORBITAL CELLULITIS (Table 2–1) Infection posterior to the septum often with proptosis, pain, EOM restriction, possibly decreased VA or APD; may have fever, sweats, nausea, or vomiting. Most cases (44%) are pediatric (0–20 years old), but also middle age (40%), and elderly (16%). Consider endogenous infection or malignancy. *Staphylococcus aureus* is leading cause, also *Streptococcus* species and anaerobes. In children, consider *Haemophilus* (rarely caused by HSV, HZV, *Aspergillus*, or *Mucor*). Usually contiguous

TABLE 2–1
Clinical Grouping of Orbital Cellulitis

Group 1	Inflammatory edema, preseptal, clear demarcation line at the arcus marginalis
Group 2	Orbital cellulitis, postseptal, EOM restriction; may have decreased VA
Group 3	Subperiosteal abscess; surgical debridement usually necessary
Group 4	Orbital abcess, systemic symptoms, abaxial displacement; urgent surgical debridement usually necessary
Group 5	Cavernous sinus thrombosis (no backflow valves in orbital veins) or orbital apex syndrome; bilateral orbital signs, dusky eyelids, profound CNS signs and symptoms; usually in an ICU setting

spread from sinusitis, most commonly ethmoids (thin perforated walls pneumatized at birth, whereas maxillary open by age 2–4 years old, frontal by 7–15 years old; sphenoid sinus is last to pneumatize). CT may show sinus opacification, diffuse orbital infiltration, ground-glass appearance, possible abscess formation, but CT findings lag the clinical picture (especially if the patient is clinically improving).

- Hospitalize and treat with IV antibiotics for at least 72 hours, then outpatient PO antibiotics for 14 days. In children, cover for *Haemophilus influenzae* and sinusitis organisms (e.g., vancomycin plus ceftazidime). Usually a very sick child; see patient several times per day. Blood culture is positive in 40% of children but not adults. In adults, cover gram-negative organisms and anaerobes (e.g., Unasyn or Cefepime plus clindamycin). Monitor vision, proptosis, motility, pupils, and CNS function. Lack of progression is good; if patient improves, then plateaus, consider abscess formation.
- Subperiosteal abscess: usually superomedial adjacent to ethmoids/frontal sinuses. Subperiosteal space is poorly vascularized (antibiotics poorly penetrate; thus, it is a surgical disease). Usually forms in a stable or improving patient who then deteriorates. May have nonaxial proptosis, ON atrophy, exposure keratitis, central retinal artery occlusion, cavernous sinus thrombosis, meningitis, and brain abscess. CT immediately; may see "ring" sign, or may have intraorbital loculi from septae of Koornneef. Treat with IV antibiotics and drainage. Children <9 years old can be medically treated up to 72 hours before considering drainage (83% improve medically, and only 17% who are drained have positive cultures; thus, it is usually a sterile phlegmon). Older children and adults need drainage (75–100% have culture-positive abscess after drainage). Urgent surgical intervention if ON compression (decreased VA, APD) or retinal compromise.
- Mucormycosis: facultative anaerobe causing obliterative vasculitis, pain, proptosis, bloody chemosis, and cavernous sinus syndrome. Usually presents in poorly controlled diabetes (70%), other immunosuppressed (18%), renal disease (5%), leukemia (3%), and no systemic illness (4%). Rapidly progressive with 6 to 8 hour window to begin treatment.
    - Get tissue biopsy (may see black eschar on conjunctiva, nasal or palate mucosa; if not, take some mucosa anyway). Pathology: large nonseptate hyphae with right angle branching on hematoxylin and eosin stain (H & E) or silver stain.
    - Treat with local surgical debridement until tissue freely bleeds (exenteration may be necessary if infection is extensive). Amphotericin B IV and local irrigation increase survival from 6% without treatment to 73% with treatment. Patients with diabetes do better because they have a treatable disease (reverse their ketoacidosis).
- Aspergillosis: chronic indolent orbital cellulitis with history of allergy, asthma, and sinusitis. Most patients are otherwise healthy; although

may be seen in patients with AIDS. CT may show allergic "aspergilloma," and pathology shows septate hyphae on H & E. Usually does not invade. Debride sinus, and treat with steroids.

PRESEPTAL CELLULITIS Acute onset of pain, tenderness, erythema, tense swelling but no proptosis, EOM restriction, APD or decreased VA and no pain with eye movement. Most common risk factor is skin trauma; may also be from chalazion, upper respiratory infection, sinusitis, or dental work. Usually from staphylococcus, streptococcus, or *Haemophilus influenzae.*

- Most adults can be diagnosed and treated clinically, but if unsure whether orbital involvement or in pediatric patient, then get complete blood count (CBC), blood culture, and CT.
- Oral antibiotics 7–10 days (e.g., Augmentin 500 mg 3 times per day or Keflex 500 mg 4 times per day). If failure to respond, then rule out abcess or foreign body. Sinus drainage if needed, warm compresses for 20 minutes 6 times per day. If <4 years old, hospitalize and use IV antibiotics (neonates are usually nonbacterial as they are protected by maternal Ab, but young children in general are more susceptible because of immunologic naivete, especially against encapsulated organisms due to poor splenic opsonization).
- Differential diagnosis: pseudotumor has "boggy" pink skin, not erythematous or indurated; no sinus disease or abscess. If diagnosis is uncertain, okay to admit for IV antibiotics; if no improvement in 48 hours, begin steroid treatment for pseudotumor.

TRACHOMA Chlamydial antigen in conjunctiva causes severe inflammatory reaction, resulting in posterior lamella shortening with entropion, keratitis sicca, and trichiasis. See Chapter 3.

TRICHINOSIS Nematode *Trichinella spiralis* from poorly cooked pork with encystment of muscles, eosinophilia. Treat with thiabendazole.

Neoplastic, Eyelid: Benign Cystic Lesions

EPIDERMAL INCLUSION CYST (EIC) Unilocular, solitary, slow-growing lesion from sequestered epithelium beneath epidermis, with epithelium cells facing lumen that secrete keratin. Milia are small multiple EIC.

HIDROCYSTOMA (SUDORIFEROUS CYST) Sweat gland origin (eccrine) with clear fluid (transilluminate), unilocular, and on pathology show arborization with cuboidal bilayer facing lumen.

- Apocrine hidrocystoma: from Moll's glands near lid margin; less common, pigmented (blue); arborizing lumen, apical "snouting" typifying apocrine secretion, and double epithelium layer on histology.

SYRINGOMA Most common adnexal eyelid tumor, from ductal eccrine sweat gland origin; benign; yellow, waxy, tadpole appearance. Syringocystadenoma (papilliform).

Neoplastic, Eyelid: Benign Growths

AMYLOID Periorbital cutaneous deposition usually with nonfamilial primary amyloidosis or secondary to systemic plasma cell dyscrasia (rarely with familial primary or other types of amyloidosis).

CHALAZION Obstruction of sebaceous apparatus with foreign body reaction around lipid, sterile, chronic lipogranuloma with multinucleated giant cells. Treat with hot compresses; if not resolved, then incision and curettage. If recurrent, differential diagnosis includes sebaceous cell CA.

HORDEOLUM Internal hordeolum, also called internal chalazion, is usually sterile. The acute external (anterior lamella) Zeis' glands, stye, is usually from staphylococcal infection.

JUVENILE XANTHOGRANULOMA (JXG) Benign nodular granulomatous disorder with multiple red-orange skin masses; iris xantholomas may cause spontaneous hyphema. Pathology shows Touton giant cells.

KERATOACANTHOMA Form of pseudoepitheliomatous hyperplasia (also seen in inverted follicular keratosis) that is an inflamed nodule with a central ulcer of keratin with very rapid onset and growth in an elderly patient. May resolve spontaneously but is usually excised, as it is difficult to distinguish from squamous cell carcinoma (SCC). Pathology shows "shoestring" sign (if you figuratively pull a string taut across the basement membrane of the histology slide, the lesion is always above the BM).

PHAKOMATOUS CHORISTOMA, ZIMMERMAN'S TUMOR Rare pediatric tumor of lenticular origin (lens in eyelid).

SEBACEOUS ADENOMA Rare benign tumor, seen as small yellow nodules usually on the face.

- Muir-Torre syndrome: multiple sebaceous adenomas with 50% incidence of visceral cancer (especially colon). Male to female ratio = 2:1, autosomal dominant with high penetrance; may also have multiple keratoacanthomas.

SQUAMOUS PAPILLOMA, SKIN TAG, ACROCHORDON Sessile or pedunculated proliferation of benign epidermis. Pathology shows apical keratosis with a fibrovascular core and red blood cells in the horn, as well as "hand in glove" appearance. May treat with excision or oral high-dose histamine-2 receptor blockers (e.g., Tagamet 4–5 g/day)

SEBORRHEIC KERATOSIS (SK) Variant of squamous papilloma with greasy "stuck-on" appearance. Pathology shows basaloid acanthosis, intraepithelial horn cysts, and variable hyperkeratosis. Is not CA, and basal cells are above the plane of the epidermis.

- Dermatosis papulosa nigra: multiple pigmented SK; common on facial skin of darkly pigmented patients.
- Inverted follicular keratosis: irritated SK, another form of pseudoepitheliomatous hyperplasia (as with keratoacanthoma). Lid margin is the primary body site for inverted follicular keratosis.

VERRUCA VULGARIS, COMMON WART Nontender, elevated, firm papule from human papilloma virus (HPV) infection. Pathology shows elongated acanthotic papillae that look like "church spires" and vacuoles in upper squamous layer that contain virus. Excision with cryotherapy to the base.

XANTHELASMA Symmetric, flat, yellow lesions that typically begin nasally in the upper eyelid. Pathology shows foamy histiocytes in the dermis with extruded lipid engulfed by macrophages. Usually normal serum lipid level (check if the patient is <40 years old) and also associated with diabetes. Excise (although may have deep extension), or use CO_2 laser or 100% trichloroacetic acid (TCA). Recurrence common.

Neoplastic, Eyelid: Hair Follicle Tumors ("Tricky" Tumors)

TRICHOEPITHELIOMA Most common benign hair follicle neoplasm with fleshy nodules that resemble BCC; usually presents in children and young adults, and may be inherited in autosomal dominant fashion.

TRICHOFOLLICULOMA Rare in periorbital skin but has firm nodule with central pore with white hairs.

TRICHILEMMOMA Nodular or fleshy malignant tumor from outer hair sheath (*lemma* = rind or sheath).

- Cowden disease: multiple facial trichilemmomas associated with occult neoplasm (especially breast or thyroid CA) and other hamartomas (keratoses, oral papillomas); autosomal dominant.

Neoplastic, Eyelid: Premalignant Lesions

ACTINIC KERATOSIS Most common precancerous lesion, with scaly papillary appearance. Pathology shows solar elastosis like pterygium; also has cellular atypia (but no anaplasia like CA), and demonstrates parakeratosis. Twelve percent become CA. Treat with cryotherapy, or excise with topical 5-fluorouracil (5-FU).

BOWEN'S DISEASE Is full thickness carcinoma in situ or intraepidermal SCC. Larger lesion than actinic keratosis, solitary; usually sun-exposed skin with "windblown look" on histology. If on non-sun-exposed skin, consider occult cancer (Rulon-Helwig syndrome) or arsenic ingestion.

Neoplastic, Eyelid: Malignant Lesions

BASAL CELL CARCINOMA (BCC) Most common lid cancer (87% of eyelid CA). Primary site is lower lid (50–60%), followed by medial canthus (25–30%,) and upper lid (10–15%). From UV exposure and solar keratosis. Often underestimated size by its appearance; great masquerader (like sebaceous gland CA). Early signs are telangiectasia and skin smoothing.

- Nodular is the most common type, with pearly raised nodule with central umbilication. May also present as nodulo-ulcerative, adenoid, pigmented, superficial, keratotic, cystic, or follicular, all of which are more benign. Infiltrating, morpheaform, or sclerosing/fibrosing types are less common but much more aggressive, often subclinical, increased recurrence; may have lash loss.
- Pathology shows "blue and below" (bluish-colored tumor cells that are below the BM), retraction artifact, peripheral palisading (also seen with other adnexal cancers), and desmoplasia. Morpheaform variant also has peripheral radiating cords ("Indian filing").
- Tumors at high risk for recurrence: sclerosing BCC and poorly defined tumors, "H" zone of face (down both temples and cheeks and across nose), cosmetically sensitive areas, young age, large size, digit or medial canthus location, and prior recurrent CA.
- Treat with excision, radiation therapy, or cryotherapy. May recur locally; unlikely to metastasize but can have perineural invasion. Medial canthus area may have a worse prognosis with a dumbbell-shaped tumor that extends into orbit because septum is discontinuous due to spiral configuration of the bone and because surgeons undercut while trying to spare the canalicular system (thus, may send to Mohs' surgeon, who may have less regard for the lacrimal drainage system). If medial canthus is involved, avoid DCR for at least 1 year to rule out recurrence.
- Basal cell nevus syndrome (Gorlin's syndrome): autosomal dominant with multiple BCC associated with cardiac, sternal, and other bony abnormalities (jaw cysts, bifid ribs). Do not give radiation therapy.

ERDHEIM-CHESTER DISEASE Rare multisystem disease characterized by lipogranulomas in the liver, heart, kidneys and retroperitoneal fibrosis. May have bilateral xanthelasma-like eyelid lesions or proptosis from orbital masses or bony lesions. Pathology shows Touton giant cells. Poor prognosis.

KAPOSI'S SARCOMA Red-blue dermal mass usually in HIV patients. Spindle-cell tumor from endothelial cell origin with extravasated blood in slitlike spaces on pathology. Excise.

LACRIMAL SAC TUMORS Signs include epiphora, irreducible swelling of the sac (classically above the MCT), bleeding with probing, and secondary dacryocystitis. Primary malignancies are rare but are most often papillary carcinoma; may also be squamous cell, transitional cell, or mixed cell type. Treat with local excision. Second most common lacrimal sac tumors are lymphomas; treat with radiation therapy after biopsy and systemic evaluation.

MERKEL CELL CARCINOMA Rare, highly malignant red "plum" tumor in older patient that may mimic chalazia and spreads via lymphatics. Pathology looks like small-cell lung CA, from neuroendocrine, amine precursor uptake and decarboxylation (APUD) cell. Wide excision with radiation therapy.

NECROBIOTIC XANTHOGRANULOMA Older patients with nodular yellow, inflamed skin lesion (may be mistaken for xanthelasma), with Touton multinucleated giant cells full of lipid and foci of necrosis on pathology. Twenty-six percent have plasma cell malignancy.

PILOMATRIXOMA, BENIGN MALHERBE'S CALCIFYING EPITHELIOMA, PILOMYXOMA, MATRIXOMA Calcified epithelioma of childhood that presents as a solitary mobile, firm, blue-red nodule with hair cortex and basophilic epithelial cells and shadow cell calcification. May be multiple on upper arms.

SEBACEOUS ADENOCARCINOMA 3% of eyelid CA that arises from meibomian glands; thus, primary site is upper lid (two thirds of cases), followed by lower lid. Yellow color, diffuse mass; a great masquerader that may present as recurrent chalazion or unilateral blepharitis with madarosis. Pagetoid spread may cause conjunctival fibrosis like OCP or Arlt's line in adult inclusion conjunctivitis.

- Older patients: 15% mortality due to delayed diagnosis; rare in other body sites (thus, general pathologists often not familiar with this diagnosis).
- Pathology: bizarre atypical cells with frothy cytoplasm, desmoplastic reaction. May be BRST-1 positive (breast tumor marker) especially with pagetoid spread.
- Full-thickness biopsy; submit in formalin for fat stains (Oil Red O), and get frozen sections to establish margins.
- Treat with wide excision, possible exenteration.

SQUAMOUS CELL CARCINOMA (SCC) 8% of eyelid CA (BCC is 40x more common); most common site is upper lid. Presents as a red, scaly, fast-growing lesion, pain from perineural invasion, dyskeratosis, waxy or glassy appearance, and inflammation at the base. Can arise from AK; also associated with HPV. Other risk factors include sun exposure, fair skin, red hair, family or personal history of skin CA, inherited DNA repair defect, and albinism.

- Pathology: pink-colored tumor cells that have violated and are above the basement membrane (mnemonic: Pink and above); can have metastatic spread. Look for actinic keratosis at margin (good prognosis, metastasis in <0.5%).
- Xeroderma pigmentosa: autosomal recessive defect of DNA repair with increased risk of SCC and BCC.
- Treat with excision, 5-FU, cisplatin, or radiation therapy.

Neoplastic, Eyelid and Orbital: Pigmented Lesions

CUTANEOUS MALIGNANT MELANOMA Rare on eyelid (<1% of eyelid CA); slowly growing pigmented lesion (may be amelanotic) that is highly malignant. One third of cases arise de novo, one third from preexisting nevus or oculodermal melanocytosis (ODM), and one third from conjunctival primary acquired melanocytosis (PAM). Frequently metastasizes, with high mortality. Treat with wide excision with permanent sections and possible sentinel node exploration. Biopsy all new pigmented lesions in patients >40 years old.

- Superficial spreading: 80% of cutaneous melanoma.
- Nodular: most common of eyelid melanomas but least common overall (only 10% of melanomas); vertical spread >1.5 mm; worse prognosis (unlike BCC, where nodular form is better prognosis than morpheaform).
- Giant congenital nevus: >10 mm horizontal size; 10% risk of malignant melanoma (MM).
- Lentigo maligna (Hutchinson's freckle): pale brown macule with irregular borders usually in elderly patients; see best with Wood's light. Ten percent become lentigo maligna melanoma.

EPHELIS, FRECKLE Common, benign pigmented macule. Pathology shows no increased number of melanocytes, but increased melanosomes from resident dendritic melanocytes (inoculated into neighboring keratinocytes for storage).

LENTIGO SIMPLEX Small brown macules on skin and mucous membranes. Peutz-Jeghers syndrome has multiple lesions associated with gastrointestinal polyps.

NEVI Flat to raised pigmented lesion that represent a collection of melanocytes. If cystic on pathology, then is a benign nevus (cysts form as the epidermal melanocytes attempt to return to their neural crest origin, dragging epithelial cells into the dermis, which then create cysts). Nevi often show pigment exhaustion with time.

- Junctional: nests of nevus cells in epidermis; well-defined, darkly pigmented macules. Lowest malignant potential.
- Compound: cell clumps in the lower epithelium and dermis; less dark and slightly elevated. Some malignant potential from the intradermal portion. Most congenital nevi are compound type.
    - Dysplastic nevus: compound nevus with architectural disorder and atypia, present in 5% of all Caucasians. Multiple lesions present in familial dysplastic nevus syndrome (B-K mole syndrome). Can transform into MM.
- Intradermal: blue cells (specialized melanocytes, not the common dendritic melanocyte) with less nesting; confined to dermis with clear band separating it from the epidermis, and clear intranuclear spaces. Lesions are pale-tan color, more elevated (may be mistaken for squamous papilloma or wart), and may contain hair. Highest malignant potential.
- Blue nevus: embryonic melanocytes that never completed their journey to the epidermis and remain trapped within the dermis; blue from the Tyndall effect because they are deeper and not superficial.
- Ocular melanosis (if dermal, called Ota's nevus): dendritic melanocytes trapped in dermis; unilateral. More common in Asians. Risk for melanoma.

PRIMARY ACQUIRED MELANOSIS (PAM) Conjunctiva melanoma in situ, occuring primarily in adults; unilateral; waxes and wanes. Excise with wide margins with random conjunctival biopsy; look for junctional pathology indicating nevus versus atypia. Risk for MM. See Chapter 3.

PRIMARY ORBITAL MELANOMA Usually from meninges; slightly increased risk of choroidal melanoma. Risk factors: Caucasian, ocular melanocytosis.

Neoplastic, Orbital: Lacrimal Gland Tumors

GENERAL Comprise 13% of orbital neoplasms. In a comprehensive practice, approximately 25% of lacrimal gland lesions are epithelial tumors (mostly pleomorphic adenoma, followed by adenocystic carcinoma, and pleomorphic adenocarcinoma). The other 75% of nonepithelial lacrimal gland lesions are mostly lymphoid hyperplasia, dacryoadenitis, lymphoma, and rarely plasmacytomas. In a referral practice, about 50% of lacrimal lesions are inflammatory or lymphoid, and 50% are epithelial neoplasms. Approximately 50% of these epithelial tumors are pleomorphic adenomas, and 50% are malignant tumors. Of these malignant tumors, about 50% are adenocystic carcinoma, and 50% of these are basaloid subtype.

- Ask about duration of symptoms; check VA, proptosis, palpation, and image. On CT, epithelial tumors are likely to be round, with bone indentation or erosion if malignant with irregular margins. Lymphoid or inflammatory lesions are usually oblong, "pancake" like.
- Adenocarcinoma: rare but is the second most common malignant lacrimal tumor; not ductal; spread via lymphatics to lung. Usually fatal within 6 months.

ADENOCYSTIC CARCINOMA (ACC), CYLINDROMA Although a rare tumor, it is the most common malignant tumor of the lacrimal gland; increased incidence in males, with poor prognosis. Painful from perineural invasion (lacrimal nerve from CN V_2) and bony destruction with rapid proptosis; symptoms duration <6 months. CT shows irregular bony erosion.

- Pathology patterns: cribriform ("purple Swiss cheese" appearance), basaloid (solid pattern; 50% of ACC, worse prognosis), comedocarcinoma (central necrosis), or tubular (ductal formation).
- Incisional biopsy through lid; when confirmed by permanent pathology sections (never based on frozen sections alone), classically offer radical exenteration (2% cure), with or without chemotherapy. However, nonradical excision, then high-dose radiation therapy (e.g., proton beam) without chemotherapy or exenteration, is just as good. Overall 10-year mortality is 80% (1-year mortality without treatment is 100%).

INFLAMMATORY LESIONS May be from pseudotumor (hypocellular pathology), sarcoid (usually asymmetric but bilateral), and others. Typically short history; no bony involvement, oblong gland appearance on imaging, and involving orbital and palpebral lobes of lacrimal gland.

MALIGNANT PLEOMORPHIC ADENOMA, MALIGNANT MIXED CELL TUMOR Malignant transformation of pleomorphic adenoma with proliferating ductal epithelium in a tubular formation. Wide excision with radiation therapy recommended. More lethal than ACC; tendency for lung metastases, not intracranial spread.

PLEOMORPHIC ADENOMA, BENIGN MIXED CELL TUMOR Most common epithelial lacrimal tumor. Painless, slow growing, usually >9 months history of gland enlargement; superotemporal mass, ptosis, proptosis. Usually found in middle-aged females, with bony remodeling, not destruction.

- Typically is a well-differentiated, well-circumscribed homogeneous mass with ductal proliferation and myoepithelium cells on pathology. Does not arise from acini; the ducts have cuboidal bilayer with inner mucinous cells and outer cells that differentiate into epithelium.
- Excise entirely (excisional biopsy) because tumor may have areas of malignant transformation. Recurrence if capsule intact 3% (31% if

capsule violated); increased malignant potential in recurrent tumors (10% risk of recurrence per decade).

PRIMARY LACRIMAL GLAND LYMPHOMA Enlarged gland with hypercellular pathology and rubbery consistency (no collagen), molding or putty-like on CT, short- or long-standing history of lacrimal gland swelling. See below.

Neoplastic, Orbital: Lymphoproliferative Lesions

GENERAL Comprise 18% of orbital neoplasms and are the most common intraorbital malignancies in adults (most patients are 60–90 years old). Tumors mold to structures in orbit. Lymphoproliferative lesions are a spectrum of disease, including B cell lymphoma (67%), lymphoid hyperplasia (16%), myeloma or Waldenström's macroglobulinemia (9%), and histiocytosis (7%).

- World Health Organization (WHO) classification of lymphomas: B cell neoplasms (primary interest of ophthalmologists), T cell neoplasms, and Hodgkin's lymphoma.
- Biopsy and send for flow cytometry: if T cells are predominant, then likely orbital inflammation; if mixture of T and B cells, then likely benign lymphoid hyperplasia; if majority are B cells, then diagnosis is likely lymphoma.

BENIGN LYMPHOID HYPERPLASIA Polyclonal (50% B cells, 50% T cells), may make follicles; overall 25% have systemic disease. Treat with steroids or may use chemotherapy if atypical cells are seen on pathology.

- Benign reactive: 6% 5-year mortality, 15 to 25% systemic risk.
- Atypical reactive: 19% 5-year mortality, 40% systemic risk

HISTIOCYTOSIS Also known as histiocytosis X or Langerhans' cell tumors (Langerhans' cells contain Bierbeck granules; do not confuse with Langhans' multinucleated giant cells of foreign body granuloma). Spectrum of the following diseases (increasing severity alphabetically):

- Eosinophilic granuloma: most common and benign histiocytosis affecting the orbit; slow growing orbital mass, usually superotemporal location. Presents by end of first decade with pain, proptosis, and lid swelling. No visceral involvement (usually skull bones involved and not systemic).
    - Patient looks good, but CT looks bad (lytic bony lesions). Pathology shows monoclonal histiocytic proliferation with many eosinophils.
    - Excisional biopsy is often curative. Use local curettage for isolated lesion or radiation therapy 400–600 cGy for multiple or inaccessible lesions. Chemotherapy (chlorambucil) is recommended for systemic involvement (more likely with Letterer-Siwe disease).

- Hand-Schüller-Christian disease: lytic skull lesions, diabetes insipidus, age 20–40.
- Letterer-Siwe disease: young, sick patients with systemic, visceral lesions (gastrointestinal system most often involved, and orbit rarely involved). High mortality; worst prognosis of the histiocytoses.

LYMPHOMA Painless proptosis, slow growth, solid but diffusely infiltrative mass; may mold but not erode bone. Orbit is the most common extranodal site for lymphoma.

- CT shows "pregnant pancake" appearing mass. Echography shows low internal reflectivity. Consider systemic work-up with whole-body CT and bone marrow biopsy.
- Biopsy; send in formalin for light microscopy, and send fresh tissue for flow cytometry. Pathology shows Dutcher bodies (intranuclear) and Russell's bodies (cytoplasmic inclusions); vast majority are monoclonal (>60% B cells).
- Treat with radiation therapy 1500–2000 cGy and chemotherapy (not concurrent with radiation therapy), but usually do not excise. Follow CBC and serum protein electrophoresis (SPEP) every 6 months for 5 years.
- Most important prognostic factor is extent of disease at time of presentation: 86% with stage 1E (involvement of single extralymphatic site) have benign indolent course. No prognostic significance whether unilateral or bilateral involvement. If eyelid is involved, there is a 67% risk of systemic lymphoma (because of lymphatics), 35% risk for orbital lymphoma; if conjunctiva are involved, there is a 20% risk.

Neoplastic, Orbital: Mesenchymal Tumors

GENERAL Diverse group of tumors that comprise 11% of orbital lesions. Ewing's sarcoma makes up 29% of orbital mesenchymal tumors, rhabdomyosarcoma 29%, fibrous dysplasia 26%, fibrous histiocytoma 11%, and fibrosarcoma 2%.

EWING'S SARCOMA Primitive tumor usually arising from the long bones and pelvis with peak incidence 10–20 years old. Orbit is secondarily involved.

FIBROSARCOMA OR OSTEOSARCOMA Slowly growing orbital mass usually from sinuses; associated with Gardner's syndrome (colon polyps).

FIBROUS DYSPLASIA Relatively common slow growing bony mass from abnormal bone maturation, typically in childhood. May cause proptosis, globe ptosis, compressive optic atrophy and pain. CT shows "ground glass" appearance. Debulk, but difficult to excise completely.

- Albright's syndrome: ossifying fibroma (aggressive fibrous dysplasia), with sharply demarcated sclerotic rim; F > M. Associated with precocious pubertys; café au lait spots, strabismus.

FIBROUS HISTIOCYTOMA, DERMATOFIBROMA Relatively common orbital mesenchymal tumor usually in young adults. May cause congestive proptosis (like a hemangiopericytoma). Generally benign (2% are malignant, usually defined as five mitotic figures per high-powered field), well circumscribed with storiform pattern of spindle and histiocyte cells on pathology and vimentin (+) and S100 (−). Excise completely, as they have a tendency to recur, with a greater chance of malignant transformation.

RHABDOMYOSARCOMA Most common malignant orbital tumor in children (average age: 7 years old), with male predominance. Characterized by new onset rapid proptosis, conjunctival injection, edema, usually no pain or decreased vision, and palpable lid mass (25%); may have incidental history of trauma that confuses the diagnosis. A-scan shows low internal reflectivity (dense, compact tumor cells). Schedule prompt biopsy if suspicious.

- Pathology shows "bubble gum and raisins" appearance of dark cells with pink connective tissue, which is the tumor trying to make smooth muscle. May be desmin +, muscle specific actin (MSA) (+). Phosphotungstic acid-hematoxylin (PTAH) or Masson trichrome stains may show cross-striations (best seen with pleomorphic variant; in the embryonal variant, striations are usually seen only with electron microscopy).
- Four variants:
  - Embryonal (75%): most common, usually superonasal orbit; may demonstrate cross-striations on pathology.
  - Botryoid: involves mucosal surfaces usually from the sinuses into conjunctiva and eyelids.
  - Alveolar (15%): most aggressive, usually involves inferior orbit (alveolar "near the lungs"); second most rare.
  - Pleomorphic: most rare and most benign.
- Treat with debulking surgery, then radiation therapy 5000 cGy over 6 weeks (may cause hypoplastic orbit, radiation retinopathy) and chemotherapy to eliminate microscopic cellular metastatic cancer (typically VAC: vincristine, actinomycin D, cyclophosphamide). Historically, all cases were exenterated. Group 1: local disease; group 2: regional disease; group 3: distant metastatic cancer.

Neoplastic, Orbital: Metastatic and Invasive Tumors

GENERAL Metastatic and invasive tumors account for 9% of orbital lesions, 25% of orbital tumors; usually hematogenous spread. In children, cancer usually metastasizes to the orbit; in adults, it often spreads to the uvea. Female patients are more likely to have a breast or lung primary cancer; males patients, usually lung or prostate. Most common lesions are breast CA, lung CA, sarcoma, gastrointestinal tract, and prostate CA, and extension from eyelid, intraocular, brain (sphenoid wing meningioma), and sinus tumors.

EYELID TUMOR EXTENSION Incidence rates are BCC (67%), sebaceous cell carcinoma (22%), melanoma (7%), and SCC (4%); is less common due to lower incidence but especially prone to extend to orbit via perineural spread. Usually presents with a "lumpy-bumpy" muscle or nerve appearance on imaging (multifocal).

INTRAOCULAR TUMOR EXTENSION Via emissary vessel or scleral extension; two thirds of cases are melanoma, one third retinoblastoma (in Africa, RB is leading cause of childhood orbital malignancy).

METASTATIC BREAST CANCER Scirrhous variant may cause enophthalmos.

METASTATIC MALIGNANT MELANOMA If metastatic, usually to EOM; extrascleral extension from choroid in 7% of choroidal MM (early exenteration gives a 97% 5-year survival; late surgery 62%; if no exenteration, 0% survival).

METASTATIC NEUROBLASTOMA Most common metastatic tumor to the orbit in children; usually from adrenals (50%), retroperitoneal (25%), mediastinum, and neck. Overall 20% have ocular involvement. Bilateral in 60%; may have abrupt ecchymotic proptosis (tumor erosion through blood vessels). May present as paraneoplastic opsoclonus-myoclonus-ataxia syndrome; if from thorax, may have Horner's syndrome. Mean age 2 years old (90% are <5 years old); prognosis is age-dependent and poor in general but considerably better if <1 year old (72% survival). Treat with emergent radiation therapy and chemotherapy.

METASTATIC PROSTATE CA Osteoclastic bony mass with a predilection for the superior orbit.

NASOPHARYNGEAL CA Higher incidence in males (2–3x) and Asian patients. Typically causes nasal obstruction, rhinorrhea, epistaxis, otitis media, proptosis, and ipsilateral dry eye.

ORBITAL GRANULOCYTIC SARCOMA, CHLOROMA Orbital tumor that precedes or occurs simultaneously with leukemia. Average age 7 years old, M > F. Characterized by rapid growth; grossly has a green color.

SINUS TUMOR EXTENSION 72% are maxillary sinus SCC with proptosis, vision loss, and eyelid edema; 17% are from ethmoid sinus.

Neoplastic, Orbital: Neurogenic Tumors

GENERAL 24% of orbital neoplasms.

MALIGNANT GLIOMA Rare tumor arising from CNS astrocytes; in the orbit is usually a class IV astrocytoma (glioblastoma multiforme). More common in older patients; one third of cases are unilateral, two thirds are bilateral. Characterized by vision loss; half have disk edema. One hundred percent in chiasm and 50% in optic tracts at diagnosis; poor prognosis.

MENINGIOMA Tumor arising from the meninges (in the orbit usually from the sphenoid bone). 60% female, average age 40 years old (for bilateral tumors, the average age is 12 years old); only 6% are bilateral. Has BCC-like activity (slow growing, local extension, rare metastasis). Of orbital meningiomas, two thirds are from brain extension, and one third are primary from the ON. Pathology demonstrates psammoma bodies (from Greek *psammos*, "sand").

- ON sheath meningioma: accounts for only 10% of all meningiomas, but is the most common primary meningioma of the orbit. Typically presents with unilateral painless vision loss, optic atrophy, axial proptosis, and optociliary shunt vessels in a middle-aged female. Most are tumors of the meningoepithelial cells from arachnoid villi and benign. May infiltrate fat and muscle and show "tram tracking" on CT. Most are isolated; however, there is a slight association with NF, especially in children, where it is more aggressive. Observe if clinically stable; rarely biopsy. May also treat with radiation therapy, chemotherapy, RU-486, or excise if progressive growth (be prepared to excise up to the chiasm).
- Sphenoid-wing meningioma: more common than sheath meningioma; invades orbit from intracranial space and encroaches on ON or chiasm with decreased VA, proptosis, and optociliary shunt vessels. CT usually shows hyperostotic sphenoid bone but may be lytic. Debulk; cannot completely excise. Increased risk with NF 1 and NF 2.

ON GLIOMA, JUVENILE PILOCYTIC ASTROCYTOMA (JPA) Accounts for two thirds of neurogenic orbital tumors; benign tumor but with potentially serious consequences. Ninety percent occur within the first decade (mean age 8.5 years). Presents with painless axial proptosis, vision loss, ON atrophy (two thirds of cases), ON edema (one third of cases), optociliary shunt vessels. Fusiform pattern on CT; MRI shows tumor that is iso- or hypointense to the ON with T1 weighting and hyperintense to ON with T2.

- Pathology: should not see histology because treatment is usually observation, but will show arachnoid hyperplasia, central liquefaction necrosis. Rosenthal fibers are present as for all astrocytomas and have "hairlike" appearance (thus the name *pilocytic*). If associated with NF 1 (30%), the pathology of ON glioma is different and has component of meningioma with arachnoid or meningoepithelial hyperplasia.
- Treatment: observe if stable. When it begins to grow toward chiasm (39% progress), surgical excision is curative; may need chemotherapy and radiation therapy.

- Mortality: 0% if orbital only, 33% if orbital and intracranial, 47% if it involves chiasm (50% of gliomas). Overall 10% lifetime mortality; half of patients have stable vision, and half have vision loss.

SCHWANNOMA, NEURILEMMOMA Encapsulated tumor that arises from sensory nerve sheaths (in the orbit usually from the short posterior ciliary nerves; thus, typically found in the superior orbit). Presents with quiet proptosis (like neurofibroma and cavernous hemangioma) and is associated with NF 2. Pathology shows Antoni A (abundant tightly packed spindle cells) or B pattern (fewer cells, myxoid matrix).

Neoplastic, Orbital: Structural Lesions

GENERAL 30% of orbital masses are structural lesions or cysts.

DERMOID CYST Most common orbital structural lesion that presents as a slow-growing mass; may have abaxial proptosis. It is formed embryologically as the two waves of neural crest migrate over the face and scalp and meet at bony suture lines and pinch a little ectoderm downward, causing a subdermal nest of surface ectoderm. Thus, all three germinal layers are present (choristoma), and the superotemporal orbit is the primary site because of the frontozygomatic suture (followed by superonasal location at the frontoethmoidal) suture. If it is not freely mobile, consider CT to rule out intracranial extension ("dumbbell" shaped), encephalocele or mucocele from the frontal sinus.

- Generally remove after 6 months of age, when the patient has lower anesthesia risk. If ruptured attempt to remove intact. May incite an inflammatory reaction mimicking cellulitis.
- Do not confuse with limbal dermoid, which is a solid growth associated with Goldenhar's syndrome.

EPIDERMAL INCLUSION CYST (EIC) Second most common orbital structural lesion. Cyst forms from keratin-producing epidermal cells misplaced in the dermis from an embryologic rest of cells or nest of epidermal cells secondary to trauma or surgery.

MUCOCELE OR MUCOPYOCELE Third most common orbital structural lesion resulting from sinus outflow obstruction (sinuses are lined with respiratory epithelium and thus fill with mucus if not draining). In adults, often presents as a fluctuant mass that is soft and compressible; usually located superomedially, with painless proptosis and down and out displacement from the frontal sinus. Usually from the frontal sinus or ethmoids in a patient with history of sinusitis or trauma. May cause ON compression, and may increase with URI. CT shows that the orbital walls are displaced inward with bony dehiscence but not erosion. A-scan may show spike behind globe with low internal reflectivity. Treat with sinus exenteration; fat obliteration.

ORBITAL MENINGOCELE Protrusion of cranial meninges or brain tissue (encephalocele) through defect in orbital wall, usually superomedial. Often presents as a bluish mass above the medial canthus. Important to consider it in the differential diagnosis of orbital cysts, especially in a child.

TERATOMA Congenital massive proptosis from large tumor that is cystic, encapsulated, with all three germ layers present. Needs careful local dissection.

Neoplastic, Orbital: Vascular Lesions

GENERAL 18% of orbital lesions.

CAPILLARY HEMANGIOMA Most common benign orbital lesion in children, resulting from proliferation of endothelial cells. Appears shortly after birth; >90% resolve by age 7. May be superficial or deep in orbit with progressive proptosis, strabismus, astigmatism, or amblyopia (visual deprivation or astigmatic). Increases with Valsalva, enhances with CT contrast, and is high flow on Doppler ultrasound.

- Best to observe unless lesions are large or if visual complications are present. May use intralesional steroids (e.g., Kenalog or Celestone), which may be complicated by skin hypopigmentation or thinning; rarely CRAO from retrograde flow through valveless veins. May also treat with interferon α-2, laser, and oral steroids, or, lastly, excise if well localized.
- Potential life-threatening complications:
    - Kasabach-Merritt syndrome with thrombocytopenia from sequestration of platelets in a large capillary hemangioma
    - High output cardiac failure
    - Visceral lesions may cause gastrointestinal bleeding or respiratory compromise (20%), or orbital capillary hemangiomas may have facial or tracheal hemangioma (listen for wheezing).

CAVERNOUS HEMANGIOMA Most common benign neoplasm in adults. Well-circumscribed, low-flow vascular hamartoma; most common in middle-aged females. Frequently involves orbit (usually intraconal) without bony erosion, causing slowly progressive proptosis (may increase rapidly in pregnancy), and may have retinal striae, hyperopic shift, ON compression, increased IOP, strabismus. CT enhances with contrast and may show calcification; echography demonstrates medium to high internal reflectivity. Typically easy to excise because of its pseudocapsule.

HEMANGIOPERICYTOMA Uncommon encapsulated vascular tumor with rapid circulation from arteriole pericyte proliferation. Middle age, M > F. Pathology shows "staghorn" vascular spaces; best seen with a reticulin stain. Fifteen percent are malignant and can metastasize, and the recurrence rate is 25%; thus, ensure wide excision.

LYMPHANGIOMA Benign nonproliferating congenital venous malformation hemodynamically isolated (not in direct communication with the venous system, unlike a varix). Classified as a vascular choristoma, although some debate that there are lymphatics in the orbit (if so then is a hamartoma). Not well defined, diffuse, infiltrating mass; develops "chocolate cysts" if bleeding into tumor. May present as bluish mass in children and cause rapid proptosis or ON compression; increases in size with URIs because of the lymphoid tissue. Twenty-five percent have noncontiguous CNS vascular malformations.

- CT enhances with contrast. Echography shows low internal reflectivity.
- If superficial, may debulk (often requires repeated excision); also CT-guided aspiration and intravenous steroids. If deep, debulk, but can never totally eradicate; thus, avoid intervention if possible.

VARICES Dilation of preexisting venous channels, which may have transient proptosis with position change or Valsalva's maneuver and may stimulate oculocardiac reflex and cause orbital hemorrhage; 15% have ON atrophy and decreased VA. Imaging shows irregular mass, often with phlebolith (calcification); may erode bone. Consider conservative treatment, as excision is difficult; avoid surgery unless there is hemorrhaging, vision loss, or cosmesis.

Metabolic and Degenerative Disease

FLOPPY EYELID SYNDROME Loose eyelids that easily evert, from decreased tarsal elastin associated with obesity, sleep apnea, and lax uvula and pharynx with risk to lose airway during surgical sedation. Treat with lid taping, lubrication, or horizontal shortening of upper lid.

INVOLUTIONAL SKIN AND EYELID LAXITY Evidenced as brow ptosis, blepharoptosis, dermatochalasis (redundant eyelid skin), steatoblepharon (bulging of fat from attenuated septum), ectropion, or entropion. See Signs and Symptoms section above.

NASOLACRIMAL DUCT OBSTRUCTION (NLDO), ACQUIRED Usually obstructed at the mid- or lower duct from chronic low-grade inflammation with fibrosis of duct walls. Treat with DCR; probing rarely effective.

Systemic and Vascular Disease

ARTERIOVENOUS SHUNTS Retrograde venous flow that when it involves orbital veins may cause congestive proptosis, ocular pulsation, orbital bruit, chemosis, corkscrew and radialization of episcleral blood vessels, blood in Schlemm's canal, increased IOP, ophthalmoplegia, and disk edema. Treat for severe proptosis, vision loss, and glaucoma. May be spontaneous in NF.

- Dural venous shunts (25%): small pial arteries in lateral dural wall bleed into cavernous sinus, usually in an elderly hypertensive patient. Low flow. Thirty to 40% resolve spontaneously. Treat with embolization, springs, or adhesives.
- Carotid-cavernous shunt (75%): high-flow anastomosis from ICA into cavernous sinus, usually in younger patients with a history of trauma. Forty to 50% have vision loss. Treat with carotid artery ligation or balloon embolization.

SARCOIDOSIS Characterized by noncaseating granulomatous inflammation, most frequently of the lungs; however, ophthalmic findings are the second most common presentation (50% of patients have ocular involvement). The most frequent eye finding is band keratopathy (due to chronic inflammation), but also may have Descemet's thickening, nummular keratitis, and granulomatous uveitis with mutton-fat keratic precipitates (KP). Eyelid or conjunctiva nodules may be present, and lacrimal involvement may cause secondary keratoconjunctivitis sicca (KCS). The main fundus finding is periphlebitis; also may have cystoid macular edema (CME), RD or ON involvement.

Physical Disease

PENETRATING ORBITAL TRAUMA First determine if patient is stable (advanced trauma life support [ATLS]/advanced cardiac life support [ACLS]); if globe is intact, always suspect a foreign body. Typically, make patient nothing per os (NPO), shield eye, document the injury (in children, suspect abuse; in women, 35% of orbital fractures are from sexual assault or domestic abuse), obtain medical history (e.g., myocardial infarction, hypertension, HIV, diabetes, bleeding disorder), and obtain informed consent. Remember to check VA and pupils; do not miss a canalicular laceration (weakest part of the lids is the MCT in the area of canaliculi). Consider use of absorbable sutures in the event that the patient is lost to follow-up.

- Type of trauma determines time of repair: immediate surgery to rule out a ruptured globe; lid or canalicular lacerations can usually wait 24 to 48 hours; fractures can often wait 1 week (for ZMC fracture) or 2 weeks (floor or medial wall fracture).

- Intraorbital foreign body: imaging localization (superficial or deep, intraocular, transorbital) with CT (not MRI) or ultrasound (metallic foreign body amplifies B-scan unlike other masses that are echolucent). Try to determine composition (organic or not, corrosive or inert). Rule of thumb and forefinger: if you can palpate it, remove it; if not palpable, you can probably observe if no functional deficit is present (e.g., diplopia, ptosis, optic neuropathy).

RETROBULBAR HEMORRHAGE Orbital bleeding from trauma or postoperative cases causes an orbital compartment syndrome with rise of orbital and possible intraocular pressures. Signs and symptoms include pain, proptosis, periorbital ecchymosis with tense lids, external ophthalmoplegia, decreased VA or APD, increased IOP, CRAO, and choroidal folds.

- CT shows proptotic "tenting" or "lollipop" globe, often with diffuse orbital stranding density. With retinal or optic nerve compromise, have maximum of 90 minutes to relieve orbital tension.
- Check finger tension of globe (do not necessarily need to confirm with tonometry). If there is a large asymmetry between globes (>40 mmHg) or decreased VA or APD, the hemorrhage is a true emergency and needs immediate lateral canthotomy and cantholysis (lower lid first, then can do upper lid if needed). If postoperative trauma from orbital or eyelid surgery, open the incision; may need to drain hematoma and control active bleeding (every orbital surgery patient should be extubated as cough can lead to orbital hemorrhage).

FACIAL BURNS Look at lashes; if they are intact, then corneal surface is probably protected. Lubricate and protect the cornea from exposure and infection; later consider reconstruction.

ORBITAL FRACTURES May be internal (i.e., blow-out) with one or two walls (usually floor and medial) or rim, which may be displaced or not (i.e., tripod fracture), or complex if >1 wall with rim is involved (e.g., Le Fort or nasal-orbital-ethmoidal fracture). Plain film Waters view shows floor and maxillary sinus, but CT is best to view bony abnormalities with 3 mm cuts or 1.5 mm cuts if optic canal injury or foreign body is suspected. Follow serial exams, monitor diplopia, check forced ductions (topical anesthesia; with two forceps at 3 and 9 o'clock, pull eye up). Use antibiotics for open fractures, large hemorrhage, or chronic sinusitis. Ice for 48 hours; patient should avoid nose blowing, lifting, and straining. Surgical repair is based on the type of fracture. Goals of surgery: (1) early intervention and (2) restore bony anatomy to provide stable support and normal globe position.

- Floor: usually "blow-out" from buckling or hydraulic forces. The floor is weakest 10–15 mm posterior to the rim and medial to the infraorbital canal. In children, "trapdoor" fracture (bone bends and breaks, allowing herniation of tissue, then rebounds, trapping tissue, like a

Volkmann's arm fracture) may be emergency, and patients may have oculocardiac reflex or nausea and vomiting, especially with upgaze.
  - Surgical repair needed for entrapment causing diplopia within 20 degrees of primary gaze or fracture that is occupationally limiting, or for >2 mm enophthalmos, >50% of floor defect (volume enlargement best seen on coronal CT), large rim defect, telecanthus, or aesthetic considerations. Usually do surgery within 7 to 14 days to limit scarring.
- Le Fort I: high transverse maxillary fracture (all Le Fort fractures involve maxillary and pterygoid plate), no orbital involvement.
- Le Fort II: pyramidal, nasal, lacrimal, maxillary bones, and medial wall and floor. May involve the NLD.
- Le Fort III: craniofacial dysjunction with floor, medial, and lateral wall fractures. May involve the optic canal.
- Naso-orbital-ethmoidal (NOE): frontal, maxillary, lacrimal, ethmoidal fractures with depressed nasal bridge, epistaxis, tearing, cerebrospinal fluid rhinorrhea, and telecanthus (>30 mm). Treat with transnasal wiring with mini-plate fixation of medial canthal tendons.
- Zygomatico-complex (ZMC): also called "tripod" fracture, which is a misnomer, as the fracture actually has four components (fractures around the frontozygomatic suture, zygomatic-maxillary suture, zygomatic-arch fracture, and floor fracture; may have an orbital rim fracture). Patients have canthal dystopia (lower lateral canthus is usually 2 mm higher than medial canthus), temporal subconjunctival hemorrhage, and features of floor fracture. Look for associated globe injuries.
- Roof: usually "blow-in" fracture with potential for cerebrospinal fluid leak or CNS herniation. May need neurosurgical evaluation.

Inflammatory and Immune Disease

IDIOPATHIC CHRONIC ORBITAL INFLAMMATION, ORBITAL PSEUDOTUMOR

Chronic, lymphoproliferative inflammation that is usually unilateral. Sixty percent of patients are age 20 to 60 (peak age 40 to 50), and present with pain, rapid onset (weeks to months) proptosis, ophthalmoplegia, and chemosis.

- Clinical presentations depend on which orbital tissue is primarily involved:
  - Anterior diffuse inflammation (28%): most common presentation; mimics cellulitis with pink "boggy" edema in anterior two thirds of orbit. Biopsy if recurrent.
  - Dacryoadenitis (17%): "S"-shaped lid. Biopsy; oral steroids are not as effective, and may debulk early. Often treated with antibiotics to first rule out infectious cause.
  - Myositis: third most common presentation. Usually affects SR and MR (opposite of Graves' disease) with tendons involved

TABLE 2–2
Comparison of Thyroid-Related Immune Orbitopathy (TRIO) and Myositis

Characteristic	TRIO (Graves' Disease)	Myositis
Pain	No	Yes
Bilateral	Yes	No
Course	Chronic	Acute
Muscles involved	IR > MR > SR > LR	SR, MR
Muscle tendons involved	No	Yes
Lid retraction	Yes	No
Loss of vision	Yes	No
Systemic involvement	Yes	No

IR, inferior rectus muscle; MR, medial rectus muscle; SR, superior rectus muscle; LR, lateral rectus muscle.

(usually spared in Graves'). (See Table 2–2 for a comparison of Graves's disease and myositis.) May be bilateral; better radiation response (less steroids needed); associated with greater rate of recurrence and systemic symptoms.
  - Sclerosing: rare form; chronic course, with tissue destruction and poor prognosis.
  - Tolosa-Hunt syndrome (7.6%): a type of parasellar or orbital apex syndrome, with pain (CN V_1) or corneal anesthesia, diplopia or ptosis (CN III, IV, VI), chemosis, venous congestion, Horner's syndrome, ON swelling, and optic atrophy. Usually affects males; unilateral but may be bilateral. Differential diagnosis: anything that involves the cavernous sinus (meningioma, pituitary adenoma, glioma, chordoma, mucocele, etc.). Treat with long-term steroids.
- Pediatric patients are more likely to have bilateral inflammation and have constitutional symptoms (nausea, vomiting, headache, and photophobia), poorer prognosis; more likely associated with uveitis, ON involvement, scleral thinning, muscle infiltration, Tenon's space edema, increased erythrocyte sedimentation rate (ESR), and eosinophilia. Rule out rhabdomyosarcoma and cellulitis. Good response to steroids; avoid radiation therapy.
- Differential diagnosis: lymphoma is the most common diagnosis; this is often confused with pseudotumor and may be steroid responsive. Lymphangioma with bleeding, Wegener's granulomatosis and vasculitis may be painful. Also consider metastatic carcinoma, TRIO, and lacrimal gland tumors.
- CT shows "dirty fat" appearance in the orbit; may have bony remodeling. On MRI the lesion is often isointense to fat on T2 (lymphoma is hyperintense).

- Pathology shows polyclonal hypocellular infiltrate in which T cells predominate ($T_{helper} > T_{suppressor}$). May be a spectrum with lymphoma, which is usually monomorphic with more B cell predominance, and higher proliferating cell nuclear antigen (PCNA). If benign, then more likely to have Dutcher bodies, macrophages, and vascular pattern. Pathologic subtypes:
  - Vasculitis: more aggressive treatment needed, rule out Wegener's granulomatosis.
  - Eosinophilic: uncommon, usually in children; associated with vasculitis.
  - Sclerosing: more fibrosis.
  - Granulomatous: uncommon, Tolosa-Hunt type; rule out foreign body, tuberculosis, syphilis, or fungal causes.
- Treat initially with oral steroids 60–80 mg daily with 4–6 week taper. Seventy-eight percent of patients have good response, often immediate (92% improve if ON involved), and 37% are cured; however, 52% of cases recur. Radiation 1500–2000 cGy, but many fail radiation therapy, especially myositis variant. May try cyclophosphamide, methotrexate, cyclosporine, and azathioprine. Consider surgery for atypical or recurrent disease or to debulk dacryoadenitis. A delay in treatment leads to decreased response, increased recurrence, and more biopsies. Surgical risks include: inflammation exacerbation (60%), residual proptosis (60%), muscle restriction (50%), ptosis (7%), and loss of the eye (3%).

THYROID-RELATED IMMUNE ORBITOPATHY (TRIO), GRAVES' DISEASE

Autoimmune disease of retrobulbar tissue. Trio of involvement: muscle enlargement, optic neuropathy, and keratopathy.

- Graves' thyroid disease: idiopathic hyperthyroidism, 2% incidence; female to male ratio is up to 7:1, onset age 20 to 30 (affected males are slightly older). Symptoms include weight loss, increased appetite, sweating, heat intolerance, tremor, fatigue, palpitations, and irritability. Graves' original triad: thyroid enlargement, palpitations, and exophthalmos. Classic clinical triad: hyperthyroidism, orbitopathy, and pretibial edema.
- Thyroid orbitopathy: affects 30 to 70% of patients with Graves' disease; male to female ratio = 1:4, onset age 50; more severe in smokers. Typically presents within 18 months of thyroid dysfunction but may occur anytime. Twenty-five percent of orbitopathy patients develop thyroid dysfunction within 1 year, 50% within 5 years; overall 70% of euthyroid orbitopathy patients eventually develop thyroid dysfunction.
- Pathogenesis: antigen against thyroid follicular cell circulates and cross-reacts with orbital tissue. Antithyroid antibodies mainly target orbital fibroblasts, which increase in number and activate local immune

reaction. Cytokine production is especially upregulated, which further stimulates fibroblast proliferation (is thus self-propagating).

- o Increased incidence with family history, humoral immunity (Ab to thyroid-stimulating hormone [TSH] receptor, long-acting thyroid stimulator [LATS], thyroid-stimulating immunoglobulin [TSI]), and cell-mediated immunity, human leukocyte antigen (HLA) DW-3 and B-8, and associated with other autoimmune diseases (up to 10% of patients may have myasthenia gravis).
- o Orbital volume is increased due to increased glycosaminoglycans from fibroblasts and thus increased orbital fluid volume (TRIO worse after sleeping on back), increased muscle size (younger patients tend to have less muscle enlargement than older Graves' patients), fibroblasts, and fat proliferation. Chemosis may also be from hypertrophy of smooth muscle in infraorbital groove (Müller's muscle of the orbit) compressing venous outflow.

- Signs and symptoms: gradual and insidious course; 80 to 90% are bilateral. Werner classification of presentation (does not represent the sequence of the disease in all patients; mnemonic: NO SPECS):
  - o **N**o signs and symptoms
  - o **O**nly signs, no symptoms: eyelid retraction (Dalrymple's sign; most common finding), eyelid lag on downgaze (Graefe's sign), lagophthalmos, temporal flaring of lids (lid peak normally medial to pupil), edema, festoons, vascular injection.
    - Superior limbal keratoconjunctivitis (SLK): velvety injection of the superior conjunctiva and peripheral cornea that stains with Rose Bengal; treat with silver nitrate solution (not sticks).
  - o **S**oft tissue signs and symptoms (mnemonic: RELIEF):
    - **R**esistance to retropulsion
    - **E**dema of conjunctiva
    - **L**acrimal gland enlargement
    - **I**njection over the horizontal rectus muscles insertions
    - **E**dema of eyelids, lymphedema
    - **F**ullness of lids
  - o **P**roptosis: minimal 21–23 mm, moderate 24–27 mm, severe >28 mm
  - o **E**OM involved: IR affected more than MR > SR > LR, differential IOP (>6 mmHg) with upgaze. Muscle involvement is considered minimal if there is restriction only in extremes of gaze, or moderate if obviously limited ductions, or severe if frozen globe is present. Spares tendon (unlike pseudotumor). Diplopia typically worse with vertical or lateral gaze.
  - o **C**ornea involved: considered minimal if only superficial punctate keratitis is present, moderate if ulcerated, or severe if perforated. Exposure keratopathy may be from proptosis (inadequate closure),

lid retraction (poor blink), or IR restriction (poor Bell's phenomenon).
    - Sight loss: decreased vision, disk edema, pallor, VF defects, dyschromatopsia, or APD. Considered minimal if VA is 20/20–60 or better, moderate if 20/70–200, or severe if 20/200 to no light perception (NLP). Optic neuropathy (present in 2.5% of cases) may be secondary to inflammation, apical compression by enlarged muscle, apex fat prolapse, or proptosis stretch. May also have gaze-evoked amaurosis. Treat actively with steroids until definitive treatment.
- Clinical presentations:
    - Type I: symmetric proptosis and lid retraction, minimal congestion and inflammation, less myopathy with fatty infiltrate only.
    - Type II: more congestion and chemosis, increased myositis, restrictive myopathy, inflammation, and ON compression (smoking increases risk and severity of type II presentation).
    - Lipogenic variant: little EOM involvement, mainly just increased fat with increased risk of globe subluxation.
- Medical management: treat early with tears, lubrication, taping at night, elevated head of bed, prisms for diplopia, and prednisone 40–100 mg every day for 4 weeks, then taper (best for inflammatory features; no effect on proptosis, retraction, or myopathy). Radiation therapy 2000–3500 rads in 10 fractions for 2 weeks to the posterior orbit, targeting lymphocytes and fibroblasts; has similar effect as steroids but effect is delayed 3 weeks, so continue steroids during treatment. Prednisone and radiation therapy are contraindicated in vasculitis. Also treat coexistent hyperthyroidism usually with thyroid ablative therapies. And 10% of patients have orbitopathy flare with I-131 treatment; thus, consider prednisone 40 mg every day for prophylaxis during radioactive iodine treatment.
- Surgical treatment: treat early for malignant proptosis or optic neuropathy; otherwise, wait 1 year (or at least until disease is stable for 6 months). Order of surgeries: (1) orbital decompression, (2) strabismus surgery, (3) eyelid retraction repair, and (4) dermatochalasis or skin resurfacing.
    - Decompression: fat decompression if this is the predominant component of orbitopathy. Often only 2–6 mm of decreased proptosis with fat removal only. If bony decompression is indicated, determine how many walls to decompress by imaging (CT scan). Types: two wall (orbital floor and medial wall), "balanced" two wall (medial and lateral wall), three wall (medial wall, floor, and lateral wall), and four wall (add roof removal; often performed with neurosurgeon). Apical decompression is best obtained with medial wall removal, either external or transnasal endoscopic (higher incidence of diplopia).

- o Strabismus: never resect thyroid muscles; consider IR/MR recession with adjustable sutures.
- o Lid surgery: for upper lids, do either Müller recession/myotomy (internal) or levator recession/myotomy (external). For lower lids, recess retractors with spacer graft.
- o Skin excess: do blepharoplasty (conservative to avoid recurrent retraction), excision of festoons, and CO_2 skin resurfacing for postinflammation pigment changes.

Eyelid Surgery

GENERAL Local anesthetic standard eyelid mix is often 50:50 lidocaine 1% with epinephrine plus bupivacaine 0.75% with Wydase in a 10 cc syringe with a 26 gauge needle. Place a drop of tetracaine in each eye. Postoperative regimen for most patients includes ice packs 20 minutes every 2 hours for 48 hours, increased head of bed, antibiotic ointment 4 times per day for 4 days; consider oral antibiotic (e.g., Levaquin 500 mg PO every day for 7 days) for reoperations. Most patients are seen for a 1-week follow-up, but ptosis patients are often seen in 4 to 5 days in case surgical adjustment is needed.

BLEPHAROPLASTY Indicated for dermatochalasis with or without steatoblepharon.

- Upper lid blepharoplasty: mark skin along lid crease, usually 8–10 mm from eyelid margin centrally and ~5 mm nasally and temporally. Laterally follow the laugh crease, and medially make a downturn and go about 5 mm medial to the punctum to prevent webbing. Then mark the upper incision line according to the amount of skin to be removed: centrally always maintain at least 10 mm distance from the inferior eyebrow to the eyelid crease, or 15 mm if the patient has high arched brows. Incise skin with #15 blade, then excise the myocutaneous flap with blunt Westcott scissors. If the patient has significant steatoblepharon, bluntly dissect thru septum, isolate the central and nasal fat pads, and gently lift the fat pad with forceps (avoid excessive traction on the fat); use cautery for hemostasis. Close skin with 6.0 sutures. Usually no dressing is needed.
- Lower lid blepharoplasty: skin incision along a line inferior to the lashes; may debulk fat pads. Excess skin is trimmed, and skin closed as above.
    - o May injure the IO or cause lower lid retraction (from lower lid retractor or septal scarring or excessive skin removal if performed transcutaneously).

- Retroblepharoplasty: blepharoplasty and fat removal via transconjunctival approach in the lower lid to avoid visible scar but does not allow for skin removal. Can perform secondarily.

BROW PTOSIS Males have flat brow, women arched. Both sexes tend to have predominant temporal brow ptosis.

- Direct brow lift: leaves a visible scar. Mark skin along the superior brow, then along a forehead crease according to the amount of skin removal desired. Incise with #15 blade, maintaining a cutting angle parallel to the eyebrow hair follicle orientation. Remove the myocutaneous flap with blunt Westcott scissors (stay superficial over the supraorbital neurovascular bundle). Close the deep layers with several 4.0 or 5.0 Vicryl interrupted sutures. Close the skin with 6.0 Prolene suture. Dress with Tefla pad.
- Coronal forehead lift: best result, but do not use in patients with a high forehead or hairline.
- Endoscopic lift: very good cosmetic result, as incisions are concealed in the hairline. Similar results as a coronal browlift, with excellent patient acceptance. Allows extirpation of procerus and corrugator muscles.
- Hairline lift (pretrichial): useful for patients with a high hairline (>6 cm) to elevate the brow and advance the hairline.

ECTROPION Treated with horizontal tightening (wedge resection, Bick procedure, LTS), reattaching retractors, or reversing Quickert sutures. Also:

- Medial spindle: excision of football-shaped area of medial palpebral conjunctiva that is closed with a vertical mattress suture that is externalized; useful for involutional ectropion of the medial eyelid associated with punctal eversion.
- Two-snip procedure: useful for medial punctal ectropion; place one blade of Vannas scissors into punctum-ampula with other on conjunctiva, and cut a V shape to allow drainage into ampulla.

ENTROPION Lower lid tightening (LTS) plus:

- Quickert sutures: plicate lower lid retractors to prevent orbicularis muscle override by forming a scar along several double-armed 4.0 Vicryl or silk suture tracts. Pass sutures 3–4 mm below lower tarsus, engage conjunctiva and lower lid retractors, turn superiorly, and exit skin 4–5 mm below lid margin. Pass second needle 3–4 mm lateral to first needle and tie tightly on bolsters, leaving for 3 to 4 weeks.
- Wies procedure: full-thickness blepharotomy with marginal eyelid rotation to treat cicatricial entropion (often used in developing countries for trachoma-associated upper eyelid entropion).
- "Kurfing": cut grooves in tarsus to allow it to bend; used to treat cicatricial entropion.

- Posterior tarsotomy: partial thickness cut across full tarsal length gives laxity to plate, and sutures are externalized and bolstered; used to treat cicatricial entropion.

EYELID LAXITY Most commonly results from involutional lateral canthal weakening. Treating lower lid laxity is a core component of entropion and ectropion repair.

- Lateral tarsal strip (LTS) procedure: do a lateral canthotomy and inferior cantholysis. Divide the lateral eyelid into anterior and posterior lamellae with #15 blade or blunt Westcott scissors (cut along the gray line to dissect between orbicularis muscle and anterior tarsus). Prepare the tarsal strip by horizontally cutting conjunctiva and lower lid retractors from inferior tarsus, remove a thin strip of lid margin from superior border of tarsus, and scrape conjunctiva on posterior tarsus. Gauge necessary amount of shortening, then cut excess tarsus. Pass suture through the anterior face of the tarsal strip superiorly and inferiorly (best to use a double-armed 4.0 permanent or Vicryl suture on a P-2 tightly curved needle). After retracting lateral orbital rim soft tissue, pass the needles along the periosteum of the inner aspect of the lateral orbital rim, wanting a slight superior overcorrection. Assess amount of excess anterior lamella and excise, then close skin (e.g., with 6.0 chromic gut).

EYELID RECONSTRUCTION General principles: complete anesthesia, sustained hemostasis, protection of globe, closure of lid in layers (anterior lamella and posterior lamella), eversion of skin edges. Avoid vertical tension (make vertical incisions), and do not debride "necrotic" tissue, as it is often viable because of good facial skin vascularization.

- Direct closure: if defect is less than one third of the total eyelid length in children or less than half in adults. May advance lid for greater amount of loss with lateral cantholysis (adds 3–5 mm), or use a semicircular flap (Tenzel). Use Vicryl for subcutaneous sutures and plain gut for skin closure.
  - Eyelid margin repair: pass suture in tarsus out gray line, then in opposite gray line out tarsus. Pass second suture through tarsal meibomian gland plane 2 mm from wound edge and 2 mm into tarsus, exiting into wound and equidistant into other tarsal segment and tie. Close tarsus with 6.0 Vicryl with knots on anterior surface. Place skin marginal sutures to align lashes with 6.0 silk, tie and leave long, and incorporate ends with skin sutures, which are removed in 7 days.
- Full-thickness lid defect: bridge flap if >50% of lid margin lost (avoid in amblyopic age group).
  - Cutler-Beard flap: upper lid defect repaired with full-thickness tissue flap from lower lid. Requires a tarsal substitute.

  - Hughes tarsoconjunctival flap: lower lid defect closed by bridge flap of tarsus and conjunctiva transposed into the lower lid defect with full-thickness skin graft or advancement flap to replace anterior lamella.
- Partial-thickness lid defect: reconstruction is based on replacing anterior lamella (skin, muscle) or posterior lamella (tarsus or other tectonic support and conjunctiva or other mucous membrane).
  - Anterior lamella: may use a flap or a free graft.
    - Flaps for anterior lamellar reconstruction: advancement flap (can decrease tension with Burow's triangle), rotation flap, or transposition flap.
    - Free skin graft: best source is the other eyelid; also may use retroauricular, preauricular, supraclavicular (can harvest up to 8 × 6 cm), and medial inner arm skin.
      - Eyelid skin graft: make a superficial incision (skin only, not muscle, as in blepharoplasty), then dissect down to dermal vessels and rete pegs between skin and muscle. Measure defect, then harvest graft 30% larger than defect, as shrinkage occurs.
  - Posterior lamella: mucous membrane grafts may be obtained from conjunctiva, buccal, or hard palate mucosa (the epithelium side glistens and tissue curls toward basement membrane side). Also, free tarsal grafts can be obtained (can take tarsus ~5 mm wide × ~12 mm long).
- Lateral canthotomy and cantholysis: using local anesthetic, cut skin horizontally with Stevens or blunt Westcott scissors, separate conjunctiva and muscle, point scissors inferonasally and strum the inferior crus, then cut while pulling the eyelid margin outward with forceps (will feel a "give" when the crus is released).

LID RETRACTION

- Gold weight: three-point fixation to superior tarsal plate with permanent suture. Cover implant with skin-muscle flap to lessen risk of extrusion.

PTOSIS SURGERY Always evaluate Herring's effect on contralateral lid if unilateral ptosis.

- Levator advancement: for good function (LF >8 mm), mild to moderate ptosis. For children, use the difference in levator height + difference in levator function + 4 mm. Drape so that both eyes are exposed. Mark skin crease and infiltrate with small amount (1.0–1.5 cc) of local anesthetic (postoperative adjustments can often be performed without local anesthetic until after the incision is teased open and the adjustments are made). Incise skin with #15 blade, then tent up wound edges and snip down through orbicularis muscle. Gently dissect subcutaneous tissue with blunt Westcott scissors (point scissors toward brow, spread open, and bluntly dissect). Open septum, push fat back, and find levator aponeurosis (may have fatty infiltration). Trim a small amount of orbicularis muscle off the tarsal face to expose the superior tarsal margin. Place a central partial-thickness suture (e.g., 6.0 Prolene) while gently lifting tarsus with forceps (tell the patient he or she may experience some discomfort), then pick up the edge of the aponeurosis and pass the needle through the edge of the levator aponeurosis. Throw a temporary tie, and have the patient open his or her eyes to compare the eyelid positions for symmetry; adjust the suture or tie permanently. Repeat for a nasal limbus suture and possibly a temporal limbus suture. Overcorrect 1–2 mm because epinephrine stimulates the Müller's muscle and lidocaine paralyzes the orbicularis muscle. Close skin to skin unless reforming eyelid crease, in which case incorporate some aponeurosis with every other suture pass. Postoperatively, if over- or undercorrected or asymmetric contour, adjust within 5 to 7 days or wait a few months.

- Posterior lamella resection: good function, minimal ptosis, no dry eye. May be tarsoconjunctival (Fasanella-Servat; removes a portion of normal tarsus) or conjunctival Mullerectomy (Putterman-Urist procedure). Preoperatively, use 2.5% phenylephrine to activate Müller's muscle to estimate postoperative lid position.
- Levator muscle resection, supra-Whitnall's resection: unilateral fair to poor function (LF 5–7 mm), with adequate Bell's phenomenon and tear function. Use difference in MRD + difference in LF + 5 ("fudge" factor) = amount of resection.
- Frontalis suspension or sling: best for very poor or absent function (LF < 4 mm). Used especially for complete CN III or congenital myogenic ptosis; contraindicated in good-fair function ptosis. Autogenous fascia lata has the best and most lasting results but may use donor fascia lata (lasts longer than silicone), temporalis fascia, Supramid (may have extrusion but less than silicone), silicone rods (higher extrusion rate), Gortex, or other donor materials (e.g., bovine pericardium, such as Perigard, or banked fascia lata).

TRICHIASIS All treatments may have depigmentation, scarring, herpetic viral activation, and recurrence.

- Electrohyfrecation: local, focal trichiasis treated with radiofrequency unit needle placed into hair shaft; activate and see bubble form. Twenty to 50% recurrence.
- Cryoablation: local anesthesia; double-cycle freeze-thaw to −20°C (compare with −30°C needed for cancer cell death and −40°C for normal cell death), then epilate in 1 week (cilia should pull out without resistance). Twenty to 40% recurrence.

- Surgical excision: full-thickness wedge resection for focal trichiasis or excision of individual internal bulbs; highest success rate.
- Laser ablation: argon red 700 mW, 0.5 second, 200 μm, is least effective treatment.

Lacrimal Surgery

CANALICULODACRYOCYSTORHINOSTOMY (CDCR) Useful for focal distal (i.e., common) canalicular obstruction with NLDO.

CANALICULAR TRAUMA Repair all recent lacerations before scarring (may wait a few days to decrease edema), and use silicone stent intubation with microanastomosis of the lacerated canalicular system. The longer the silicone stents remain, the greater the chance of permanent patency. Fifty percent of monocanalicular patients have symptomatic epiphora, so attempt repair or refer.

CONJUNCTIVODACRYOCYSTORHINOSTOMY, JONES TUBE Canalicular system is disrupted and inadequate for tear flow; a second passage is created from the conjunctiva into the lacrimal sac and stented with a Jones tube.

DACRYOCYSTORHINOSTOMY (DCR) Osteotomy created at middle meatus (often within 10 mm of the cribriform plate), and the lacrimal sac is divided and secured to the nasal mucosa. Very high surgical success rate (>90%). The most common reasons for failure is obstruction at the common canaliculus or bony ostomy site.

NASOLACRIMAL DUCT PROBING Enter punctum with probe vertically, then turn horizontally and pass into the lacrimal sac until a hard stop is felt. Swing the probe vertically, hugging the brow, and drop down into the NLD; may feel pop through obstructing membrane. Confirm placement in the nose with a second probe into the nares under the inferior meatus. May combine with silicone sent intubation (i.e., Crawford tubes), which are passed through the superior and inferior puncta into the nose; the ends of the tube are retrieved from the nose and tied together. The stent is left in place typically 6 to 12 months before removal.

Orbital Surgery

GENERAL Consider intraoperative steroids (e.g., dexamethasone 10 mg IV) and Ancef for orbital cases.

ANOPHTHALMIC SOCKET Loss of the eye causes loss of one sixth of the VF, loss of depth perception, fear of losing the other eye, job concerns, and increased rate of accidents. Psychological issues: patients are dealing with loss of eye, fear of the normal eye, and self-image problems (especially children). Five percent of blind painful eyes harbor tumor.

- Net orbital volume deficit of 0–6 cc: globe removal (7.0–7.5 cc) – fat atrophy (0–4 cc) + orbital implant (2–4 cc) + prosthesis (2.0–3.5 cc). To optimally replace volume and improve prosthetic motility, maximize orbital implant size and minimize prosthesis size.
- Implants: usually made of porous polyethylene (Medpore), hydroxyapatite (HA), or polymethylmethacrylate (PMMA); 16 mm size replaces 2 cc of orbital volume, and 18 mm gives 4 cc. May coat implant with sclera or Ocuguard to provide a smooth surface, increase volume, allow muscle suturing to the implant, and may help to prevent posterior migration. Can also place a motility peg in the orbital implant to maximize prosthesis motility.
- Prosthesis: should be large enough to have good retention, but if the prosthesis is too big, it will have poor motility and cause more weight on lower lid and more drag on the upper lid.

DECOMPRESSION May be bony decompression, usually two wall (floor and medial wall), "balanced" (medial and lateral wall), three wall (medial and lateral wall and floor), or all four walls; also fat decompression (intraconal and orbital fat posterior to the globe). The sphenoid wing is thin in the inferior orbit and thicker higher up; thus, burr but do not infracture (may get cerebrospinal fluid leak).

ENUCLEATION Globe removed; Tenon's capsule and muscles remain. Goals: remove pathology, preserve volume, retain conjunctival fornices, and achieve prosthetic movement.

- Indications: large primary intraocular tumor, palliation for large tumor, blind painful eye, severe ocular trauma, and cosmesis of disfigured blind eye.
- Procedure: perform 360-degree conjunctival peritomy under Tenon's capsule (point scissors posterior), and isolate Tenon's and muscle insertions. Detach the extraocular muscles, and cut the ON, remove the globe, and pack the orbit with cold-soaked gauze. Place ocular implant (with or without a covering), and suture the muscle tendons to the implant cover in a "splayed out" fashion (to allow anterior ciliary arteries to ingrow); close Tenon's capsule and conjunctiva with interrupted sutures every 2 mm. Ensure that bleeding vessels are cauterized and that closure is free of tension to prevent exposure and make watertight. Place conformer (smallest that fits), pressure patch for 5 days, antibiotic ointment, and follow up in 4 to 6 weeks. At that time may consult for prosthesis fitting and request that the ocularist vault the prosthesis (do not want the posterior surface in contact with the wound edge).

- If intraocular tumor is present, use a "no touch" technique with gentle peritomy; do not hook the rectus muscles or clamp the ON; may use cryotherapy around the base of the tumor if there is extension to emissary veins.

EVISCERATION Use in endophthalmitis and as an alternative for enucleation. Advantages: local anesthetic may be used, simpler than enucleation, and no muscle or fat manipulation. This technique may provide better prosthesis motility. Evisceration is contraindicated with intraocular tumors. Disadvantages include risk of sympathetic ophthalmia.

- Procedure: perform 360-degree peritomy, incise sclera 2–3 mm from limbus to enter behind scleral spur, and remove cornea and entire uveal tract in one piece. Swab sclera with absolute alcohol, irrigate, then place implant (may need scleral relaxing incisions). Close sclera, followed by Tenon's capsule, then conjunctiva, and place conformer. Socket looks like enucleation.

EXENTERATION Remove eye, lids, and intraorbital contents, with or without removal of the bony walls. Indications include extrascleral extension of intraocular tumor, intraorbital malignancy, severe infections (e.g., *Mucor*), and severe inflammatory orbits. A limited anterior exenteration uses a subciliary incision to remove the posterior globe, sparing a portion of the lids. May use skin graft or leave orbit open to granulate, packing for 10 days with daily peroxide cleaning. Radical exenteration removes periorbital skin and eyelids and will need mulage prosthesis.

FLOOR FRACTURE REPAIR Transconjunctival or subciliary approach with subperiosteal dissection. Dissect along the floor with a Freer-type elevator to find the posterior wall of the maxillary sinus (usually 4–6 mm anterior to the orbital apex). Reduce herniated soft tissues, repair defects with orbital implants supported on all sides by stable bone, and close periosteum without incorporating septum.

PHTHISICAL EYE Small, shrunken blind eye that is the end result of various pathologies; often an indication for enucleation. Pathology shows squaring of the posterior pole due to EOM position and thickened posterior sclera.

Other Surgery

BOTULINUM TOXIN TYPE A (BOTOX) Chemical muscle denervation by toxin binding to acetylcholine receptors of the motor nerve terminal. Effects last several months, but with chronic use, some patients may develop antibodies that decrease efficacy. Lyophilized toxin should be kept frozen until time of use and reconstituted with unpreserved saline. Maximize concentration, and minimize the volume of injection. Use ice several minutes pre- and postinjection to aid in comfort and decrease spread of botulinum toxin.

- Blepharospasm: 30 gauge needle on tuberculin syringe, 2.5–10.0 units per 0.1 cc subcutaneous injection superficially between skin and orbicularis (see rete pegs with formation of a small vesicle). Typically five to eight injection sites around each eyelid to cover distribution of spasms, especially junction of preseptal and orbital orbicularis muscle, just within the confines of the bony rim, avoiding the levator muscle, IO, and lid margin (may also inject into corrugator and procerus muscles; inject deeper into the muscle). Used also in dystonias with multiple superficial injections.
- Chemical tarsorrhaphy as in Bell's palsy: orbicularis injection with 30-gauge needle, deep through septum (do not want to see a good bleb, as in superficial injections for blepharospasm).
- Rhytids (wrinkles): common request for cosmetic concerns. Inject superficially in glabella and lateral "crow's-feet."
- Overall 96% response rate; maximum effect 3 to 5 days, usual duration 3 to 6 months. Effects for benign essential blepharospasm last an average of 13 weeks, Meige's syndrome 12 weeks, and hemifacial spasm 20 weeks. Gradual decreased effectiveness with multiple injections over time (may need to change concentration or injection sites). Lethal dose is several thousand units (much greater than the doses used for local injection).
- Complications: ptosis, dry eye from lagophthalmos, photophobia, diplopia, epiphora, ectropion, or entropion.

CN VII PALSY MANAGEMENT (See Chapter 8); results in loss of orbicularis tone with decreased blink response, lagophthalmos, dry eye, failure of lacrimal pump, and paralytic ectropion. Treatment stages:

- Supportive: find etiology (trauma, tumor, infection, HSV or HZV neuritis) or most often idiopathic Bell's palsy. Treat with ocular lubrication and drops, no patching; may tape lower eyelid up or use moisture chamber.
    - Bell's palsy: 75% of CN VII palsy; 85% regain function within 3 to 6 months. Image if not better by 6 months or if there are signs and symptoms of vestibular or hearing defect.
    - Treat Bell's palsy with prednisone 1 mg/kg/day for 7 to 10 days plus acyclovir or valacyclovir 1 g PO 3 times per day for 7 days (many think Bell's is not idiopathic but is actually a herpes viral infection).
- Facial reanimation: if patient is an appropriate candidate, may perform cross facial nerve graft surgery followed 8 to 12 months later by muscle and neurovascular bundle graft from the gracilis, lateral dorsi, or

TABLE 2–3
Fitzpatrick Skin Types

Type	Skin Color	Response to Sun Exposure
Type 1	White	Always burn, never tan
Type 2	White	Usually burn, tan with difficulty
Type 3	White	Sometimes burn, average tan
Type 4	Medium brown	Rarely burn, tan with ease
Type 5	Dark brown	Rarely burn, tan very easily
Type 6	Black	Never burn, tan very easily

pectoralis minor muscle; may improve facial tone (does not improve blinking).

- Lower eyelid and canthal resuspension with or without suborbicularis oculi fascia (SOOF)/midface-lift with free hard palate mucosal graft (HPMG) or ear cartilage graft.
- Passive upper lid animation: gold weight aids gravity-dependent closure.
- Dynamic lid animation: Morel-Fatio palpebral sling, arion silicone sling or temporalis muscle transfer.
- Soft tissue repositioning: brow lift, blepharoplasty if no dry eye or keratopathy.
- Residual treatments: management of synkinesis due to aberrant regeneration and hypertonicity, blepharospasm, or crocodile tears. Treat with botulinum toxin or surgery.

LASER SKIN RESURFACING Best in Fitzpatrick types 1–3, caution in types 4–6 (Table 2–3). Consider pretreating with hydroquinone 4% cream.

- Carbon dioxide laser: 10.6 μm with HeNe aiming beam. Laser energy is absorbed by water, and increased temperature causes cell destruction. Able to remove small tissue increments.

SUBORBICULARIS OCULI FASCIA (SOOF) LIFT Midface lift; SOOF is contiguous with superficial musculoaponeurotic system (SMAS) of the face. Levator labi superficialis muscle lies over the infraorbital nerve.

TEMPORAL ARTERY BIOPSY (TAB) With small incision, find artery, then open wound for full exposure. Pass 3.0 silk for double tie proximally then distally. Remove artery distally then proximally; close with 5.0 Vicryl subcutaneously and chromic suture or staples for skin.

CHAPTER 3

Cornea and Conjunctiva

Anatomy and Physiology

EMBRYOLOGY The cornea begins to form when the lens cup separates from the surface ectoderm (7–9 mm embryo at about 33 days), consisting of one to two rows of epithelial cells resting on a thin basal lamina with a cluster of mesenchymal cells near the lip of the optic cup just posterior to the corneal basal lamina. During the following week, some of these mesenchymal cells grow centrally between the basal laminae of the lens and corneal epithelia. At about 40 days the epithelium has a basal cuboidal and a superficial squamous cell layer. Posterior to the basal lamina, the mesenchyme has produced a double row of flattened cells, the future endothelium. By 22–24 mm, migrating mesenchymal cells of neural crest origin invade the space between the epithelium and the endothelium from the periphery to form stroma and sclera.

At 2 months (about 35 mm), the cornea has an epithelium of outer squamous and basal columnar cells resting on a basal lamina with a stroma of about 15 layers of cells with rapidly developing collagen fibrils, most in the posterior portion. At 3 months, the endothelium of the central area consists of a single row of flattened cells that rest on an interrupted basal lamina, the first indication of a thin Descemet's membrane. Collagen fibril formation is preceded by a gradual change from the randomly dispersed stellate fibroblasts to spindle-shaped cells with their long axes parallel to the corneal surface beginning in the posterior layers (in contrast, the sclera develops homogeneously, not in layers, as does the cornea). Although the lamellae are superimposed upon one another, each continues to grow by the addition of collagen fibrils from keratoblasts. Bowman's layer arises relatively late during the fifth month, formed by the most anterior fibroblasts of the stroma.

Fiber formation is preceded by synthesis of ground substance, and late in the sixth fetal month keratan sulfate is detectable and increases in amount. The early fetal corneal stroma is hydrophilic and translucent rather than transparent, and condensation begins in the posterior stroma until about the time that the most anterior lamellae are formed when corneal transparency reaches adult quality. By the fifth month, nerve endings are distributed in the epithelium. The diameter of the cornea is determined by the size of the retinal cup; if the eye fails to grow to a normal size, the cornea is also dwarfed, but it is qualitatively normal.

CONJUNCTIVA Composed of nonkeratinized stratified columnar epithelium (keratinization seen as leukoplakia is often a sign of neoplasia). More wing cells are present than in the cornea, thus conjunctival epithelium is 10 to 12 cells in thickness. Goblet cells in the epithelium are important for mucus production (lost with inflammation = dry eye) and more abundant nasally, in the fornix and the caruncle (most goblet cells are about 4 mm from the limbus called the glands of Manz). Melanocytes and Langerhans' cells are found among basal cells. Substantia propia has collagen type 1 matrix and a normal chronic lymphocytic infiltrate with IgA present (mucosa-associated lymphoid tissue like Waldeyer's ring in the throat or Peyer's patches in the gastrointestinal tract).

- Episcleral vascular plexus: superficial and deep episcleral network. Episcleritis has edema that separates deep and superficial episcleral vessels with retained scleral contour (in contrast, edema from scleritis distorts scleral contour with retained relation between deep and superficial network).
- Normal flora: *Staphylococcus epidermidis*, *Corynebacterium* species, *Propionibacterium acnes*

LIMBAL STEM CELLS Progenitor cells of the corneal epithelium located in the deep basal layers at the pallisades of Vogt. The G_1 cell cycle S-gate, which remains closed in normal epithelial cells, is stimulated to open and allows cell mitosis in the stem cells.

CARUNCLE Contains epithelium, goblet cells, hair, adipose, and pilosebaceous units. Do not excise; if it contains a pigmented lesion, it is always a nevus.

TEAR FILM 7 μm thick, pH 7.4, hyposmolar (302 mOsm/L), 6.5 μL volume, produced 1.2 μL/minute; thus, turnover every 5 minutes. Functions to smooth surface of epithelium (which has 0.5 μm elevated microvilli), provides O_2 to cornea, and provides IgA, lactoferrin, lysozyme, beta-lysin, complement, trophic proteins, and growth factors. Classically three tear layers are present:

- Inner mucinous layer with mucopolysaccharides (MPS): carboxylated mucin from holocrine goblet cells, sulfinated mucin from conjunctiva epithelium; 0.02–0.05 μm thick, adherent to glycocalyx.
- Middle thick aqueous layer from Krause's and Wolfring glands (basal tear secretion) and lacrimal gland (reflex secretion).
- Outer oil layer: 0.1 μm thick (about the wavelength of light); there is 15× greater aqueous evaporation without it, from Zeis' (holocrine), Moll's (apocrine sweat glands), and meibomian (holocrine) glands.

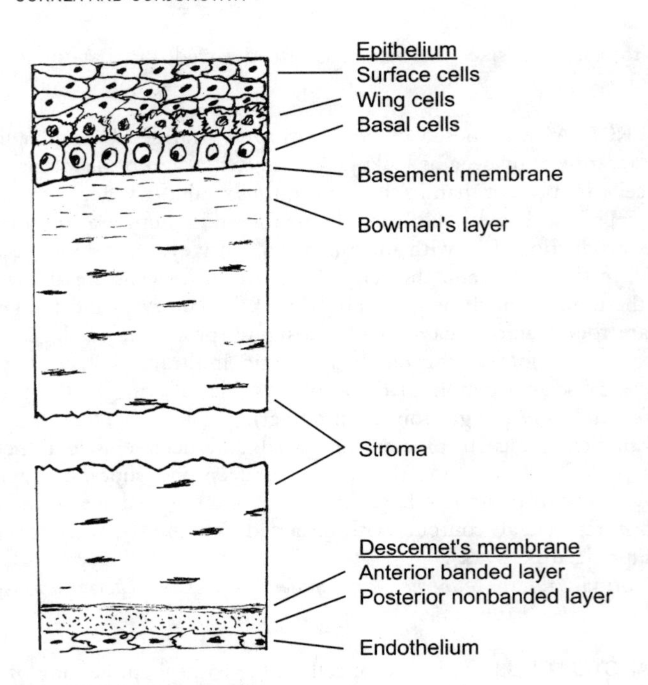

Figure 3–1 The five layers of the cornea in cross section.

CORNEA (Fig. 3–1) Derived from surface ectoderm, 500 μm central thickness, 800 μm peripheral. It is 11 × 12 mm anteriorly (a horizontal oval that points toward the LR, due to a more superficial corneoscleral limbus superiorly and inferiorly), but posteriorly it is circular. The cornea is naturally avascular (receives O_2 and nutrition from tears and aqueous) and dehydrated (but still 78% water). It has about 40D refractive power (mainly from the air-tear interface). The sensory nerve pathway is from CN V via the gasserian ganglion to V_1 nasociliary nerve through the ciliary ganglion without synapse then the long ciliary nerve to the ciliary body, iris, and cornea. Cornea nerves enter the anterior one-third stroma mostly at 3 and 9 o'clock and have naked nerve endings at the epithelium BM.

EPITHELIUM 50 μm thick, four to five cellular layers (deep basal columnar cells undergo mitosis to middle wing cells, then superficial squamous cells desquamate) with a true BM (not Bowman's layer), and arise from stem cells at the limbus. It turns over approximately every 7 days. BM takes several months to reattach firmly if traumatized.

BOWMAN'S LAYER Not a membrane but is condensed acellular anterior stroma 15 μm thick composed of randomly arranged compact collagen lamellae. Binds certain growth factors (e.g., anti–fibroblast growth factor). Scars when disrupted, does not heal, and is nonrenewable.

STROMA 90% of corneal thickness; composed of approximately 250 regularly spaced collagen lamellae that contain 600 Å fibrils that extend across the entire cornea. Keratocytes and glycosaminoglycans (keratan sulfate and chondroitin sulfate) are clear because the wavelength of visible light is about 5000 Å. Nonrenewable.

DESCEMET'S MEMBRANE Basement membrane of endothelium, 10–12 μm thick. Anterior third is the fetal band, and the posterior nonbanded portion continues to grow with age. The posterior may become banded with diseased endothelium (e.g., Fuchs' dystrophy has banded posterior Descemet's membrane in the patient's teenage years even though guttae is often not present until age 40). Site of guttae and peripheral Hassall-Henle bodies.

ENDOTHELIUM From neural crest, nonrenewable cellular monolayer. Controls hydration by pump function (not a good mechanical barrier). Endothelial cells do not multiply: cell density is about 3500 cells/mm^2 at birth and decrease gradually throughout life at about 0.6% per year and about a 10% loss per intraocular surgery. Corneal edema develops if cell density drops below 500–1000 cells/mm^2; thus, with normal aging we have about an 80% reserve of endothelial cells. A Na^+/K^+/ATPase and bicarbonate pump in the lateral membrane pumps Na^+ and bicarbonate into the aqueous. Cells are joined by zonula occludens (closes posterior intercellular space toward the AC) and macula adherens.

CORNEAL HYDRATION The epithelium to endothelium ratio to electrolyte diffusion resistance is about 200:1 (i.e., epithelium is a good water barrier). Stromal GAG ground substance (polyanionic charges) is a "dry sponge" and wants to absorb water (swelling pressure = imbibition/oncotic pressure + IOP) balanced by endothelial pump and epithelium evaporation (only 5%). Earliest symptom of corneal edema is morning vision clouding from microcystic epithelium edema from decreased evaporation overnight. Stromal edema and Descemet's folds occur when corneal thickness reaches about 0.6 mm, and epithelial edema and bullae form when the cornea is about 0.7 mm.

- Acute glaucoma with increased IOP pushes more water into the cornea, but with a normal endothelium, the stroma can still be dehydrated. Thus, only epithelial edema is seen because high epithelium resistance to water causes the excess corneal water to collect subepithelially (microcystic edema) and has greatly decreased VA.
- In contrast, endothelial damage (e.g., PBK of Fuchs' dystrophy) has more stromal edema (water displaces orderly collagen) but less decreased VA than epithelial edema.

Signs and Symptoms

BLUE SCLERA (Mnemonic: GNOME-P): **G**oltz syndrome (focal dermal hypoplasia), Ota's **n**evus (oculodermal menlanocytosis), **o**steogenesis imperfecta type I (decreased type I collagen, autosomal dominant), **M**arfan syndrome, **E**hlers-Danlos syndrome type VI (autosomal recessive; rule out cardiac disease), **p**seudoxanthoma elasticum (also may have keratoglobus)

BLEPHARITIS (Table 3–1) May be anterior (staphylococcus or seborrheic), posterior (meibomian seborrhea or posterior meibomitis), or mixed ("triple S" syndrome: staphylococcus, seborrhea, and sicca). Patients often have keratoconjunctivitis sicca, tylosis (irregular lid margin), poliosis (lash whitening), madarosis (lash loss), distichiasis, or trichiasis. Treat all types with lid scrubs and warm compresses; may need antibiotic ointment.

- Staphylococcal lid disease (SLD): characterizd by collarettes; seen mainly in younger patients, 50% of whom have tear deficiency. May cause punctate epithelial erosions (PEE), peripheral infiltrates, and phlyctenulosis (leaves a triangular scar at limbus). Ninety-five percent of normals are culture positive for *Staphylococcus epidermidis*, but 50% of staphylococcal blepharitis patients are culture positive for *Staphylococcus aureus* versus 10% of normals.
- Seborrhea: characterized by scurf on lashes; coexistant seborrheic dermatitis with oily, flaky skin. Thirty-threee percent of patients have keratoconjunctivitis sicca (KCS).
- Meibomian gland dysfunction (MGD): characterized by rapid TBUT, papillary reaction, and PEE; 60% of patients have rosacea. May be meibomian seborrhea with foamy tears, or posterior meibomitis with "toothpaste-like" secretions composed of increased cholesterol esters with increased melting point and increased free fatty acids.
- *Demodex follicularum*: characterized by "sleeves" present on lashes from hair mite.
- Angular blepharitis: *Staphylococcus aureus* is the leading cause, but classically it is from *Moraxella*; also *Candida* and HSV.

BULBAR FOLLICLES Chlamydia, sarcoid, lymphoma

CONGENITAL CORNEAL OPACIFICATION (Mnemonic: glaucoma + STUMPED): **g**laucoma, **s**clerocornea, **t**ears in Descemet's membrane (e.g., forceps delivery or other trauma), **u**lcer (HSV, interstitial keratitis, rubella), **m**ucopolysaccarides (MPS-1; Hurler's syndrome), **P**eters' anomaly, **e**ndothelial or stromal dystrophy (CHED < CHSD, PPMD; bilateral), and **d**ermoid. Also chromosomal abnormalities 21, 18, 13, and XO.

CONJUNCTIVAL GRANULOMA Parinaud's oculoglandular syndrome (usually from *Bartonella*/cat-scratch disease in North America, tuberculosis

TABLE 3–1
Types of Blepharitis

Characteristic	Staphylococcal	Seborrheic	Meibomian Gland Dysfunction
Location	Anterior eyelid	Anterior eyelid	Posterior eyelid
Lash loss or whitening	Frequent	Rare	Rare
Eyelid margin	Hard, fibrinous scales; matted crusts	Oily or greasy crusting	Inspissated meibomian secretions
Lid ulcers	Occasional	No	No
Conjunctivitis	Papillary with mucopurulent discharge	Papillary with mild injection	Papillary tarsal reaction with mild injection
Tear deficiency	50%	33%	Frequent
Keratitis	Inferior PEE (up to 33%); may have marginal infiltrates	Inferior PEE	Inferior PEE, marginal infiltrates, vascular pannus
Rosacea	No	Occasional	Present in 34 to 66%

elsewhere), sarcoidosis (discrete noncaseating granulomas), fungal, parasitic (increased eosinophils), syphilis (vessel in middle of granuloma), foreign body reaction, and chalazion

CONJUNCTIVAL HYPEREMIA Inflammation (infection, allergy, toxicity, neoplasm), irritation (foreign body, eyelash), reflex (eyestrain, crying), vasodilation (alcohol use, increased oxygenation, carcinoid), autonomic dysfunction (sympathetic paresis, sphenopalatine ganglion syndrome), and vascular engorgement (venous obstruction, hyperviscosity)

CONJUNCTIVAL PIGMENTATION (Mnemonic: like a dirty "damp apron"): **d**rugs (e.g., chlorpromazine, adrenochrome from epinephrine), **A**ddison's disease, **m**elanoma, **p**regnancy, **a**rgyrosis, **p**rimary acquired melanosis (PAM), **r**adiation, **o**cular or oculodermal melanocytosis (congenital, blue, episcleral), **n**evus

CONJUNCTIVAL TELANGIECTASIAS Louis-Bar's syndrome (ataxia telangiectasia; associated with cerebellar and immunologic abnormalities), or HIV

CONJUNCTIVAL ULCERATION Stevens-Johnson syndrome (SJS), OCP, factitious conjunctivitis, *Bartonella* infection

CONJUNCTIVITIS, CICATRIZING OCP, SJS, Lyell's disease, toxic epidermal necrolysis (TEN), trauma (e.g., chemical injury foreign body), HZV, trachoma, sarcoid, prior infection (epidemic keratoconjunctivitis, diphtheria), primary Sjögren's syndrome, atopic keratoconjunctivitis (AKC), rosacea, certain drugs (e.g., practolol and glaucoma medications), malignancy (e.g., CIN, SCC, sebaceous gland CA, fibrosarcoma, lymphoma, melanoma), porphyria cutanea tarda, and lichen planus

CONJUNCTIVITIS, ACUTE FOLLICULAR Pharyngeal conjunctival fever (adenovirus), herpes simplex virus (HSV), EKC (adenovirus), hemorrhagic viral (coxsackievirus, enterovirus), chlamydia (acute trachoma or adult inclusion conjunctiva), Newcastle disease (poultry handlers), molluscum contagiosum (may also cause Parinaud's oculoglandular syndrome) or medications (e.g., dipivefrin). Follicles are small "lymph nodes" in the conjunctiva.

CONJUNCTIVITIS, CHRONIC FOLLICULAR (Mnemonic: Passing tough tests mostly means late cramming): **P**arinaud's oculoglandular syndrome (cat-scratch disease), **t**rachoma, **t**oxins (miotics, neomycin, gentamycin, atropine, Iopidine, propine), **m**olluscum, ***M**oraxella*, **L**yme disease, **c**hlamydia.

CONJUNCTIVITIS, HEMORRHAGIC Most cases are coxsackieviruses; also caused by enteroviruses and Newcastle disease (found in poultry workers). Conjunctivitis with subconjunctival hemorrhage.

CONJUNCTIVITIS, MEMBRANOUS Bacterial infection (streptococcus, pneumococci), ligneous conjunctivitis (true membranous), adenovirus, HSV, chemical reaction, and diphtheria (true membranous). Exudation that adheres to conjunctiva epithelium; causes bleeding when removed.

CONJUNCTIVITIS, PAPILLARY The result of infections (bacterial, chlamydia), allergic or vernal conjunctivitis, foreign body, many medications (especially glaucoma), giant papillary conjunctivitis (GPC) from contact lens wear. Papillae are inflamed mounds formed from conjunctival septae and contain a central blood vessel.

CONJUNCTIVITIS, PSEUDOMEMBRANOUS Chlamydia in newborns, SJS, superior limbal keratoconjunctivitis (SLK), OCP, and bacteria (e.g., gonococci and staphylococcus). Characterized by exudation that congeals on the conjunctiva surface; can be removed without bleeding.

CONJUNCTIVITIS, VESICULAR HSV, HZV, varicella, erythema multiforme, and OCP

CORNEAL ABRASION, RECURRENT CORNEAL EROSIONS Trauma, HSV, EBMD, stromal dystrophies, diabetes, and microcystic edema. Treat with 5% NaCl, 40% glucose ointment, bandage soft contact lens (BSCL), eyelid taping, debridement, stromal puncture, or PTK.

CORNEAL DYSTROPHIES VERSUS DEGENERATIONS Dystrophies are familial (all autosomal dominant except macular, lattice type III, and CHED type II, which are autosomal recessive), appear early in life, and are avascular, bilateral, symmetrical, central, and slowly progressive. Degenerations are acquired mid- to late life, vascularized, unilateral, asymmetric, peripheral, and frequently associated with systemic or other disease.

CORNEAL EDEMA, ACUTE (Mnemonic: THICK): **t**rauma (epithelial defect, surgery), **h**igh pressure, **i**nflammation (e.g., infection or graft rejection), **c**ontact lens hypoxia, **k**eratoconus hydrops (ruptured Descemet's membrane). Acute edema is often a barrier problem.

CORNEAL EDEMA, CHRONIC PPMD, iridocorneal endothelial syndrome (ICE), trauma, toxins, failed graft, PBK, ABK, and Fuchs' dystrophy. Chronic edema is usually an endothelial pump problem.

CORNEAL EDEMA, CONGENITAL Glaucoma, CHED, PPMD, and birth trauma (forceps delivery)

CRYSTALS IN CORNEA Schnyder's crystalline dystrophy, interstitial crystalline keratopathy (from *Streptococcus viridans*), Bietti's crystalline dystrophy, multiple myeloma, gout, uremia, cystinosis, indomethacin or chloroquine (crystals in epithelium), and calcium oxalate deposits from *Dieffenbachia* plant sap

DENDRITIC KERATITIS (Mnemonic: HAZE ETC): **H**SV, ***A**canthamoeba*, **z**oster, **e**pithelial healing defect, **E**pstein-Barr virus, **t**yrosinemia II, and **C**LW

DESCEMET'S MEMBRANE BREAKS OR SCROLL Keratoconus, trauma (vertical striaė usually seen with forceps delivery), and congenital glaucoma (horizontal Haab's striae)

DISCIFORM KERATITIS HSV, HZV, mumps, varicella, chemical injury; rule out bacterial or fungal keratitis and anesthetic abuse

DRY EYE, KERATOCONJUNCTIVITIS SICCA (KCS) Hyperosmolar tears from aqueous deficiency or evaporative loss (MGD). Symptoms typically worse at the end of the day, with foreign body sensation, punctate keratopathy, interpalpebral exposure pattern seen best with 1% rose bengal stain, and filamentary keratopathy (mucous strands). Treat with artificial tears, lubrication, punctal occlusion, oral pilocarpine (not proven to increase tear secretion), or acetylcysteine 10% for mucolytic.

- Sjögren's syndrome: diagnosis requires xerostomia or coexistent connective tissue disorder. Work-up includes rheumatoid factor (RF), autoantibodies against Sjögren's syndrome antigen A (SS-A/Ro; present in about 70%), and Sjögren's syndrome antigen B (SS-B/La; present in about 50%), antinuclear antibodies (ANA), and rheumatology consult. In primary Sjögren's, 90% have HLA-B8 autoantibodies. The disease is called secondary Sjögren's syndrome if another connective tissue disorder is identified.
- Non–Sjögren's syndrome:
  - Congenital: Riley-Day syndrome (familial dysautonomia), alacrima, Adie's syndrome
  - Acquired: Shy-Drager syndrome (idiopathic autonomic dysfunction), CLW
  - Secondary lacrimal dysfunction from inflammatory disease, trauma, anticholinergic medications, and neuroparalytic hyposecretion. Common after bone marrow transplant. Risks for KCS following bone marrow transplant include increased age, chronic graft versus host disease, female sex, and use of methotrexate.

- Meibomian gland dysfunction (MGD): characterized by lipid deficiency, increased evaporation, foreign body sensation, injection, papillary reaction, punctate erosions on inferior cornea, foamy tears, and increased TBUT. Sixty percent of cases are from rosacea; also from oral retinoids. Treat with lid hygiene.
- Delayed tear currents: often coexistent with dry eye from poor pump or tear clearance (e.g., punctal plugs) and exacerbated by preservatives in many eyedrops, often with morning symptoms. Treat with non-preserved steroids.
- Loss of conjunctival goblet cells from OCP, SJS, or chemical burn
- Vitamin A deficiency (xerostomia): characterized by Bitot's spots (foamy gray triangles on bulbar conjunctiva), keratomalacia, nyctalopia
- Darier's disease (keratosis follicularis): rare autosomal recessive disorder of vitamin A metabolism causing decreased desmosomes. Presents with keratotic eyelid plaques, belpharoconjunctivitis, corneal opacities (central, whorllike), pannus, and retinitis pigmentosa (RP)–like retinal changes with flat electroretinogram (ERG) and cataract. Treat with vitamin A, isoretinoin, or steroids.
- Ichthyosis: characterized by eyelid scaling, ectropion, conjunctiva thickening, and corneal opacities. Vulgaris is the most common, autosomal dominant form. Also Sjögren-Larsson syndrome, Rud-Conradi syndrome, and congenital vascularizing keratitis-icthyosiform-deafness (KID) syndrome. Worsens with Retin-A. Also seen in Refsums disease and congenital hemidysplasia with icthyosiform erythroderma and limb defects (CHILD) syndrome.
- Xeroderma pigmentosum: autosomal recessive defect in DNA repair after it is damaged by UV light. Presents with photophobia, tearing, blepharospasm, and KCS, leading to exposure keratitis or ulceration. Eleven percent of patients have ocular neoplasms: SCC (primary), BCC (secondary).

EOSINOPHILS IN CONJUNCTIVA Allergy, parasite, leukemic eosinophilic granuloma, and Kimura's disease (eosinophilic granulomas of the soft tissues, usually in Asian patients)

GRANULOMAS, CLASSIC ASSOCIATIONS Caseating = tuberculosis; non-caseating = sarcoid; vessel in middle = syphilis; eosinophilic = parasitic

HYALINE IN CORNEA Granular dystrophy, Salzmann's nodules

HYPHEMA (Mnemonic: hemorrhages too numerous to count): **H**SV or **H**ZV iritis (causes a vasculitis), **t**rauma or surgery, **n**eovascularization (Fuchs' HIC, neovascularization of the iris, PDR, retinopathy of prematurity, Coats' disease, persistent hyperplastic primary vitreous), **t**umor (juvenile xanthogranuloma, RB, leukemia, intraocular lymphoma), **c**lotting disorder or blood dyscrasia

HYPOPYON (Mnemonic: CLUE HIT): **c**ontact lens too tight, **l**ens reaction (intraocular lens or retained lens proteins), **u**lcer (bacterial, fungal, or viral keratitis), **e**ndophalmitis, **H**SV, **i**ritis (any severe hyperacute uveitis, especially Behçet's or B-27–related, including Reiter's syndrome and ankylosing spondylitis), **t**umor (pseudohypopyon from intraocular tumor necrosis can be seen with RB, leukemia, and large cell lymphoma).

INTERSTITIAL KERATITIS (IK) 90% of cases from syphilis (87% congenital and 3% acquired; also called Grayson's disease). Other causes include HSV, Cogan's disorder (hearing loss, IK; associated with polyarteritis nodosa), onchocerciasis, tuberculosis, HZV, mumps, leprosy, *Acanthamoeba*, psoriasis, and inflammatory bowel disease. Signs: ghost vessel, stromal scarring.

KERATIC PRECIPITATES, CHARACTERISTICS Arlt's triangle (sarcoid, inferior between 4 and 8 o'clock), diffuse (Fuchs' HIC, HSV, cytomegalovirus retinitis, Vogt-Koyanagi-Harada disease), "greasy" (sarcoid, syphilis), stellate (HSV, Fuchs' HIC, toxoplasmosis, sarcoid), geographic (tuberculosis, syphilis). Represent collections of inflammatory cells that settle on the corneal endothelium.

KERATITIS, BILATERAL (PREFERENTIALLY) Leprosy, syphilis (congenital), phlyctenulosis, Cogan's disorder, mumps, sarcoidosis, collagen vascular diseases, systemic vasculitis, onchocerciasis, psoriasis, and inflammatory bowel disease

KERATITIS, UNILATERAL (PREFERENTIALLY) HSV, HZV, bacterial or fungal keratitis, *Acanthamoeba*, syphilis (acquired), and tuberculosis

LEUKOCYTES IN THE CORNEAL EPITHELIUM SLK, acute infection

LIMBAL CELL DEFICIENCY OCP, aniridia, SJS, chemical injury, multiple endocrine neoplasis (MEN) syndrome, pterygium surgery

LYMPHANGIECTASIA Dilated lympatics on bulbar conjunctiva; may be developmental or acquired from trauma or inflammation. Treat with excision.

MARGINAL LESIONS OR INFILTRATES Staphylococcal blepharitis, Herbert's pits (trachoma), Horner-Trantas dots (vernal keratoconjunctivitis), periperal ulcerative keratitis (long differential diagnosis)

MAST CELLS IN CONJUNCTIVA Allergy (especially AKC), OCP, pterygium, NF

NEUROTROPHIC ULCER Trigeminal nerve palsy or inflammation, HSV, HZV, surgery, strokes, tumors, chemical burn, anesthetic abuse, and diabetes. Usually oval-shaped, inferior cornea with rolled edges and stromal loss. Treat with lubrication, antibiotics, patching, lid taping, punctal occlusion, or tarsorrhaphy.

ORGANISMS THAT CAN PENETRATE AN INTACT EPITHELIUM *Neisseria gonorrhoeae* and *meninigitis Corynebacterium diphtheriae*, *Haemophilus aegyptius*, *Listeria*, *Shigella*. Note: *Pseudomonas* is not on this list.

ORGANISMS SEEN ON H & E STAIN Bacteria plus *Acanthamoeba* and *Mucor*

PANNUS (Mnemonic: LAB VERSUS PORCH): **l**imbic (SLK micropannus), **a**niridia (limbal stem cell deficiency), **b**urns (chemical), **v**ernal KC, **s**taphylococcal hypersensitivity, **p**hlyctenule, **o**verwear or tight CL (superior pannus), **r**osacea, **c**hlamydia (superior pannus from trachoma or adult inclusion conjunctivitis), **H**SV. Pannus is anything that is between Bowman's layer and the epithelium; if Bowman's layer is not intact, it is a degenerative pannus.

PERIPHERAL CORNEAL THINNING Collagen vascular disorder (rheumatoid arthritis or systemic lupus erythematosus, usually ulcerated), Terrien's marginal degeneration, Mooren's ulcer, pellucid marginal degeneration ("shaggy cone," epithelium intact), furrow degeneration (peripheral to arcus), dellen, dry eye, vernal KC, rosacea, inflammatory bowel disease, neurotrophic cornea, surgery, and leukemia.

PERIPHERAL ULCERATIVE KERATITIS (PUK) Blepharitis-associated marginal infiltrates, ulcerative keratitis connective tissue disease (RA, SLE, etc.), Mooren's ulcer (autoimmune, chronic, progressive), HSV, and hepatitis C–associated

PIGMENT LINES IN THE CORNEA Hudson-Stähli (physiologic, lower lid apposition to cornea), Ferry's (filtering bleb), Stocker's (pterygium), Fleischer ring (keratoconus, iron in epithelium), Kayser-Fleischer ring (Wilson's disease, copper in Descemet's membrane), Waring (along radial keratotomy incisions)

PROMINENT CORNEAL NERVES (Mnemonic: $LMNR_2A$): **l**eprosy, **MEN** IIb (pheochromocytoma, medullary thyroid CA, conjunctival and mucosal neuromas), **N**F, **R**efsum's disease, **R**iley-Day syndrome, and ***A****canthamoeba*

- More visible nerves: keratoconus, ichthyosis, Fuchs' corneal dystrophy, corneal edema, congenital glaucoma

PUNCTATE EPITHELIAL EROSIONS (PEE) Dry eye, atopic KC, and topical toxicity

PUNCTATE EPITHELIAL KERATITIS (PEK) HSV, adenovirus, and Thygeson's superficial punctate keratitis

RING CORNEAL INFILTRATE *Acanthamoeba*, HSV, *Pseudomonas*, topical anesthetic abuse, and *Moraxella*

STROMAL SCARRING HSV (by far the most common), HZV, and syphilis

SUBCONJUNCTIVAL HEMORRHAGE, BLOODY TEARS Trauma, conjunctivitis, Valsalva's maneuver, febrile illness, vascular fragility, clotting disorder, and thrombocytopenia

SYMBLEPHARON (Mnemonic: ACID STORE): **A**topic KC, **c**hemical burns (especially alkali), **i**nflammation of any type, **d**rugs, **S**JS, **t**rauma, **O**CP, **r**adiation, **E**KC

VASCULAR CAUSES OF A RED EYE Lymphangioma, orbital varices, and hemangioma

VERTICILLATE, WHORL-LIKE CORNEAL EPITHELIAL OPACITY (Mnemonic: FIT CAP): **F**abry's disease, **i**ndomethacin or Naprosyn, **t**amoxifen, **c**hloroquine, **a**miodarone (vortex keratopathy; may also cause anterior ischemic optic neuropathy or striate melanokeratosis), and **p**henothiazines. Whorl appearance is due to the pattern of epithelium migration from the limbus.

WHITE, LEUKOPLAKIC LESIONS OF CONJUNCTIVA Associated with SCC, CIN, Bitot's spots, benign hereditary intraepithelial dyskeratosis (BHID), papilloma, amyloid, pinguecula, and amelanotic nevus or melanoma

Exam and Imaging

SCHIRMER'S TESTING Schirmer's I—nonanesthetic; Schirmer's II—anesthetic plus irritate the nasal mucosa

SPECULAR MICROSCOPY Mean endothelial cell count 2400/mm^2, coefficient of variation <0.3 (smaller indicates more uniform cells), pleomorphism <50% (cells that are not the normal hexagonal shape)

- Polymegatheism caused by: CLW (causes release of arachidonic acid via the cP450 system, which is changed into hydroxyeicosatetraenoic acid [HETE], which in turn changes the cell cytoskeleton and increases endothelial cell size), inflammation, diabetes, and LASIK.

TOPOGRAPHY

- Placido's ring topography (conventional): usually gives axial topography, which is the average of all points compared with the center of the corneal radius of curvature, and thus smooths over localized defects
- Tangential topography: compares one point to adjacent point and thus shows local defects more accurately.
- Scanning slit topography (i.e., Orbscan): looks at light scatter from the cornea like a slit lamp. Based on the elevation of the corneal surface, not the radius of curvature. Determines the "best fit sphere" for the entire cornea, then maps if any areas are elevated above this ideal sphere (warm color) or are below the best fit (cool color). Standard four-frame printout shows: upper left—anterior surface elevation; upper right—endothelial surface elevation; bottom right—thickness (anterior minus posterior surface height); bottom left—standard keratometric topography. Posterior float >50 μm is suggestive of keratoconus if associated with corneal thinning.

Congenital and Genetic Disease

ANIRIDIA Central corneal vascularization and clouding after age 2 from limbal stem cell deficiency. Poor visual prognosis with limbal transplants or penetrating keratoplasty (PK). See Chapter 9.

CORNEA PLANA Small, thin, flat corneas (similar radius of curvature as sclera: keratometry measurements are <42, usually 20–30 D), diameter about 9 mm; cornea looks like dense arcus. Associated with, hyperopia, early cataract, and angle-closure glaucoma (ACG). Patients usually of Finnish descent. An autosomal recessive abnormality of chromosome 12q21 causes defective keratan sulfate (part of the ground substance of normal stroma). May also be autosomal dominant with other anomalies.

KERATOECTASIA Intrauterine infection and perforation with bulging opaque cornea (like anterior staphyloma) protruding through palpebral fissure at birth. Usually vitamin deficient.

LIGNEOUS CONJUNCTIVITIS Pseudomembranous conjunctivitis in children from heritable defect in plasminogen gene; patients have deep fibrin "woody" infiltrate of conjunctiva and lids. May have similar exudative membranes in trachea, vagina, and elsewhere.

MEGALOCORNEA Bilateral, nonprogressive corneal enlargement >12 mm diameter at birth (normal ~ 10 mm) or >13 mm after age 2. X-linked recessive, 90% male. Associated with cataract and ectopia lentis; 20% have open-angle glaucoma (exclude congenital glaucoma). May also be isolated or rarely associated with craniosynostosis, dwarfism, facial hemiatrophy, and Down, Marfan, or Alport's syndromes.

MICROCORNEA <10 mm corneal diameter from fetal developmental arrest in the fifth month. Autosomal dominant; hyperopic with a flat cornea. Associated with ACG, cataract, coloboma, and PHPV.

MICROPHTHALMOS Small, disorganized eye, 1:2000 incidence; axial length <20 mm in adult (usually 17 mm in newborn). Seen with trisomies, especially chromosome 13; also associated with cataract, coloboma, PHPV, basal cell nevus syndrome, and odontogenic jaw cysts.

NANOPHTHALMOS Small "functional" or "normal" eye, axial length <20.5 mm. Associated with hyperopia, uveal effusions, and possible serous retinal detachment and ACG (usually at age 40–60). Disorder of abnormally arranged scleral collagen that becomes thickened and obstructs venous outflow. Avoid intraocular surgery. Needs laser peripheral iridotomy (LPI), maybe vortex vein decompression.

SCLEROCORNEA Noninflammatory, nonprogressive scleralization of cornea with an ill-defined limbus and corneal vessels and loss of transparency; 80% of patients also have cornea plana. Ninety percent bilateral; no sex predilection; 50% sporadic.

ANTERIOR SEGMENT DYSGENESIS

- Axenfeld-Rieger: bilateral neurocrestopathy, autosomal dominant from chromosome 4q25 and 13q14 RIEG gene mutation with abnormal solurshin protein leading to mesenchymal changes (anterior iris structure is missing). Sixty percent of patients have glaucoma (8% congenital, 50% by second decade). Spectrum of clinical presentation:
    - Axenfeld's anomaly: bilateral anterior displaced Schwalbe's ring (posterior embryotoxon), iridocorneal adhesions; 50% of patients have juvenile glaucoma.
    - Axenfeld's syndrome: above anomaly plus skeletal anomalies (hypertelorism, facial asymmetry)

- Rieger's anomaly: above Axenfeld's syndrome plus anterior stromal iris atrophy, corectopia, ectropion uvea, peripheral anterior synechiae (PAS); glaucoma in >50% of cases.
- Rieger's syndrome: above Rieger's anomaly plus skeletal anomalies such as malar hypoplasia, prominence of lower lip, hypodontia, hypospadias, heart defects; umbilicus button does not resorb. Associated with oculocutaneous albinism.

- Peters' anomaly: corneal leukoma (central corneal opacity, peripherally clear) with posterior corneal defect with thinning or absence of endothelium and Descemet's membrane. May have adhesions between lens and cornea, anterior polar or cortical cataract, microspherophakia, and anterior lens displacement. Fifty percent of patients have trabeculodysgenesis glaucoma. Cornea may be perforated at birth with loss of lens. Usually sporadic but also autosomal recessive; PAX 6 gene defect from failure of neural crest cell migration that normally separates the surface ectoderm of the cornea and the developing lens. Eighty percent are bilateral; may be associated with many other ocular defects, malformations, and fetal alcohol syndrome. Called Peters'-plus anomaly if cardiac, skeletal, or clefting abnormalities are present. Treat with PK usually at age 2–3 weeks.
  - Circumscribed posterior keratoconus: unilateral, nonprogressive, nonfamilial localized posterior cornea crater-like defect. F > M. Descemet's membrane and endothelium intact. Normal vision.
  - Internal ulcer of von Hippel: posterior keratoconus with cloudy cornea following intrauterine inflammation
- Posterior amorphous corneal dysgenesis: bilateral, limbus-to-limbus opacity; autosomal dominant
- Posterior embryotoxon: thickened and anteriorly displaced Schwalbe's ring. Autosomal dominant; present in 8 to 30% of normals; may be part of Axenfeld's anomaly.

ANTERIOR CORNEAL DYSTROPHIES

- Epithelial basement membrane, map-dot-fingerprint, Cogan's microcystic dystrophy: disorder of the basement membrane and loss of epithelial cell polarity. Characterized by geographic plaques of thickened BM (maps), intraepithelial debris and pseudocysts (dots), "mare's hairs" reduplications of BM (fingerprints), and recurrent corneal erosions (in 10% of patients, but is the cause of 50% of all recurrent corneal erosions). Autosomal dominant with incomplete penetrance; 6 to 18% prevalence, typically females age >50. Treat acute RCE, then try 5% NaCl ointment and lubricants, or BSCL 4–6 weeks, epithelial scraping, stromal puncture (cure 90%, may scar in visual axis; better for traumatic RCE), or PTK; avoid LASIK.
- Meesman or juvenile epithelial dystrophy: rare disorder that presents at young age with central, mainly interpalpebral, tiny bubble-like

intraepithelial vesicles and fine microcysts containing "peculiar substance." These coalesce with age, and cysts begin to rupture usually about age 40 to 50, causing severe RCE. Autosomal dominant, with 60% penetrance from defect of keratin 3 gene (chromosome 12q13) and keratin 12 (chromosome 17q12). These gene mutations cause defective cytokeratins that are part of the intracellular cytoskeleton. Treat RCE; BSCL often helpful.

- Reis-Buckler's dystrophy: autosomal dominant, strong penetrance, defect of the keratoepithelian gene (βig-h3 gene) found on chromosome 5q31 (like granular and lattice dystrophies). Bowman's layer is replaced with superficial geographic or honeycomb gray-white granular material centrally. Multilaminar eosinophilic deposits beneath the epithelium stain red with Masson-trichrome, like granular dystrophy. Onset is age 10 to 20, with frequent recurrent corneal erosions. Treat with PTK; recurrence after PK common.
    - Type 1: rod-shaped bodies; same gene as granular dystrophy; has decreased corneal sensation.
    - Type 2 (Thiel-Behnke): most frequent type, has curly fibers, chromosome 10q24 gene defect. Presents in early childhood with recurrent corneal erosions; normal corneal sensation.

STROMAL CORNEAL DYSTROPHIES (Table 3–2)

- Central cloudy dystrophy of François: autosomal dominant, nonprogressive; faint deep central shagreen, with normal VA.
- Congenital hereditary stromal dystrophy (CHSD): very rare, autosomal dominant, bilateral, nonprogressive feathery central corneal clouding, periphery normally clear. Normal Descemet's membrane and endothelium but abnormally aligned collagen. No corneal edema and normal thickness (unlike CHED), no photophobia or tearing.
- Fleck or pre-Descemet's dystrophy: rare, nonprogressive, faint disorder of excessive GAG and lipids in cornea. VA preserved, diagnosis of exclusion.
- Gelatinous-droplike dystrophy: autosomal recessive primary familial amyloidosis, defect of chromosome 1p; found mainly in Japan.

TABLE 3–2
Major Stromal Dystrophies and Histologic Stains

Stromal Dystrophy	Deposited Material	Histologic Stain
Macular	Mucopolysaccharide	Alcian blue
Granular	Hyaline	Masson-trichome
Lattice	Amyloid	Congo red

- Granular dystrophy: autosomal dominant disorder of transforming growth factor-beta-induction gene (βig-h3); also known as keratoepithelin gene found on chromosome 5q31 (like Reis-Buckler's and lattice dystrophies). Second most common dystrophy and the most benign stromal dystrophy. Characterized by anterior stromal, discrete, crumblike or granular focal opacities with intervening clear spaces. Pathology shows hyaline material that stains with Masson-trichrome (mnemonic: Cells are red, collagen blue, Masson-trichome is the stain for you). Cornea has an irregular BM, and Bowman's layer is thin or absent. Uncommonly have recurrent corneal erosions. Onset is early in life, although symptoms occur much later. Granular dystrophy is disciform in teens and not to limbus. Treat with PTK or PK late; often recurs after transplant.
  - Groenouw's type I: most benign and most frequent type.
  - Groenouw's type II: second decade onset; fewer and larger opacities with clear spaces; VA good.
  - Groenouw's type III: onset in infancy with erosions (like Reis-Buckler's).
  - Avellino: combined granular (appears first) and lattice (latter) dystrophies with subepithelial deposits in older patients. Same gene but different location; autosomal dominant with high penetrance. Treat with BSCL or PTK; may recur after PK.
- Lattice dystrophy: autosomal dominant disorder of chromosome 5q31 gene. Most common stromal dystrophy, with onset in first decade. Characterized by refractile lines of amyloid deposition; best seen with retroillumination, and stains with Congo red. Severe, frequent recurrent corneal erosions. Graft recurrences most common of all the dystrophies. PTK may reduce erosions, improve VA, and delay PK.
  - Type I (Biber-Haab-Dimmer): localized to cornea, deposition of nonimmunoglobulin amyloid-associated (AA) protein, classic; symptoms appear by end of first decade; autosomal dominant, keratoepithelin gene.
  - Type II (Meretoja): unilateral ocular involvement with systemic amyloidosis; symptoms appear around age 30; usually seen in persons of Finnish ancestry; autosomal dominant, chromosome 9q34, gelsolin gene. Patients often have masklike facies, blepharochalasis, pendulous ears, dry, lax skin, and nerve palsies.
  - Type III: midstromal, amyloid pentagonal (AP) component; chromosome 1p31, autosomal recessive; symptoms appear around age 30.
  - Type IIIA: autosomal recessive, keratoepithelin gene; symptoms appear around age 50.
- Macular dystrophy: autosomal recessive, chromosome 16q22 defect synthesizing keratan sulfate (can consider it a localized MPS disorder).

The unsulfated keratan (GAG) accumulates within the endoplasmic reticulum and deposits beneath the epithelium, within stromal cells and the endothelium. Clear cornea at birth but cloudy by age 3 to 9, with focal gray-white superficial opacities that progress to full thickness and periphery with late guttae and erosions. Stains with colloidal iron or alcian blue. This is the least common but most severe dystrophy, with no clear spaces and total cornea involved. Most patients require PK by age 30 to 40; frequently recurs after transplant.
- Schnyder's central crystalline dystrophy: autosomal dominant disorder with fine needle-shaped cholesterol crystals in anterior stroma with dense arcus. Crystals are not indicative of a certain lipid level, but rule out hyperlipidemia. Often symptomatic with good VA.

POSTERIOR CORNEAL DYSTROPHIES

- Congenital heridiitary endothelial dystrophy (CHED): bilateral "ground glass" corneal opacification to limbus with epithelial and stromal edema (may be 4× normal thickness; adult cornea can only swell to about 1.4×). No glaucoma, guttae, or associated ocular or systemic disease.
    - Type 1: autosomal dominant, progressive; presents around age 1 to 2 (no nystagmus) with corneal clouding, pain, photophobia, and tearing.
    - Type 2: autosomal recessive; more common than type 1; stationary; presents at birth with clouding, sensory nystagmus, and amblyopia. Defect on chromosome 20q11-cen, like PPMD.
- Fuchs' endothelial dystrophy: autosomal dominant, variable penetrance; F > M 2:1, usually postmenopausal. Affected females have 2.5× more guttae and 5.7× increased incidence of edema than males. Fuchs (1910) described a triad of stromal edema, subepithelial scar, and bullae and thought the condition was epithelial dystrophy.
    - Caused by accelerated apoptosis (programmed cell death) of endothelial cells (normally decrease 0.5% per year; thus, usually have enough for 150 to 200 years). Remaining endothelial cells spread out to cover the posterior cornea and demonstrate polymegathism and pleomorphism.
    - Early guttae (thickening and excrescences of Descemet's membrane) with pigment dusting, followed by microcystic edema with decreased vision in the morning that improves during the day as H_2O evaporation increases tears' hypertonicity. Later may develop bullous edema, recurrent corneal erosions, pannus, pain from ruptured bullae, with secondary infection and beaten metal appearance to endothelium. Up to 20% of patients have glaucoma (may be ACG with increased incidence of hyperopia).
    - Treat with hyperosmotic solutions and ointments; use hair dryer in the morning to dry cornea, and consider lowering IOP. Treat

ruptured bullae with patching or BSCL. Common cause for transplant. If cataract is visually significant, consider triple procedure (PK/cataract extraction/IOL) if pachymetry >620 μm centrally (normally about 520 μm) or cell count <1200. However, if patient is asymptomatic without edema or morning symptoms, go ahead with best phacoemulsification through scleral tunnel, with generous use of viscoelastic.

- Posterior polymorphous membrane dystrophy (PPMD): autosomal dominant or recessive, chromosome 20q11-cen (like CHED type 2) defect of endothelial cells that behave like epithelial cells (similar to ICE syndrome except PPMD is bilateral and congenital). "Nests" of endothelial cells look like "snail tracks" with vesicular gray lesions and opacities in Descemet's membrane and on endothelium. Onset is at birth to age 1; bilateral but asymmetric, usually asymptomatic. Open- or closed-angle glaucoma seen in 15% of cases. Epithelial-like cells in endothelium have desmosomes, microvilli, and keratin staining. VA usually normal; rarely requires PK but can recur after graft.

Infectious Disease

ACANTHAMOEBA Ubiquitous protozoan found especially in stagnant, contaminated water, nonsterile contact lens solution, and hot tubs. Typically inoculated, with corneal trauma causing a keratitis with pain out of proportion to the corneal ulcer, PEE or epithelial irregularity (may mimic HSV), multifocal stromal infiltrates and late ring infiltrate, radial neuritis with prominent corneal nerves, and hypoesthesia. Can also cause meningitis from diving into contaminated water, with transmission through the cribriform plate.

- Usually first treated as a bacterial keratitis, but when it is suspected, do culture or biopsy and stain with H & E and periodic acid. Look for mobile trophozoite (active) or double-walled cysts (inactive). Can also stain with Calcoflour white (not clinically practical, as fluorescent microscope is needed to see stain binding to cell wall; also positive for fungi). Culture cornea and CL case or lenses; may see tracks of the trophozoites on *Escherichia coli* nonnutrient agar. May need corneal biopsy at border of infiltrate and normal tissue.
- Treat with debridement, oral ketoconazole, polyhexamethylene biguanide (PHMB) 0.02% (made from swimming pool cleaner), acridene orange, 0.01% propamidine (Brolene; available in Europe), or Neosporin. Requires months of topical treatment, and often requires systemic treatment. May require palliative PK if infection is nearing the limbus or to debulk infectious burden; otherwise, wait 6 months after infection clears for PK.

ADENOVIRUS Predominantly follicular conjunctivitis with preauricular lymphadenopathy in 50% of cases. May have subconjunctival hemorrhage or membranes.

- Epidemic keratoconjunctivitis (EKC): serotypes 8, 11, and 19 (mnemonic: $8 + 11 = 19$); symptoms peak 5 to 7 days; mixed papillary and follicular conjunctivitis. Progresses from diffuse PEE, to diffuse PEK (day 3), to deep focal PEK (day 7), to subepithelial infiltrates (day 15), and finally to gray epithelial infiltrates (day 17). Give supportive care, and avoid steroids, as prolonged taper is often necessary to prevent the recurrence of subepithelial infiltrates. The developing world is especially prone to pandemics of acute follicular conjunctivitis—set up mass screening clinics utilizing "no touch" exam techniques and provide supportive care.
- Pharyngeal conjunctival fever (PCF): adenovirus serotypes 3, 4, 7 (mnemonic: $3 + 4 = 7$); EKC with fever and pharyngitis. Provide supportive treatment.

BACTERIAL KERATITIS Predisposed by trauma, preexisting corneal disease, eyelid abnormalities, steroids, CLW (extended CLW has 5× risk of daily CLW, which has 2× greater risk than rigid gas-permeable contact lens wear) mostly from poor lens case hygiene, anterior segment surgery (RK and AK have 0.25 to 0.70% incidence, photorefractive keratectomy 1.2%), and smoking. Most cases occur from staphylococcus, streptococcus, or *Pseudomonas* associated with CLW. May also be from:

- *Actinomyces*: filamentous bacteria, obligate, anaerobic, not acid-fast. Grows on vitamin K–dependent blood agar; may also cause canaliculitis. Sensitive to penicillin.
- Atypical mycobacterium: indolent "cracked windshield" infiltrate associated with trauma or foreign body. Grows on acid-fast stain and Lowenstein-Jensen medium. Treat with amikacin plus erythromycin.
- Interstitial crystalline keratopathy (ICK): colonization along corneal lamella from *Streptococcus viridans* with crystalline or feathery appearance; usually occurs in a corneal graft while patient is on steroids or after LASIK.
- *Moraxella*: gram-negative diplobacilli; dumbell shaped with flat ends. Grows on Löffler's medium or 5% CO_2 at 37°C blood agar; may cause opportunistic infection in alcoholic or debilitated patients.
- *Nocardia*: typically from trauma or foreign body; mimics fungal keratitis. Treat with Polytrim.
- Sterile infiltrates associated with CLW: small multiple infiltrates, usually peripheral, with intact epithelium, no cell in AC, minimum pain.

CHLAMYDIA Cause of trachoma (serotypes A–C; mnemonic: trA-Choma), adult inclusion conjunctiva (types D–K), and lymphogranuloma venerum (types L1–L3). Obligate intracellular organism that demonstrates intracytoplasmic inclusion bodies.

- Trachoma: a major cause of preventable blindness in the world from chronic conjunctival reinfections with upper lid scarring, entropion, secondary bacterial keratitis, and eventual corneal scarring. Endemic in the Middle East and spread by houseflies and fomites.
  - Diagnosis made by two of these: conjunctiva follicles on superior tarsus, limbal follicles, superior pannus, Herbert's pits (scarred remnants of involuted limbal follicles), Arlt's line (linear conjunctival scar across superior tarsus). Culture to confirm diagnosis (need to scrape and break cells open).
  - Staging: MacCallan staging describes course—immature follicles, mature follicles, conjunctival scarring, and inactive. World Health Organization (WHO) staging describes severity based on five signs—conjunctival follicles, diffuse conjunctival inflammation, tarsal conjunctival scarring, trichiasis, and corneal opacification.
  - Treat with erythromycin or tetracycline 500 mg tid for 3 weeks and topical. Large populations can prevent infection by washing hands and face at least once a day (do not even need soap).
- Adult inclusion conjunctivitis (AIC): sexually active direct or indirect contact with follicular conjunctivitis, superior micropannus, and no membranes, unlike neonatal chlamydia infection. Course waxes and wanes for 1 to 2 weeks after exposure. Diagnose with chlamydia immunofluorescence (take sample before applying fluorescein), culture, or Giemsa stain. Treat with macrolides (e.g., Zithromax 1 g single-dose or erythromycin) or tetracycline for 3 weeks. Considered a sexually transmitted disease; thus, rule out gonorrhea and syphilis, and recommend treatment for partner.

CONJUNCTIVITIS, BACTERIAL Constitutes only 5% of conjunctivitis cases; papillary reaction with purulent discharge, slow onset. Most cases resolve spontaneously; patients usually have other risk factors (immunocompromised, trauma, etc.).

CONJUNCTIVITIS, NEONATAL, OPHTHALMIA NEONATORUM Gram stain and culture to confirm organism.

- Chemical: onset within 24 hours of use of irritating agent, usually silver nitrate; few to no polymorphonuclear leukocytes (PMNs).
- Bacterial: usually *Streptococcus viridans*. Treat with topical antibiotics except *N. gonorrhoeae* (rare, but may have disseminated infection such as proctitis, rhinitis, or meningitis); also treat with IV antibiotics.
- Chlamydial: no follicles but may have membranes, unlike adult inclusion conjunctivitis. Intracytoplasmic inclusion bodies seen on Giemsa stain. Treat with erythromycin topical and PO for pneumonia usually 3 to 13 weeks later (not covered by silver nitrate).

- Herpetic: onset within 2 weeks after birth if infant was inoculated during delivery. Use IV acyclovir to treat concurrent pneumonitis, and use topical antiviral ointment or drops. No follicles are present, as infants are immunologically incompetent.

DEMODEX Normal commensal mites on hair follicles and in meibomian glands. Ubiquitous; causes itchy eyes, may see "sleeves" on lashes. Treat with lid scrubs, metronidazole topical gel.

FUNGAL KERATITIS Predisposed by trauma, foreign body (especially vegetable matter), immunocompromised, CLW. Indolent, severe pain when established; infiltrate characterized by rough textures, elevated borders, feathery margins, satellite lesions, descemetatrophic, endothelial migration. In northern United States, most likely *Candida* (mnemonic: near Canada); in southern United States, most likely *Fusarium*.

- Culture on Sabaroud's medium: 54% positive culture in 24 hours, 83% in 72 hours, 97% in 1 week (thus, hold culture at least a week even if there is negative initial growth).
- Treat based on initial potassium hydroxide (KOH) preparation or fungal stain, and modify depending on culture results:
  - Filamentous hyphae (often *Fusarium, aspergillus*): treat initially with topical natamycin and oral fluconazole. May also use itraconazole (suspend 100 mg tablet in 10 cc saline) or topical Betadine.
  - Yeast or pseudohyphae (often *Candida*): treat initially with amphotericin B 0.1% or natamycin plus fluconazole oral 400 mg load.

HERPES SIMPLEX VIRUS (HSV) The leading cause of corneal blindness; caused by DNA virus that after primary infection remains latent in the trigeminal ganglion (and maybe in cornea). Pathology shows intranuclear inclusion bodies (Lipschütz bodies or Cowdry type A).

- Primary infection presents as unilateral follicular blepharoconjunctivitis with membranes, vesicles, and preauricular lymphadenopathy. Two thirds of cases have PEK or dendrites; <10% develop stromal keratitis or uveitis. Ten percent are bilateral; consider work-up for immunosuppressed or atopic conditions if bilateral. Treat cornea prophylactically with drops even if infection is confined to the conjunctiva.
- Recurrent infection presents with dendritic keratitis, which are true ulcerations rather than epithelial swelling and elevation, as seen in HZV (active viral replication in epithelial cells produce sloughing and stain well with fluorescein, and epithelial cells neighboring the dendrite are full of virus and stain well with rose Bengal). May also have geographic ulcers, disciform stromal keratitis, necrotizing keratitis with destruction of Descemet's membrane (may have a foreign

body–like reaction to Descemet's), ring KP, iridocyclitis, iris atrophy with transillumination defects, and increased IOP (trabeculitis). "Backdoor" infection does not need primary ocular infection (latent reactiviation after primary V_2).

- HSV may be implicated in ICE, Posner-Schlossman syndrome, and Fuchs' HIC.
- Epithelial HSV: geographic defect or dendritic ulcer. Treat with Viroptic 9× per day (use limited by its epithelial toxicity), acyclovir 400 mg 5× per day; consider epithelial debridement. If the cornea becomes trophic (nonhealing), stop topicals, change to orals, lubricate, and consider BSCL.
- Stromal HSV: immune reaction to viral antigens, not active viral replication, with intact epithelium, stromal infiltrate, and edema; often see ring KP. Treat with steroids; consider prophylactic antivirals, PTK for corneal scarring (HSV may reactivate).
- Herpetic Eye Disease Study (HEDS): use acyclovir 400 mg (do not need Viroptic) bid for 1 year for those with recurrent stromal keratitis. Hold steroids until epithelial process resolved. Three arms of study found that:
    - Acyclovir is not proven for stromal keratitis (but is often used) and has a benefit for iritis.
    - Topical steroids increase resolution of stromal keratitis, decrease progressive and persistent keratouveitis by 68%, but no change seen in visual outcome at 6 months compared with controls.
    - Acyclovir for keratitis does not prevent subsequent stromal keratitis or iritis.

HERPES ZOSTER VIRUS (HZV), VARICELLA ZOSTER VIRUS (VZV) DNA poxvirus that causes chickenpox, shingles, and herpes zoster ophthalmicus. In all body dermatomes, affects 24% of adults, with pitting scars. Ocular involvement is possible with trigeminal nerve infection. Hutchinson's sign (vesicle at side of the tip of nose) indicates that nasociliary nerve is involved and ocular infection is likely. Unusual in young patients; thus, rule out malignancy or immunosuppression. Recurrent disease is common.

- Epithelial infection demonstrates raised dendrites that stain best with rose Bengal (swollen and heaped up in HZV versus sloughing in HSV), corneal hypoesthesia (more pronounced than in HSV with greater risk for neurotrophic cornea). Disciform keratitis is often bilateral. May have iritis with increased IOP from trabeculitis and prominent iris atrophy. May also cause acute retinal necrosis (ARN) and Ramsay Hunt syndrome (CN VII palsy). May present with ocular symptoms without skin rash.
- Treat with oral acyclovir (not topicals) 800 mg 5 times per day (higher dosage than for HSV) or Famvir 500 mg 3 times per day, or IV if

immunosuppressed. Disciform keratitis and iritis are treated with topical steroids. Prednisone decreases postherpetic neuralgia.

- Vaccination for HZV for those not previously exposed: single dose age 1 to 12 years old or two doses 4 to 8 weeks apart if over 12 years old; contraindicated in pregnancy, and no salicylates within 6 weeks (risk of Reye's syndrome).

HUMAN PAPILLOMA VIRUS HPV (types 16 and 19) causes papilloma. Treat with observation, cryotherapy, excision with minimal manipulation, intralesional alpha-interferon, or oral cimetidine. Sessile variant in adults, usually single, at the limbus.

INTERSTITIAL KERATITIS (IK) Stromal inflammation and vascularization with later ghost vessels and scarring.

- Leprosy (Hansen's disease): may cause neurotropic keratitis or peripheral IK. Treat with dapsone or thalidomide. Two types:
  - Lepromatous: organism grows at room temperature; thus, anterior eye (corneal scarring), tip of nose, and skin, more affected.
  - Tuberculoid: grows at higher temperature; thus, internal organs affected.
- Syphilis: interstitial keratitis from inflammatory response to treponemal antigen; patients typically present at age 7 to 17. Eighty percent are bilateral, and most cases are congenital infection or rarely acquired (60% of these are unilateral). Classic Hutchinson's triad if infected in utero: IK, notched incisors, and deafness. May also have anterior uveitis, glaucoma, saddle nose, saber shins, and rhagades (linear scars around the mouth). IK typically presents as a painful red eye as a child with corneal edema and vascular "salmon patch" for weeks to months (patient may give a history that he or she had to stay in a dark room for several weeks), which then resolves; usually see only ghost vessels thereafter. Whenever syphilis is diagnosed for the first time, it needs to be treated with penicillin IV for 10 days. Microhemagglutination—*Treponema pallidum* (MHA-TP) remains positive forever; rapid plasma reagin (RPR) is positive only with disease activity.
- Tuberculosis: unilateral, sectoral, peripheral IK

LOA LOA Mango fly (*Chrysops* genus) that has subcutaneous or subconjunctival migration.

MORAXELLA Classically causes angular blepharitis, but also conjunctivitis and keratitis. Slow-growing aerobic bacterium that grows best in blood agar, 5 to 10% CO_2 at 37°C.

NEISSERIA GONORRHOEAE Hyperacute onset of conjunctivitis or keratitis; can penetrate corneal epithelium. Treat with topical and PO antibiotics. Also treat for chlamydia.

ONCHOCERCIASIS A roundworm larva that causes river blindness. Ninety percent of cases are in Central or West Africa; however, it also can be found in Central and South America. Infections occur in 10- to 15-year cycles and are caused by *Onchocerca volvulus* carried by the *Simulium* black fly. The fly incubates in aerated, fast-moving water (most infections are in villages within 1 mile of a river); the worm larvae enter the host and travel to subcutaneous nodules (look like buboes). The nodules are mating male and female worms, and larvae are found mainly in the skin but also in the eye. If not taken up by the black fly in a blood meal, the larvae die in the host (straighten and stiffen) and cause sclerosing keratitis, optic neuritis, or choroiditis. To examine, have the patient keep his or her head down for 30 minutes to better see the larvae in the aqueous at the slit lamp. The disease is preventable with ivermectin every 6 months for 10 years, which is a dog heartworm pill that neuters female worms but does not kill the adults.

PARINAUD'S OCULOGLANDULAR SYNDROME Chronic follicular conjunctivitis (lymphoid follicles without germinal centers) with lymphadenopathy; often from *Bartonella henselae* (cat-scratch disease) or tuberculosis if from endemic area, plus many other causes.

PHTHIRUS PUBIS Crab louse that prefers lashes and pubic hair due to the spacing of cilia; transmitted by sexual contact. Treat by mechanical removal or with bland ointment or pilocarpine gel. Physostigmine ointment is effective as a respiratory poison against the louse but has ocular side effects.

PICORNAVIRUS Enterovirus 70, coxsackievirus; causes hemorrhagic conjunctivitis.

STAPHYLOCOCCUS SPECIES May cause conjunctivitis, keratitis, phlyctenulosis, and marginal corneal infiltrates (hypersensitivity to staphylococcal exotoxins released from staphylococcal blepharitis and meibomianitis with lucent area separating from limbus; use mild steroid drops).

Neoplastic Disease: Benign Masses

AMYLOID Unilateral, yellowish, flat eyelid or conjunctival lesion that hemorrhages when eye is rubbed (amorphous substance laid down like concrete; scratching ruptures the encased blood vessels); usually seen in young females.

COGAN'S PLAQUE Scleral pigment spot around Axenfeld's nerve loop (melanocytic cyst); benign.

CONJUNCTIVA LYMPHOID HYPERPLASIA Mixed T and B cell polyclonal (heavy and light chains) increase in lymphoid cells; spectrum with conjunctiva lymphoma and appears as fleshy pink mass

DERMATOLIPOMA Choristomas (tissue in an abnormal location)

- Lipodermoid, dermal lipoma: yellow-tan nodule composed of adipose tissue. Superotemporal conjunctiva location may extend deep into orbit; thus, excision with caution. If superotemporal, may be associated with Treacher Collins–Franceschetti.
- Solid limbal dermoid: keratin-filled nodule with pilosebaceous units and thick epithelium that looks like skin. Characterized by inferotemporal limbus with lipid in adjacent corneal stroma. May cause amblyopia and astigmatism. May be difficult to excise, as it involves Bowman's membrane and thus scars. Usually sporadic or associated with Goldenhar's syndrome.
- Episcleral osseous choristomas: superotemporal plaque of mature bone; may be complex with other tissue (adipose, cartilage, etc.).

EPIDERMAL INCLUSION CYST (EIC) Conjunctival lesion that often arises after trauma or surgery; usually excise.

BENIGN HEREDITARY INTRAEPITHELIAL DYSKERATOSIS (BHID) Bilateral bulbar leukoplakic lesions without dysplasia; characterized by parakeratosis, dyskeratosis, and hyperkeratosis. Seen in triracial families (Haliwa Indians) from Halifax County, North Carolina.

JUVENILE XANTHOGRANULOMA (JXG) Nonneoplastic histiocytic proliferation in infants that regresses by age 5; characterized by dermatologic vascular anomalies, granulomas, fleshy tan nodules, vascularized iris lesions that may cause heterochromia or spontaneous hyphema, and secondary glaucoma. Touton giant cells and lipid-filled histiocytes are seen on pathology. Treat hyphema with steroids and IOP control.

PYOGENIC GRANULOMA Exuberant growth of granulation tissue with chronic lymphocytic inflammation that arises in areas of trauma or chalazion. Not pyogenic and not a granuloma.

SARCOID GRANULOMA Usually millet-seed granulomas on the conjunctiva with giant cells (epithelioid histiocytes). Diagnosis is a clinical-pathological correlate (no special stains to prove sarcoid); thus, must rule out other granulomatous causes with tissue biopsy for Gram stain, acid-fast stain, silver stain for organisms, and foreign body. Lacrimal gland is most commonly involved ocular tissue, followed by conjunctiva.

SQUAMOUS PAPILLOMA Sessile or pedunculated fleshy growth with fibrovascular core that may be viral or nonviral in origin. Viral cases tend to be pedunculated, recur after incomplete excision, and regress spontaneously. May be multiple or recurrent in children or immunocompromised patients (e.g., HIV). Rare malignant potential. Careful when excising to avoid viral spread.

- Sessile: seen in older patients, usually HPV 16, 18; higher malignant potential.
- Pedunculated: seen in younger patients, most commonly HPV 8, 11.

Neoplastic: Malignant

BASAL CELL CARCINOMA (BCC) In conjunctiva found only on caruncle (only normal conjunctival site with pilosebaceous units).

CONJUNCTIVAL INTRAEPITHELIAL NEOPLASIA (CIN) Thickened epithelium replaced by dysplastic, atypical cells arising from basal layer. Typically limbal leukoplakic lesion in interpalpebral fissure with abrupt transition.

- Be suspicious of a lesion that turns from red to white, from flat to elevated, or from bulbar conjunctiva to limbus, and presence of a feeding blood vessel.
- Predisposing factors: HPV 16 or 18, older patient, smoker, actinic damage, and petroleum exposure.
- Pathology: faulty maturation and polarity, basilar unrest, shouldering, dysplasia, basement membrane intact. Mild if <50% thickness; severe if >50%. Called carcinoma in situ (CIS) if it is full thickness and the BM is intact, or squamous cell carcinoma (SCC) if it violates the BM. Mucoepidermoid variant has poor prognosis.
- Diagnose and treat with excisional biopsy with or without cryotherapy. Is a local disease (no metastatic potential, as no blood vessels are in the epithelium), but excise any lesion invading the limbus or cornea or that is leukoplakic.

CONJUNCTIVAL LYMPHOMA "Salmon patch" or "fish flesh" neoplastic growth that arises from resident conjunctiva lymphocytes (i.e., follicles from mucosa-associated lymphoid tissue: no large collections of lymphocytes in the orbit except in the lacrimal gland). Monocellular diffuse B cell monoclonal infiltrate with plasmacytoid (Dutcher) bodies without germinal centers. Biopsy for permanent sections and send fresh tissue for flow cytometry. Treat with radiation therapy.

- Most benign of all lymphomas; usually a local disease. Decreasing risk of systemic involvement (lid-orbit-conjunctiva [LOC]): 66% of eyelid lymphoma patients have systemic lymphoma, 33% if orbit is affected, and 20% if conjunctiva is involved.

CONJUNCTIVAL RHABDOMYOSARCOMA Embryonal variant (botryoid "grapelike" appearance).

KAPOSI'S SARCOMA Red lesion usually in HIV/AIDS patients with extravasated blood on pathology. Treatment usually is not necessary unless the lesion is causing a functional problem; can be excised or treated with chemotherapy or radiation therapy.

MULTIPLE ENDOCRINE NEOPLASIA IIB (Also known as MEN III, Sipple-Gorlin syndrome): characterized by enlarged corneal nerves, pheochromocytoma (check urine vanillylmandelic acid [VMA]), medullary thyroid carcinoma (check serum calcitonin), and mucosal neuromas.

ONCOCYTOMA, OXYPHILIC ADENOMA Benign, glandular tumor of caruncle (also found on nasal conjunctiva and lacrimal gland); pathology shows big pink cells with cytoplasm full of mitochondria.

SEBACEOUS CELL CA Pagetoid spread from eyelid into conjunctiva; identified with oil red O stain; best seen with fresh frozen tissue.

SQUAMOUS CELL CA (SCC) Most common malignancy of the conjunctiva, which presents as a leukoplakic lesion, locally invasive but rarely invades the orbit or globe (malignant epithelial ingrowth usually via lymphatics or surgical wound). Pathology: well differentiated, "pink and below" tumor that violates BM, cytokeratin+. Risks include age, alcohol use, CIN, AIDS, UVB (damages p53 tumor suppressor gene). Excise and consider cryotherapy, or if large, then biopsy, image; may need to exenterate.

- Spindle cell variant: aggressive, faster cell turnover (vertical nuclei).
- Mucoepidermoid variant: 4 to 6% of SCC; age >60. Very aggressive and invasive, with associated malignant goblet cells; suspect if recurrent after primary excision.

Neoplastic: Melanocytic Lesions

BENIGN, RACIAL, OR OCULAR MELANOSIS, COMPLEXION ASSOCIATED PIGMENTATION (CAP) Seen in darkly pigmented patients with increasing conjunctival pigmentation; bilateral, does not wax/wane; pigment in basal epithelial layer; no malignant potential.

CONJUNCTIVA COMPOUND NEVI Most common pigmented conjunctival lesion. Can rapidly increase in size and pigmentation, especially during puberty and pregnancy. Many are amelanotic (melanocytes are not obligated to produce melanin). Any variant can have cysts. Generally, excise all new nevi in patients over 20 years old.

- Junctional: along BM; may rarely have malignant transformation.
- Compound: junctional and stromal; have cystic inclusions in epithelium and are never malignant.
- Subepithelial: in stroma; no malignant potential.

MALIGNANT MELANOMA, CONJUNCTIVAL Arises from PAM (30%), nevus (40%), or de novo (30%) in mature adults and violates the BM. Thirty percent mortality overall, with metastases to regional lymph nodes or orbital extension. On pathology, does not have spindle A or B cells like uveal melanoma (which metastasizes preferentially to the liver and has 50% mortality). If multicentric, consider that this may be metastatic MM to the conjunctiva.

- Breslow thickness is prognostic: depth of invasion >0.8 mm has worst prognosis. Pedunculated lesion has better prognosis, amelanotic worst. HMB-45 marker is (+) in 50%; also may be S-100 (+) (as with neural crest cells).
- Excise lesion and cryotherapy; if recurrent (usually amelanotic), consider enucleation.

OCULAR MELANOCYTOSIS Typically affects Asian or African-American patients with focal melanocyte proliferation (blue nevus); half have ipsilateral skin pigmentation (Ota's nevus); increased uveal and orbital melanoma risk.

PRIMARY ACQUIRED MELANOSIS (PAM) Acquired unilateral conjunctival pigmentation in middle-aged Caucasian patients that waxes and wanes. Pathology demonstrates increased number of melanocytes confined to the basal epithelium. Different from nevi, which are larger, more diffuse, and approach the limbus. Do three incisional biopsies (one at the most elevated area, one at the transition area, and one at a random or limbal area). Melanoma is present in 32% of cases. Excise and cryotherapy entire area. Prognosis depends on whether cellular atypia is present on pathology:

- Thirty-three percent of cases are without atypia: 0% melanoma risk, just increased number of melanocytes.
- Sixty-seven percent of cases are with atypia: 46% melanoma risk, lower risk if pathology shows basilar hyperplasia. Is basically MM confined to basal layer.

Metabolic and Degenerative Disease

BAND KERATOPATHY Calcification of Bowman's layer, typically in sick eyes (leading cause is chronic uveitis or glaucoma) or from systemic chronic mercurial exposure, hypercalcemia or hyperphosphatemia (milk-alkali syndrome), kidney or liver disease. Has "Swiss cheese" appearance. Called "calcerous degeneration" if exaggerated band keratopathy. Check Ca+, phosphorus, and uric acid levels if no obvious cause. Treat symptoms with BSCL, ethylenediaminetetraacetic acid (EDTA) chelation (0.08–0.25 mol/L or a 1.5–3.0% solution), superficial keratectomy, or PTK.

COAT'S WHITE RING From foreign body breakdown.

CORNEAL ARCUS Rule out hyperlipdemia if <40 years old (arcus juvenilus); has lucid zone, starts inferiorly. If arcus is asymmetric, rule out contralateral carotid artery stenosis.

CORNEAL FARINATA Seen in older patients with "flour dust" flecks in deep stroma; not visually significant.

CROCODILE SHAGREEN Polygonal faint gray opacities with clear borders. If anterior, also known as mosaic degeneration; if posterior, is associated with central cloudy François' dystrophy.

FLOPPY EYELID SYNDROME Spontaneous upper lid eversion during sleep, often in obese patients. Associated with obstructive sleep apnea and decreased rapid eye movements (REM) sleep. Conjunctival inflammation is driven by hypoxia plus mechanical trauma and shows a fine velvety tarsal reaction. Treat with a nocturnal shield for 1 month, lid shortening procedure, or topical retinoic acid 0.01% to decrease lid keratinization.

HASSALL-HENLE BODIES Benign, age-related peripheral guttae, not a disease.

IRIDOCORNEAL ENDOTHELIAL (ICE) SYNDROME Acquired, nonfamilial, unilateral disease of epithelialized endothelium (hammered-metal appearance) that migrates across the posterior cornea, trabecular meshwork, and iris. Usually occurs in middle-aged females with a high incidence of glaucoma. May be related to PPMD, which is a bilateral inherited disorder of epithelialized endothelium; others have suggested a possible HSV etiology. Differential diagnosis: PPMD, Fuchs' endothelial dystrophy, Axenfeld-Rieger syndrome, aniridia, iridoschisis, iris nevus syndrome, iris melanoma, and NF. Treat edema with dehydration. If glaucoma is present, treat IOP; patients usually do well with trabeculectomy (if closed, may need to YAG laser trabeculectomy opening) but not argon laser trabeculoplasty (ALT). May need PK for corneal edema, but do not allow AC to become shallow, as iris sticks to endothelium. ICE syndrome is a spectrum of diseases (mnemonic: ICE):

- **I**ris nevus (Cogan-Reese syndrome): advanced ICE with pigmented iris nodules (not true nevi, but mamillations of iris pinched up in the membrane), iris atrophy, and pupillary distortion.

- Chandler's syndrome: 56% of patients have signs confined mainly to the cornea, with edema and less prominent iris findings. Presents with pupil abnormality, decreased VA, or pain (corneal edema). May have subclinical mild pleomorphism in fellow eye. Gonioscopy shows broad PAS and a cellular membrane.
- Essential iris atrophy: progression from Chandler's syndrome as the abnormal endothelium moves onto the iris, causing atrophy (stretch holes from membrane away from the PAS or ischemic melting holes in the area of the PAS), corectropia, and polycoria. More likely to have glaucoma at this stage.

KELOID More glistening and jellylike than a dermoid

LABRADOR OR SPHEROIDAL DEGENERATION, CLIMATIC DROPLET, OR RICE PADDY KERATOPATHY Solar elastosis with proteinaceous deposits in the superficial cornea; a pinguecula, or yellowish spot of proliferation, of the cornea, with pannus and band keratopathy. Usually bilateral, M > F.

LIMBAL VOGT'S GIRDLE Pinguecula of the cornea

LIPID KERATOPATHY Vascularized corneal scars (as from HSV) allow lipid to deposit. May attempt to close vessel with argon laser.

PINGUECULA Yellow, gray conjunctival thickening from UV damage. Pathology shows solar elastosis (fragmented and "cooked" subepithelial connective tissue), as seen in actinic keratosis. Verhoeff-von Gieson stain shows elastoid degeneration.

PTERYGIUM (from the Greek *pterygion*, "wing") A triangular fibrovascular growth onto the cornea, usually nasal, bilateral, and progressive. May cause astigmatism, irritation, and EOM restriction. Cannot pass a muscle hook underneath if at the limbus, unlike a pseudopterygium, which can occur after trauma. Pterygium and SCC incidence increase near equatorial climates and usually are interpalpebral (if not, think SCC).

- Etiology is the same as pinguecula. In addition, focal limbal stem cell deficiency is caused by the natural "hot spot" of UV light directed temporally across the cornea. This preferentially focuses light onto the nasal limbus, damaging the basal limbal cells that are otherwise protected from direct head-on light by the overlying epithelium. This allows secondary conjunctivalization, seen as a pterygium.
- Pathology shows elastoid degeneration (stains with elastin but does not digest with elastase). "Recurrent" pterygium is pyogenic tissue.
- Treatment: bare sclera excision has 30 to 70% recurrence; excision with primary closure (pedicle flap), 5 to 10% recurrence; with conjunctival autograft or with mitomycin, 5% recurrence.

SALZMANN'S NODULES Gray-white elevated lumps composed of hyaline on Bowman's layer, usually seen in older female patients. Most arise from sequelae to staphylococcal lid disease, old keratitis, or trauma. Treat with superficial keretectomy ("SuperK") by lifting with 0.12 forceps, and peel or scrape with Weck-Cel sponge or #15 blade or PTK.

VITAMIN A DEFICIENCY More severe ocular scarring if it coincides with measles infection. Causes decreased goblet cells, drying, and keratinization of conjunctiva (Bitot's spots) that are foamy from *Corynebacterium*, corneal scar, and central leukoma. Contributes to the cause of 70% of childhood blindness; also have nyctalopia.

DEGENERATIONS: ECTATIC CORNEAL DISORDERS

- Fuchs' marginal keratolysis: upside down Terrien's marginal degeneration (inferior location).
- Furrow degeneration: benign corneal thinning that is more apparent than real.
- Keratoconus: acquired, bilateral (often asymmetric), noninflammatory anterior ectasia. Onset after puberty, M:F = 2:1; slowly progressive for 5 to 10 years, then stable (later onset has a better prognosis). Familial pattern exists but no clear inheritance pattern; family members may have subclinical inferior steepening.
    - Many associated conditions: Down syndrome (eye rubbing is likely cause, as increased incidence of OD keratoconus with right-handed individuals and vice versa), atopy, RP, Leber's congenital amaurosis, osteogenesis imperfecta, Ehlers-Danlos syndrome, Marfan syndrome, Alport's syndrome, mitral valve prolapse, and keratosis palmaris and plantaris.
    - Ectasia causes irregular astigmatism and myopia. Clinical signs include outward lower lid bulge with downgaze (Munson's sign), shadow with tangential light illumination (Rizutti's sign), inferotemporal corneal thinning, deep vertical scars (Vogt's striae), epithelial iron ring around base of cone (Fleischer ring), and scissoring on retinoscopy. Acute edema or hydrops (break in Descemet's membrane) often resolves spontaneously after 4 to 6 weeks with scarring; degenerative pannus between Bowman's layer and epithelium may develop, and apical scarring may be nodular (easily removed with superficial keratectomy) or diffuse (needs PK).
    - Treat with spectacles, then RGP, for irregular astigmatism (fit to vault apex; may need to piggyback lenses); 90% of patients never need surgery. PK is more than 95% successful (may have persistent mydriasis after PK). Keratoconus is a contraindication to refractive surgery.

- Keratoglobus: rare nonhereditary globular rather than conical midperipheral thinning from defect in collagen synthesis. Present from birth; high myopia with K readings 55–60 D, and risk of spontaneous rupture, so prescribe safety lenses. PK is difficult.
- Pellucid marginal degeneration: noninflammatory, bilateral, peripheral thinning, usually inferior location. Usually seen in 20- to 40-year-old patients of European or Japanese descent, M = F. Causes irregular against-the-rule (ATR) astigmatism. Can be considered as keratoconus near the limbus, with a thinned inferior band 1–2 mm wide and corneal bulging superior to thinned area. May have hydrops, but no lipid or vascularization. Prescribe eye protection and RGP lenses, and consider annular lamellar keratectomy.
- Terrien's marginal degeneration: peripheral corneal thinning that begins superiorly (mnemonic: Terrien's on top, pellucid on bottom), then moves circumferentially, causing bilateral corneal steeping at 90 degrees (ATR astigmatism). Intact epithelium and usually noninflammatory quiet eye (unlike Mooren's ulcer). Usually patients are 20 to 30 years old, M > F. Typically static, with lipid deposition and fine vascular pannus, but may be inflammatory and progressive. Associated with pseudopterygium (can pass muscle hook under it, unlike a pterygium). May perforate with trauma. Treat with corneal allograft or compression sutures over thinned area (tighten to make with-the-rule astigmatism equal to amount of previous ATR astigmatism, and cut sutures over several months to regress to middle).

DEGENERATIONS: METABOLIC DEPOSITIONS

- Amyloidosis: eosinophilic hyaline material deposited in various tissues that represents chondroitin/sulfuric acid protein in a beta-pleated sheet that the body cannot degrade. At least 14 genes are involved in amyloidosis, with 3 identified types: AP if derived from alpha globulin, AL if composed of immunoglobulin, and AA for nonimmunoglobulin.
  - Characteristics (mnemonic: ABCDEF):
    - **A**utoflouresence
    - **B**irefringent: two polarizing filters block all light except that which is phase-shifted by amyloid.
    - **C**ongo-philia: stains with Congo red, and also metachromatically with crystal violet and thioflavin T.
    - **D**ichroism: changes from red to green with a filter and green light; all the tissue looks red except the Congo red–stained amyloid, which has parallel light rays and looks green.
    - **E**lectron microscopic bundles of microfilaments
    - **F**ilaments
  - Four clinical classifications:
    - Primary localized amyloidosis: most common type, characterized by conjunctival plaques. Most are nonfamilial but are

hereditary in lattice dystrophy types I and III, Avellino, granular, and gelatinous droplike dystrophies.
- Primary systemic: ophthalmoplegia (orbital and muscle infiltration), ptosis, vitreous veils, dry eye, pupil abnormalities
- Secondary localized: nonfamilial skin, conjunctival and corneal deposition secondary to many inflammatory or traumatic conditions
- Secondary systemic: rare

- Cystinosis: inability of lysosomes to excrete cystine; severity ranges from benign to nephrotic. Nephrotic cases have renal failure, rickets, salt and pepper fundus, and corneal crystals in anterior stroma, causing glare and photophobia.
  - Infantile: most severe form; autosomal recessive. Characterized by dwarfism, rickets, and renal failure. Most patients die in first decade without renal transplant.
  - Adolescent: less severe; autosomal recessive. Most patients die in second decade.
  - Adult: asymptomatic; normal life expectancy.
- Fabry's disease: X-linked glycolipidosis with corneal verticillata, tortuous conjunctival and retinal vessels, posterior spokelike cataract associated with vascular anomalies of the heart, kidney, and brain, and burning in the hands and feet.
- Hemosiderosis bulbi: iron deposited in epithelial cells; usually from hyphema with hemoglobin release or iron foreign body.
- Miscellaneous deposits:
  - Adrenochrome: epinephrine-containing medications
  - Alkali powder: airbag injury
  - Argyrosis: silver; usually silver nitrate used as infant
- Mucopolysaccharidoses (MPSs): corneal clouding, especially with Hurler's (MPS-1, mental retardation, skeletal defects), Scheie's, Morquio's, and Maroteaux-Lamy syndromes.
- Wilson's disease, hepatolenticular degeneration: copper deposited in the posterior lamella of Descemet's membrane, seen as the Kayser-Fleischer ring. Defect causes decreased production of ceruloplasmin in liver, with increased serum copper. Kayser-Fleischer ring is also seen in primary biliary cirrhosis, chronic hepatitis, and progressive intrahepatic cholestasis of childhood. Treat Wilson's disease with penicillamine, and ring will disappear; slit lamp exam can be used to monitor therapy.

Physical Disease

ANESTHETIC ABUSE Topical anesthetics are toxic to corneal epithelium and may cause nonhealing epithelial defect, stromal infiltrate, hypopyon, and perforation. Also known as "crack cornea" with drug use. Test corneal sensation in patients suspected of abusing anesthetics.

BIRTH TRAUMA Forceps delivery, especially with left occiput anterior presentantion, may cause vertical or oblique Descemet's tears and resulting corneal edema that progress over the first few days, clearing over weeks to months. Watch for amblyopia, astigmatism, or late endothelial decompensation.

CHEMICAL BURN Acid denatures and precipitates proteins, which serve as a barrier to further damage, whereas alkali damages cells through membrane saponification and thus rapidly penetrates stroma.

- Grade 1: corneal epithelial damage with no limbal ischemia. Grade 2: hazy cornea with less than one third limbal ischemia. Grade 3: total epithelial defect and stromal haze that blurs iris details, with one third to one half limbal ischemia. Grade 4: opaque cornea with greater than one half limbal ischemia.
- Treat with immediate copious irrigation with pH testing to neutralize chemical, sweep fornix, debride necrotic conjunctiva and particulate matter, and BSCL. Topical steroids may be beneficial in the acute phase; also consider topical medroxyprogesterone 1%, ascorbate citrate, metalloproteinase inhibitors, limbal autograft, or keratoprosthesis.
- Total epithelial defect: exacerbated by steroids, poor innervation (neurotrophic), dry eye (epithelium will not grow without tears), stem cell injury, diabetes, and dead keratinocytes from chemical burn (epithelium will not grow on dead bed). Treat with lubrication, tears, limbal stem cell transplant, or amniotic membrane; may consider tarsorrhaphy to create environment for epithelial growth.
- Neurotrophic cornea: innervation has a primary effect on epithelial cell health, secondary on lacrimation and blinking reflexes (CN VII). Watch for spontaneous blink (cornea gets O_2 from tears when open and lids when closed).

CONTACT LENS–INDUCED CORNEAL EPITHELIAL HYPOXIA, TIGHT LENS SYNDROME, SATTLER'S VEIL Epithelial edema from tight-fitting contact lens; usually reversible with CLW holiday.

ERYTHEMA NODOSUM, TARANTULA KERATOPATHY Fine hairs launched by spiders and some caterpillars, causing a local conjunctival granuloma or corneal inflammation.

EXPOSURE KERATOPATHY Punctate epithelial erosions in interpalpebral zone, as seen with lagophthalmos (Bell's palsy, proptosis, incomplete closure of lids, ectropion). Treat with lubrication and taping, and ensure adequate Bell's phenomenon; consider tarsorrhaphy.

HYPHEMA Blood in AC, measured in millimeters or percentage; may be total (100%) or black color, indicating deoxygenation ("black ball" hyphema). Check for sickle cell trait in patients of African-American, Hispanic, or Mediterranean ancestry. Patients are often somnolent; check VA and DFE early in case the bleeding worsens, and avoid gonioscopy and scleral depression for 2 weeks. Majority of cases are traumatic, M:F = 3:1; 60% of injuries are sports related. Patients are usually <20 years old and bleed from the major arterial circle at the root of the iris. May also be spontaneous from JXG, NVI, intraocular tumor, or sickle cell disease.

- Rebleed: 8% of cases from lysis and retraction of fibrin plug that sealed the vessel. Usually occurs within 5 days and is often worse than the initial bleed, with increased risk of secondary glaucoma and corneal bloodstaining. Risks for rebleed include recent aspirin or NSAID use, hypotony, young age, and African-American or Hispanic patients.
- Secondary glaucoma: early glaucoma may be from TM obstruction by red blood cells, pupillary block by large clot, hemolytic glaucoma, or steroid-induced. Late glaucoma causes include angle recession, ghost cell (degenerated RBCs in vitreous migrate to AC and obstruct the TM), PAS, or posterior synechia, causing iris bombe.
- Bloodstaining: 5% of hyphemas; very subtle early but takes months to clear. Watch for amblyopia in children; otherwise, wait and will clear from the periphery. Pathology shows RBC breakdown products in the cornea: hemoglobin particles, sphericles, yellow deposits in posterior stroma, or hemosiderin granules in keratocytes. May occur quickly with high IOP.
- Sickle cell disease: hyphema increases AC hypoxia, hypercarbia, acidosis, and a hyperosmolar state, all of which exacerbate sickling. The deformed RBCs obstruct the TM easier, increase IOP, increase clearance time, may cause CRAO at relatively low IOP, and make the ON and retina more susecptible to ischemia. Sickle cell patients may have spontaneous hyphema.
  - Avoid carbonic anhydrase inhibitors: cause increased aqueous ascorbic acid, leading to decreased pH and metabolic acidosis, thus increasing AC sickling.
  - Avoid epinephrine, alpha agonists and phenylephrine: cause vasoconstriction and further AC deoxygenation.
  - Avoid hyperosmotics: cause hemoconcentration and vascular sludging. Sickle cell patients may have spontaneous hyphema.
- Treatment: prevent rebleed, monitor and treat elevated IOP, stop aspirin and NSAID use, decrease activity, provide eye shield, increase angle of head of bed, and prescribe a cycloplegic and topical steroids.
  - Aminocaproic acid (Amicar 50 mg/kg every 4 hours up to 30 g/day): stimulates plasminogen formation of plasmin, which stabilizes the clot to prevent rebleed. Hospitalize patient; contraindicated in clotting disorder, hepatic disease, and pregnancy.

Watch IOP after stopping Amicar because of increased risk of clot lysis. A 30% gel will also be available.
- Surgery: for large hyphema present >10 days, total hyphema >5 days, blood staining, increased IOP refractory to treatment or treating ON or retinal perfusion, or IOP >50 mmHg for 5 days, or >35 for 7 days or a patient with sickle cell disease and IOP >25 mmHg. Use paracentesis with AC washout with peripheral iridectomy, and preserve conjunctiva in case future trabeculectomy is needed. Be careful when removing clot (debulk but do not completely remove), as it may interdigitate with the iris and attempting to completely remove it may remove entire iris.

LACERATION OR FOREIGN BODY Penetrating injury passes into a structure, perforating injuries pass through a structure.

- Close limbus first with 9.0 nylon, then cornea with 10.0 nylon (take shorter bites near center of cornea); close sclera with 8.0 nylon.
- Fibrous downgrowth: break in Descemet's membrane, allowing stromal ingrowth into globe.
- Splendore-Hoeppil reaction: Ag-Ab complexes around foreign body

OPERATIVE INJURY

- Brown-McLean syndrome: peripheral corneal edema and iridocorneal touch, with clear central cornea secondary to flat chamber and endothelial cell loss after intracapsular cataract extraction (ICCE).
- Pseudophakic bullous keratopathy: endothelial loss after intraocular surgery, especially cataract surgery, with prolonged phacoemulsification time. No guttae, but patients have edema.

THERMAL OR UV KERATOPATHY Epithelium sheds several hours after exposure; treat like a corneal abrasion.

Inflammatory and Immune Disease

ATOPIC KERATOCONJUNCTIVITIS (AKC) Types I and IV hypersensitivity reactions, which are the most severe forms of ocular allergy. Older patients are most often affected; patients have systemic atopy characterized by asthma, rhinitis, eczema (especially of flexor skin surfaces), and susceptibility to skin infections such as staphylococcus, impetigo, and disseminated skin HSV. AKC is not seasonal.

- Looks like vernal keratoconjunctivitis (VKC) with thickened lid margin, Dennie-Morgan line (infraorbital skin fold) from inferior lid edema, conjunctival subepithelial fibrosis in 58% of cases, symblepharon in 27% (mimics OCP), Horner-Trantas dots, PEK, PUK, SPK, corneal scarring and vascularization, keratoconus, and stromal melts (possible perforation). Twenty-five percent of patients have anterior subcapsular cataract (lens is surface ectoderm and is thus affected in many skin disorders). Thirty percent of patients are 20/200 or worse, mostly secondary to suboptimal treatment. Eosinophils cause the most damage (produce cation protein).

- Hyper IgE syndrome: poor PMN chemotaxis with recurrent skin, respiratory infections, atopic dermatitis and AKC; may benefit from plasmapharesis.
- Treat as VKC. Patients may need antibiotics or antivirals; systemic antihistamines are better than topicals (e.g., Claritin or Zyrtec 10 mg every day). Treat nose (e.g., Nasalcrom or Vancenase), allergen elimination; may need immunotherapy (e.g., cyclosporin) or weak steroid (e.g., Pred Mild, Vexol, Lotemax). Prescribe long-term suppression with antivirals if history of HSV.

CHALAZION Granulomatous inflammation around extravasated lipid in eyelid. Pathology shows Langhans' giant cells. Treat with warm compresses or excision, or rarely may use intralesional steroid (may cause skin atrophy or depigmentation).

COGAN'S SYNDROME Nonsyphilitic IK with hearing loss and vertigo; associated with polyarteritis nodosa (PAN).

DISCIFORM KERATITIS Immune reaction to HSV, HZV, varicella, mumps, and other infections, with corneal stromal edema, underlying KP, and mild iridocyclitis. Treat with steroids.

EPISCLERITIS Painful red eye with dilated superficial radial vessels; benign and often bilateral but nonsimultaneous. May have freely movable nontender nodule, and vessels blanch with phenylephrine. Seventy percent of cases are idiopathic; also collagen disease (13%), HSV, atopy, gout, rosacea, and syphilis. Check CBC, chem 7, urinanalysis, antineutrophil cytoplasmic antibodies (ANCA), RPR, and MHA-TP. Treat with benign neglect and no steroids (increased duration and recurrences). May use oral NSAIDs for cosmesis and artificial tears.

GIANT PAPILLARY CONJUNCTIVITIS (GPC) Types I and IV hypersensitivity to allergens on contact lens surface (95%) or other foreign body (ocular prosthesis, etc.). Symptoms: itching, foreign body sensation (FBS), tearing, redness, and discharge with upper tarsal papillae easily seen after fluorescein.

- Stage 1: subtle micropapillae. Stage 2: obvious papillae. Stage 3: large papillae. Stage 4: looks like VKC.
- Stopping CLW provides the cure (especially encourage if large number or size of papillae or apical epithelial defects on papillae). May

continue lenses with frequent enzymatic cleaning and sterilization. Eliminate preservatives, replace lenses, or use mast cell stabilizer (e.g., Patanol).

GRAFT VERSUS HOST DISEASE (GVHD) Chronic conjunctivitis and KCS from T cell infiltrate; may have lenticular opacity, retinal microangiopathy, and mucosal or skin lesions. Considered acute if <100 days from bone marrow transplant, or late onset if GVHD occurs >100 days. Needs systemic immunosuppression by oncologist.

KAWASAKI DISEASE Childhood systemic vasculitis of unknown etiology affecting skin, mucous membranes, and heart. May cause red eye with perilimbal blanching. Get echography to rule out coronary artery aneurysm, and treat with IV Ig and aspirin but not steroids (increased risk of coronary aneurysm rupture).

MOOREN'S ULCER Progressive thinning of peripheral cornea of unknown etiology with conjunctival injection, ulceration of peripheral cornea, undermined leading edge, severe pain, and photophobia. Autoimmune disease with Ig, complement and plasma cells found in adjacent conjunctiva. Treat with steroids, immunosuppressive agents, or lamellar keratectomy (LK).

- Older adults: unilateral, mild, more responsive to therapy with steroids; perforation is rare.
- Young, black males, usually patients of African descent: bilateral, rapidly progressive, poor response; associated with hepatitis C infection.

OCULAR CICATRICIAL PEMPHIGOID (OCP) Systemic autoimmune disease that is a type II hypersensitivity autoimmune reaction (IgG against the BM) in all mucous membranes. Causes cicatricial chronic conjunctivitis and severe dry eye with symblepharon formation that obliterates the tear meniscus, interferes with normal blink, and infiltrates the lacrimal gland, causing sicca, all of which lead to decreased corneal clarity. Affected tissues: mouth (90%), eye (70%, unlike bullous pemphigoid), skin (25%), larynx (20%; ask about difficulty breathing or swallowing), and genitalia (20%). Rare, 1:12,000, but underreported; F:M 3:1, average age 65; all races and geographic areas affected. Predisposition with presence of HLA-DR4, DQW3, and DQW7 has 10× risk.

- Long differential diagnosis of chronic conjunctivitis with subepithelial fibrosis: many glaucoma drops (especially miotics and epinephrine), topical antivirals, practolol, radiation, chemical burn, rosacea, SJS, postsurgical, CIN, or SCC. In young patients also consider linear IgA deposition. Contrast with pemphigoid, which has subepithelial blisters and thus scars unlike pemphigus, which has intraepithelial blisters and does not scar.

- Ocular manifestations: chronic cicatrizing conjunctivitis, trichiasis, entropion, keratinization, and MGD. Late occurrences have sicca, epitheliopathy, corneal ulcers, and scarring.
  - Stage 1: subepithelial fibrotic striae
  - Stage 2: fornix foreshortening
  - Stage 3: symblepharon
  - Stage 4: ankyloblepharon, profound sicca
- Etiology: immunoreaction to alpha-6/beta-4 integrin protein in the epithelial BM. OCP antigen molecule is an integrin hemidesmosome protein that helps bind the basal epithelium cell membrane to the lamina lucida of the BM. Antibody against this integrin protein binds and causes local cytokine production and fibroblast recruitment, producing type III collagen, leading to fibrosis. Tissue also demonstrates increased numbers of T cells, plasma cells, and lymphocytes. The T cells are dysregulated (increased CD4 versus the more normal increased CD8), interleukin-2R is upregulated, and lymphocytes are activated and express CD25 molecule (interleukin-2 receptor); if they have a prolonged state of immune activation, then serum levels of CD25 are increased.
- Diagnose with immunopathology from conjunctival biopsy (may increase inflammation), and submit in Michael's medium. Technique: inflate bulbar conjunctiva with lidocaine with epinephrine; cut long strip of conjunctiva with Vannas scissors; use steroid/antibiotic ointment postoperatively.
- Treat with chemotherapy (not topicals). If mild, start with Dapsone 25 mg bid (if G6PD is normal), and escalate to 150 mg per day as needed (monitor liver function, blood counts, and metahemoglobin). If needed, add Cytoxan next.
  - If severe start with Cytoxan and prednisone, which is tapered off within 3 months; add Dapsone if needed. Cyclophosphamide is most effective, but as alkylating agent it has many adverse drug reactions. Cytosine araboside and IV Ig are expensive and should be used last. Comanage with chemotherapist.
  - Treat lashes with epilation and lids with mucous membrane grafting if keratinized. May treat symblepharon with subconjunctival mitomycin C (MMC).

PHLYCTENULOSIS Type IV hypersensitivity to staphylococcus (primary cause) but historically seen as a reaction to tuberculosis and many other infectious diseases, including chlamydia, candidiasis, parasites, HSV, coccidioidomycosis, and rosacea.

ROSACEA Facial skin disorder of thickened sebaceous gland secretions characterized by facial telangiectasias, rhinophyma, MGD, recurrent chalazia, chronic conjunctivitis, marginal corneal infiltrates, sterile ulcers, episcleritis, iridocyclitis, and corneal neovascularization with triangular scarring. Seen in patients age 30 to 50 years old and associated with alcohol use. Treat with tetracyclines or topical metronidazole. Treat sterile ulcers or marginal infiltrates with topical steroids.

SEASONAL ALLERGIC CONJUNCTIVITIS (SAC), HAY FEVER CONJUNCTIVITIS Type I hypersensitivity with IgE to airborne allergens. Presents at any age, but usually seen in adults; if not seasonal, think of AKC (has eczema). Characterized by prominent itch with underwhelming signs including chemosis, hyperemia, allergic shiner or salute. If there is any confusion about the diagnosis, consider biopsy (pathology shows mast cells in the basal layer of epithelium; thus, scraping alone is not helpful).

- Treat with a topical antihistamine (e.g., Livostin) and, if needed, a mast cell stabilizer (e.g., Alomide) prophylactically to prevent degranulation. Combination drops are often a good choice (e.g., Patanol). Systemic antihistamines often work better than topicals (e.g., Zyrtec, Allegra).
- Do not give steroids or NSAIDs, as they only affect cyclooxygenase pathway (prostaglandin synthesis). Vasoconstrictors may be used to decrease injection and are not addictive. Most important is allergen avoidance; thus, consider allergist referral for testing, counseling, and possible desensitization.

SCLERITIS Painful, tender, red or violaceous eye with deep and nonblanching injection that is bilateral in 50% of cases. Marker for progression of collagen-vascular disease from a type III immune reaction with diffuse soluble antigen and IgM–IgM complexes in vasculature. At the posterior pole, the sclera is 1 mm thick (melts because too few fibroblasts are available to heal the inflammatory damage). Okay to biopsy sclera if diagnosis is unsure.

- Types of presentation: 98% anterior, 2% posterior
  - Diffuse anterior scleritis: painful, most benign
  - Nodular anterior scleritis: tender, immobile nodule formation
  - Necrotizing scleritis with inflammation: scleral thinning with uveal show; always associated with systemic disease (RA, PAN, Wegener's granulomatosis). Sixty percent of cases are associated with PUK, uveitis, and cataract, and 40% of patients have vision loss. Ominous diagnosis with poor life prognosis.
  - Necrotizing scleritis without inflammation: scleromalacia perforans associated with RA.
  - Posterior scleritis: may present in isolation or with anterior scleritis. Characterized by deep boring pain, especially with eye movement, and no lacrimation; associated with decreased VA from hyperopic shift, uveitis, choroiditis, retinal folds, effusion, striae,

exudative RD, angle closure glaucoma, myositis, pseudotumor, proptosis, and diplopia. Age >40 years old, M > F; unilateral, recurrent. Forty-six percent of patients have systemic disease, 30% have RA. On ultrasound may see "T" sign from Tenon's fluid and thickened sclera.

- Etiology: collagen vascular disease present in 90% of patients (often RA, Wegener's granulomatosis, polychondritis, PAN, SLE, ankylosing spondylitis, Crohn's diseasae) and infections in 7% (usually tuberculosis, syphilis, HSV, HZV, fungal infection, leprosy); also metabolic diseases (gout).
  - Wegener's granulomatosis: necrotizing granulomatous vasculitis of the upper and lower respiratory tract that involves both arteries and veins, with marked eosinophilia and giant cells. Characterized by respiratory tissue vasculitis with crescentic glomerulonephritis; 60% of patients have ocular involvement (25% of cases precede the systemic disease). Antineutrophil cytoplasmic Ab (C-ANCA) is positive in 70%. Repeat systemic evaluation if high suspicion.
  - Relapsing polychondritis: scleritis associated with cartilage destruction, such as tracheal collapse, heart valve destruction, saddle nose, and ear cartilage collapse, and kidney lesions. Scleritis is marker for disease progression and mandates change in treatment.
  - Polyarteritis nodosa: classically ANCA (–) unless microscopic PAN, then P-ANCA (+). Eighty-eight percent mortality within 5 years if not treated with oral steroids or cyclophosphamide, then 80% survival.
  - Fungal scleritis: often a farm injury with vegetable matter. Treat with topical fluconazole or amphotericin B; very difficult to eradicate.
- Work-up with chart biopsy, uveitis questionnaire, CBC (lymphopenia in SLE), urinanalysis (hematuria or casts in Wegener's granulomatosis or SLE), C-ANCA (check in every patient with scleritis or PUK; positive in 70% of Wegener's granulomatosis), P-ANCA (positive with microscopic PAN and Churg-Strauss syndrome), ESR/C-reactive protein/C25 (nonspecific inflammation and immune system activation), ANA, RF, FTA-Abs, angiotensin-converting enzyme level (ACE), hepatitis B surface antigen (positive in 40% of PAN), circulating immune complexes, purified protein derivative (tuberculin), chest x-ray, and sinus CT (to rule out Wegener's granulomatosis).
- Treat with NSAID if no systemic disease or prednisone 1 mg/kg/day, then a slow taper to 10–20 mg every other day, then decrease to every 2 weeks. Avoid depot steroids, although use is occasionally judicious and does not actually increase scleral melting.
  - If scleritis is progressive or unresponsive, begin immunosuppressive chemotherapy (always indicated for RA, Wegener's

granulomatosis, PAN, relapsing polychondritis, and SLE) such as methotrexate 7.5–25 mg/week, cyclosporine 2–5 mg/kg/day, Imuran 3 mg/kg/day, cyclophosphamide, or Cellcept.
- There is a 54% mortality rate with RA-associated necrotizing sclertitis if not immunosuppressed.

STEVENS-JOHNSON SYNDROME (SJS), ERYTHEMA MULTIFORME Systemic immune complex vasculitis from reaction to medications (especially penicillin), neoplasia, or infection (HSV, mycoplasma, etc.). Presents with target-lesion rash, bullae, mucous membrane erosions and scarring, fever, and malaise. Ocular involvement typically presents as conjunctival bullae, ulerations, scarring, and cicatricial conjunctivitis. Usually young adults, M > F; increased incidence in winter. Supportive treatment, consider high-dose steroids; mortality 5 to 20%. May need ocular lubrication, fornix sweeping, mucous membrane grafting for keratinization, 577 nm laser photocoagulation for corneal neovascularization, or gas-permeable custom scleral lens to create tear meniscus.

SUPERIOR LIMBAL KERATOCONJUNCTIVITIS (SLK) Chronic, recurrent, bilateral superior bulbar conjunctiva injection with superior limbal pannus that stains with rose Bengal. Characterized by burning sensation, FBS, and photophobia. Typically affects older women and is associated with dysthyroidism. Treat with silver nitrate solution (not silver nitrate sticks, which destroy cornea) or conjunctival excision after ruling out superior palpebral conjunctival foreign body.

SYSTEMIC LUPUS ERYTHEMATOSUS (SLE) Associated with subepithelial nummular opacities. Photosensitivity is caused by photosensitive vascular products or porphyrins, which affect nitrous oxide (NO) synthesis; the increased NO causes vasodilation.

THYGESON'S SUPERFICIAL PUNCTATE KERATITIS Bilateral (96%) recurrent punctate keratitis with otherwise quiet eye of unknown etiology. Characterized by tearing, FBS, photophobia, decreased VA with anterior corneal opacities, and clumps of granular material. Typically affects middle aged patients, F > M. Treat with lubrication, steroids (may increase recurrence), BSCL, topical cyclosporine, and no antivirals.

TOXIC EPIDERMAL NECROLYSIS (TEN) SJS-like mucous membrane scarring with cicatricial KC. Observe for neurotrophic cornea if patient is not complaining of pain.

VERNAL KERATOCONJUNCTIVITIS (VKC) Types I and IV hypersensitivity disease of children (usually ages 5 to 10). Occurs mainly in warm climates, during spring season, M > F; recurs over 4 to 10 years, and patient usually has a history of atopy. An odd disease that is potentially blinding.

- Presents with large tarsal papillae (consider GPC if CLW), PEE, itching, ropy discharge (contains mucin, proteins, and DNA from damaged corneal epithelial cells), superficial keratitis, or shallow gray superior shield ulcer. Patients also often have ptosis from giant papillae (lid edema and cytokines stimulating fibroblasts that increase the collagen and bulk of lids), and mucus-fishing syndrome. Cellular infiltrate is much more complicated than SAC, with a predominance of eosinophils that cause the most destruction.
- Two main types:
  - Palpebral vernal: lid signs predominant, with upper lid giant papillae (>1 mm) that look like cobblestones, and subepithelial fibrosis.
  - Limbal vernal: limbal signs predominant, with papillae and Horner-Trantas dots (infiltrated and degenerated eosinophils; also see in atopic KC and GPC). Mainly affects African-American and Asian patients.
- Treatment: allergen avoidance, mast cell stabilizer (e.g., cromolyn, Alomide, Patanol). Cool climate, cool compresses, and brief steroids may be necessary. Consider hospitalization if severe to remove patient from the allergic environment and to control medicamentosa and expedite allergy consult. In refractory cases, consider 2% cyclosporine or superior tarsal excision with graft.

Surgery

AMNIOTIC MEMBRANE GRAFT Used for persistent epithelial defect or to cover surgical defect. Is like conjunctiva, has a stromal side (sticky) and basement membrane side (smooth). Usually place basement membrane side up to fill a tissue defect, but can use either side up if using membrane as a biological "contact lens." May also use human processed pericardium (irradiated) that becomes rapidly reepithelialized.

CONJUNCTIVAL BIOPSY Place in glutaraldehyde for electron microscopy (EM), formalin for histopathology, saline for immunostains, and fresh tissue for polymerase chain reaction (PCR).

CONJUNCTIVAL FLAP Used for chronic ulcers, closed but unstable wounds, pain from bullous keratopathy, and phthisical eye in preparation for shell. Remove all corneal epithelium (very important), and remove Tenon's capsule from the conjunctival flap before placing graft. Flaps may be complete (Gunderson), incomplete, bipedicle, or advancement. Can also use amniotic membrane.

CONJUNCTIVAL SURGERY Close with a "primary vascular closure," pulling conjunctiva with substantia propria and Tenon's capsule that provide vascular supply. Make conjunctival incisions radially if possible to avoid severing vessels.

CORNEAL BIOPSY Punch biopsy at border of pathology and normal tissue. Use 1–2 mm dermatology punch and partial thickness trephination; remove block with spatula and send for culture and pathology.

CORNEAL PERFORATION, DESMETOCELE REPAIR May use BSCL, glue, LK, PK, or patch graft (e.g., Tutoplast). Causes include infection, corneal thinning, and trauma. Cyanoacrylate adhesive is not approved by the U.S. Food and Drug Administration (FDA) for eye use: place an air bubble or viscoelastic in the AC to push the iris back, then use thinnest drop of glue (in an emergency, can use commercial super-glue, which has one more carbon than Histocryl). Less is better when working with iris (cutting, suturing, etc.) and when applying corneal glue. Perforation >1 mm needs graft, not glue.

KERATOPROSTHESIS Complications include sterile vitritis, glaucoma, extrusion, and retroprosthetic membrane.

LAMELLAR KERATOPLASTY Partial thickness PK; excise corneoscleral rim of donor. Usually have at least two or three lines of vision loss due to stroma-stroma interface.

LIMBAL STEM CELL TRANSPLANT Peripheral corneal tissue graft that may be autologous (best) or allograft from family or cadaver (fresh, healthy donor globes without inflammatory disease or dry eye). Can store allograft in cell culture medium and use systemic or topical cyclosporin. Transplant to supply limbal stem cells for severe ocular surface disease (e.g., chemical or thermal burns, BHID, aniridia). Cells found in pallisades of Vogt. May need to use autologous serum for tear replacement.

PENETRATING KERATOPLASTY (PK) 40,000 cases per year seen in the United States alone, decreasing as incidence of PBK has decreased. Indications: PBK (26%), regraft (18%), Fuchs' endothelial dystrophy (16%), keratoconus (13%), aphakic bullous keratopathy (8%), and others. In children, primary indication is Peters' anomaly. Overall 90% graft survival, 20 to 25% lifetime chance of endothelial graft rejection. Percentage of grafts clear at 1 year: PBK (91%), keratoconus (90 to 98%), Fuchs' endothelial dystrophy (85%), and herpetic corneal scarring (86% if inactive, 67% if active disease).

- Poor candidates: inflamed eyes, connective tissue disorder, traumatic or hereditary epithelial surface disorder, poorly controlled blepharitis or KCS, and patients with unrealistic expectations. Poor prognosis: ocular surface disease, deep neovascularization (NV), poorly controlled glaucoma or intraocular inflammation, and peripheral corneal thinning.

- Donor tissue: excluded if unknown cause of death, unknown CNS disease, or known CNS infection, HIV, and hepatitis. Donor age 1 to 70 years old (graft age <6 is more flaccid and difficult, and newborn corneas will continue to grow until age 2). Ensure <12-hour death-to-preservation time. Store in Optosol (colorimetric pH indicators change color if microbial infection) up to 2 weeks but prefer to use within 5 days. Older solutions include McCarey, Dexsol, and corneal storage medium. Collaborative corneal transplantation studies (CCTS) showed that blood typing (A, B, and O) may be helpful but that HLA matching is not beneficial. Ensure endothelial cell count >2000 on specular microscopy, and coefficient of variation <0.3 (more uniform cells), pleomorphism <50%, and no polymegatheism.
- Preoperative: ensure adequate social situation, ability for postoperative care, and rule out ocular surface disease, lid malposition, trichiasis, inflammation, and glaucoma. Surgical goals are to correct corneal contour, treat thinning or perforation, relieve pain, and remove infection or scar.
- Technique: basically trephine donor, then host, then suture. First reduce positive vitreous pressure (preoperative ballottement, intraoperative vitreous aspiration, or dehydration with mannitol; remove pressure from speculum, fingers, etc., or hyperventilate if using general anesthesia). Flieringa ring may be needed for scleral support, especially for pediatric patients. Trephination may be manual (especially for corneal perforation cases), motorized, or vacuum system. Oversize donor button 0.25–0.5 mm to facilitate watertight closure, decrease glaucoma, decrease corneal flattening, and give more endothelial cells.
- Suture: 10.0 nylon (50 μm width); pass 90 to 100% depth on both donor and host. Running suture incites more inflammation, loosens easier, and does not allow selective removal of sutures; thus, always use interrupted sutures for high-risk PKs (rejections, regraft, perforation, inflammation, or infections). For running suture, ensure symmetry between bites and same depth; may be single or double running or combined with interrupted. Ideal is a 16-bite running with 8 interrupted, which can be removed for astigmatism. Most important interrupted suture is the second suture for postoperative astigmatism.
- Postoperative care: topical antibiotics until epithelium heals, resuture any wound leak >3 days, topical steroids 3 to 6 months, selected nonadjacent suture removal at 2 months, and RGP fitting at 6 months. Any broken suture needs to be removed unless buried, and if running, must remove the entire running suture.
- Children: usually use 4.5–5.0 mm trephines instead of 8.0 mm. Strip iris from cornea; may need to reform iris and angle. Remove lens; may need anterior vitrectomy. Eye wall is flaccid and requires scleral

support. Often lens–iris diaphragm bulges; thus, use a small size graft, which also reduces PAS; needs frequent postoperative follow-up, and early suture removal (as early as 2 to 4 weeks in neonates, 4 to 6 weeks in older patients) to decrease graft NV, inflammation, and rejection. Poor long-term visual prognosis: only 20% of patients are 20/100 or better; need aggressive amblyopia treatment. Glaucoma is very common and frequent cause of failure. Forty to 50% of grafts are clear at 1 year, 20 to 25% require regrafts.

- Complications:
  - Keratitis after corneal graft (or LASIK): often *Streptococcus viridans*, causing interstitial crystalline keratopathy (feathery appearance). Treat with topical vancomycin or penicillin G 100,000 units.
  - Vascularization: treat with steroids or argon laser closure.
  - Astigmatism: cut suture in steep axis, or do wedge resection in flat axis, RGP, or LASIK.
- Graft rejection: can occur anytime and is a type IV hypersensitivity reaction; if hyperacute, is due to circulating Ab. Risk factors: vascularization in at least two quadrants or history of previous graft rejection, glaucoma (30% of PK with trabeculectomy fail; consider tube shunt at the time of PK; posterior tubes generally have better outcome for graft), extensive PAS, and traumatic or hereditary ocular surface disorder. Treat rejection with topical steroids, and consider oral steroids, topical cyclosporine, or azathioprine.
  - Endothelial: more symptoms than epithelial rejection, usually with pain, photophobia, Khodadoust line of endothelial rejection (vs. Wessley ring of endothelial inflammatory cells seen with corneal ulcer). Treat with steroids.
- Epithelial: minimum symptoms, foreign body sensation, subepithelial infiltrate (SEI), and epithelium rejection line; may progress to endothelial rejection if not treated with steroids.
- Stromal rejection or combination of above types.

PTERYGIUM EXCISION Grasp superior edge of pterygium next to limbus with 0.12 forceps, and cut radially down to sclera. Repeat inferior, then undermine with a needle driver. Grasp the body of the pterygium transversely with one jaw of the needle driver under and the other over the pterygium. Cut the noncorneal side, then, using the needle drive as a handle, peel the pterygium head off the cornea, using a wiping dissection with a Weck-Cel sponge. May need to smooth the corneal surface by scraping with a blade or with corneal burr. Next, balloon the superior autograft site with balanced salt solution (BSS), measure, and undermine with quick snips (like a barber). Suture graft to the pterygium removal site with Vicryl. May also use amniotic membrane instead of autograft. Recurrence: bare sclera (75%), direct closure, advancement or rotational flap, conjunctiva autograft (5 to 10%).

SUPERFICIAL KERATECTOMY ("SUPERK") Used to peel or scrape off superficial corneal lesions (e.g., Salzmann's nodules).

TARSORRHAPHY For neurotrophic, severe dry eye; protect for exposure. Scarify superior and inferior lid margins, and close with 6.0 Vicryl tarsal sutures. Quicker than the more attractive tongue-and-groove technique.

THERMOKERATOPLASTY Burns placed on the epithelium with cautery to create a fibrovascular pannus and prevent bullae in a blind painful eye from corneal edema and bullae.

KERATOREFRACTIVE SURGERY: INCISIONAL

- Astigmatic keratotomy (AK): follow nomogram to create deep arcuate corneal incisions in the steep axis to correct astigmatism. Avoid arcuate incision greater than 90 degrees due to increased instability and decreased efficacy.
- Automated lamellar keratoplasty (ALK): flap created with a microkeratome followed by a second stromal cut. The middle layer is removed, and the superficial flap is replaced. Precursor to LASIK; leaves steep edges.
- Epikeratophakia: cornea layered on cornea; old treatment for aphakia.
- Radial keratotomy (RK): radial, nearly full-thickness depth incisions that cause midperipheral steepening with central flattening. Obtain preoperative paracentral pachymetry; thinnest inferotemporally in most patients (38% of patients), followed by temporal (28%), inferior (19%), nasal (11%), and superior (4%). After eight incisions there is little gain of myopic effect. RK shows a slow hyperopic drift of about 0.1 D/year (Prospective Evaluation of Radial Keratotomy [PERK] study).

KERATOREFRACTIVE SURGERY: LASER

This is a laser surgery used to treat refractive errors. Patients should have a stable refraction, and contact lens patients should be evaluated out of RGP lenses for at least 3 weeks and out of soft contact lenses (SCL) at least 2 weeks to ensure refraction is stable. For myopia, the laser is used to remove central corneal tissue. Munnerlyn's formula states that ablation depth = diopters of myopia divided by 3 times the square root of 0.2 mm. For hyperopia, an annular ablation area in the midperipheral cornea is performed.

- Contraindications to laser refractive surgery: uncontrolled ocular surface disease (KCS, blepharitis, etc.) and corneal anesthesia; may want to avoid surgery with patients with glaucoma and uveitis (patients may assume you made their chronic disease worse), keratoconus or ectasia, systemic immunosuppression, autoimmune diseases including RA and connective tissues disorders, irregular astigmatism, and active HSV.

- Excimer laser (*excimer* meaning "excited dimer"): a photochemical laser creating an unstable argon-fluoride dimer by applying an electrical charge to argon and fluorine gas in a cavity. As it drops to the ground state, a photon of energy is released from the charged dimer at 193 nm. Each photon has 6.4 eV of energy (high energy compared with other lasers), and carbon–carbon bonds have only 3.2 eV of bond energy. Thus, each photon from the excimer has the energy to break two bonds. The laser is of short pulse duration (14 ns), so it leaves surrounding tissue undamaged ("cold laser"). It is extremely precise: each photon removes 0.25 μm of tissue.
    - Laser characteristics: fluence mJ/cm^2 (energy delivered at energy plane), repetition rate (Hz), beam diameter (mm), and beam homogeneity (smoothness, energy consistency across the beam).
    - Broad beam: fast beam that can widen up to 6.5 mm, limited by optical quality at the edges of beam. Can vary the shape to treat myopia, hyperopia, and irregular astigmatism. Plume generation can block the central beam and cause central islands (reduced with "pretreatment" software to give extra pulses centrally). Smoothness across beam varies.
    - Scanning beam: small, high-quality beam (1 mm) that scans the corneal surface. Plume is less of an issue because of the smaller size and moving beam; thus, central islands are rare. Surfaces are smoother than broad beam. Can perform very large ablation zones: up to 8.0 mm optical zone plus blend (important for large pupils). Treatment time is increased (up to 2 minutes); requires good fixation: needs tracking device to follow eye movements.
- Laser-assisted in situ keratomileusis (LASIK): microkeratome used to cut a partial thickness corneal flap that is lifted, allowing laser stromal ablation; flap is then replaced. Most complications are related to the flap. Base the ablation on the manifest refraction, but if patient is <40 years, verify that patient is not over-minused with a cycloplegic refraction.
    - If preoperative keratometry >46 D, rule out keratoconus or corneal warpage, especially if patient is long-term RGP wearer and has an increased risk of buttonhole (use a smaller corneal ring). If keratometry is <41 D, there is an increased risk of a free cap (use a larger corneal ring).
    - Key surgical step is to create an ideal flap. Small hinge often occurs if K < 42 D, normal if 42–44, and large hinge if >44 D (hinge too close to pupil; may double ablate over the flap and induce irregular astigmatism; thus, move suction ring 1 mm nasally).
    - Always leave at least 250 μm posterior stroma to prevent posterior ectasia, endothelial polymegtheism, and Descemet's deposits. The flap is usually about 180 μm thick; add this to the 250 μm

posterior cornea, which should never be violated, to arrive at approximately 430 μm, which should be the minimal corneal thickness. Subtract this from pachymetry measurement to determine the amount of tissue available for ablation. Thick flaps have more memory and consistency and lie better. Law of thickness: flap of uniform thickness has no relative refractive power.

- Confirm adequate suction (low suction may cause thin flap, which may dislodge, buttonhole, or cause striae). Four-step check (mnemonic: ABCD): **a**pplanation tonometry (Barraquer); **b**lackout of vision confirmed by patient; **c**onsole readout of vacuum obtained (may have false reading with conjunctival laxity or debris or kinked tube); **d**ilation of the pupil.
- Complications:
  - Macrostriae: may have thick or thin flap, pain, decreased VA, epithelial downgrowth, and torqued flap. Needs immediate revision and SCL.
  - Microstriae: wrinkles, usually with thin flaps (<120 μm) and usually high correction (epithelium lying in laser divot); predisposed by air-drying or flap dehydration.
  - Thin flap: laser ablation contraindicated; reposition flap and recut in 3 months. Similar treatment for buttonhole: do not lift flap.
  - Diffuse lamellar keratitis (DLK): noninfectious; many proposed causes, including gram-negative exotoxin and keratome oil.
  - Posterior ectasia: prevention is key; treatment is difficult.
  - Flap dislocation or avulsion: replace and use BSCL.

- Photorefractive keratectomy (PRK): epithelial removal either mechanically or by laser, followed by laser stromal ablation. Longer healing time than LASIK, with potential complications related to epithelial defect early (use BSCL) and late-onset corneal haze (LOCH) from epithelial or fibroblast migration later in the course (treat with steroids). Typically use 3-month steroid taper, required to prevent haze and myopic regression. Basically, LASIK and PRK have the same visual acuity results at 6 months postop.
  - Laser-assisted in situ epithelial keratomileusis (LASEK) and other names used for the technique of PRK after lifting an epithelial flap.
  - Photoastigmatic refractive keratectomy (PARK): older technique that creates cylindric elliptical ablation (i.e., a horizontal ellipse that is steeper vertically treats WTR astigmatism).

CHAPTER 4

Glaucoma

Anatomy and Physiology

LIMBUS-ANGLE STRUCTURES (FIG. 4–1) From anterior to posterior: Schwalbe's ring (Descemet's termination), trabecular meshwork (TM), scleral spur (SS), and ciliary body (CB).

TRABECULAR MESHWORK, THREE DIVISIONS Uveal (iris processes), corneoscleral (from SS to Schwalbe's, lined by endothelium; engulf debris), and juxtacanalicular (greatest resistance to outflow; uses micropinocytosis and transcellular vacuoles to move aqueous fluid across the endothlium; likely site of primary open-angle glaucoma pathology; steroids increase GAG here).

- Endothelial cells lining trabecular beams are phagocytic and act as a "self-cleaning filter." Pigment can overwhelm the endothelial cells, which also cannot phagocytize exfoliative material. Red blood cells also pliably squeeze through the TM (except ghost cells) and pass into vacuoles or are phagocytized.
- Posterior TM is more pigmented and overlies Schlemm's canal, which drains to the aqueous veins of Ascher, then to laminated veins of the conjunctiva, then the episcleral vein, and finally into the superior orbital vein. More external collector channels are inferior and nasal.

AQUEOUS FLUID OUTFLOW The Goldmann equation shows that IOP = $(F_{formation} / C_{facility}) + EVP$. The equation can be rearranged to show that aqueous outflow is directly proportional to the net forward aqueous pressure (IOP – EVP) and inversely proportional to outflow resistance: $F_{formation} = (IOP - EVP) / R$, where R is resistance. The equation is missing uveoscleral outflow.

- Tonography: measures resistance; the inverse of resistance is known as facility (C), and is normally 0.2–0.3 μL/minute/mmHg. Low C = high resistance and pressure; for example, age-related loss of endothelial cells leads to decreased outflow and thus increased IOP.
- Some determinants of IOP: increases with age, female sex, African-American race, family history, high blood pressure, obesity, posture,

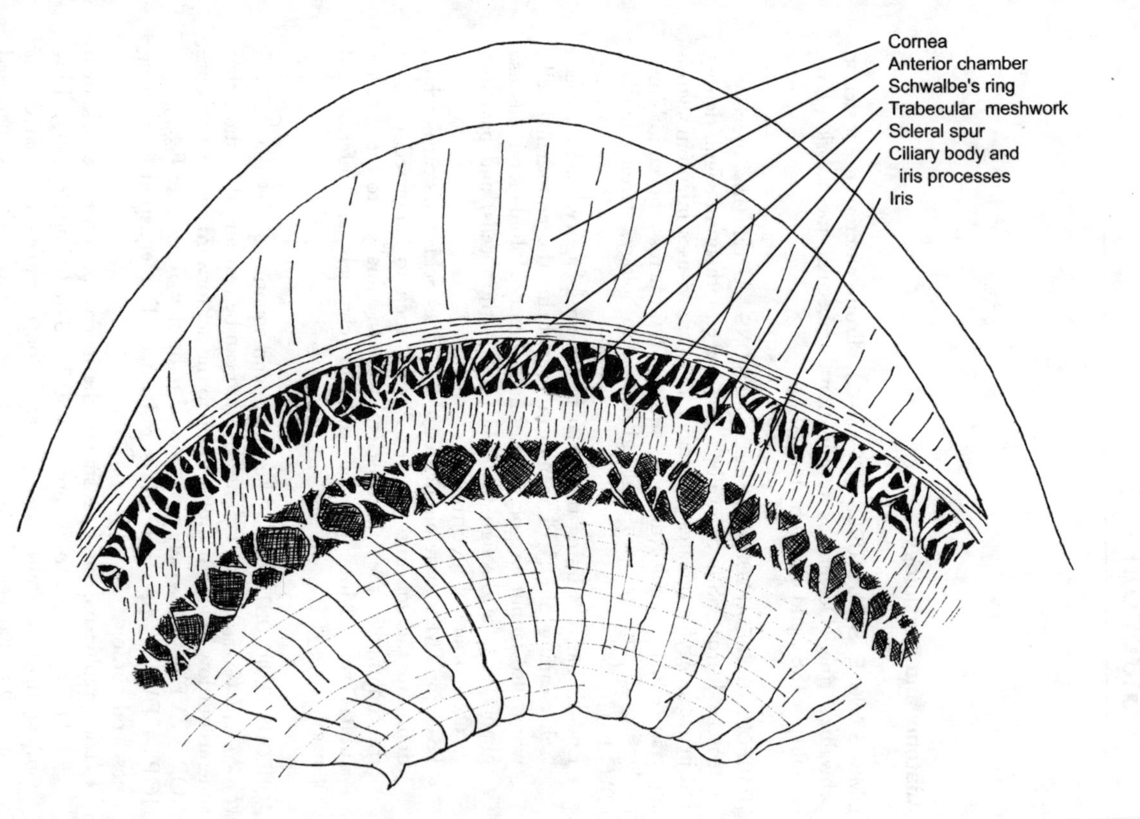

Figure 4–1 Gonioscopic view of a wide-open anterior chamber angle.

myopia, exercise, lid closure, inflammation, water imbibition, cycloplegics, steroids, ketamine, and succinylcholine. IOP is decreased with inhalational anesthesia, alcohol, and marijuana. Diurnal peak in morning from endogenous corticosteroids.

- An acute increase in the EVP (normally about 9 mmHg) increases the IOP in a 1:1 ratio (chronic EVP increases the IOP less).
- Diurnal variation: the net forward aqueous flow pressure (P) is the result of pressure in the eye minus venous pressure: $P_{outflow} = P_{IOP} - P_{EVP}$, and is normally about 5 mmHg (14 – 9). If inflow doubles (as with diurnal variation), the outflow pressure also doubles. For example, if IOP were 14 mmHg and the inflow doubles ($P_{outflow}$ that was 5 doubles to 10), then the IOP would increase to 19 mmHg (10 + 9) because the EVP remains constant. Glaucoma is characterized by large diurnal fluctuations (e.g., 22 mmHg may increase to 35 when diurnal production doubles).

- TM outflow: responsible for 80% of outflow; increased with elevated IOP, pilocarpine, epinephrine, dipivefrin, ALT, and trabeculotomy. Outflow is passive bulk flow through the TM due to hydrostatic pressure gradient. Parasympathetic tone keeps the TM open (thus cycloplegics cause TM collapse and may increase IOP).
- Uveoscleral outflow: responsible for about 20% of outflow, through the ciliary body face into the suprachoroidal space. Ouflow increases with atropine, epinephrine, alpha-2 agonists, and prostaglandin analogues, as well as a cyclodialysis cleft. Uveoscleral outflow is decreased with pilocarpine from ciliary muscle contraction and closure of spaces between muscle fibers. Unlike the TM, uveoscleral outflow is pressure-independent (if IOP < EVP, all outflow is uveoscleral).

CILIARY BODY Composed of two divisions: the pars plicata, which is the anterior 2 mm (approximately 3 mm posterior to limbus) and has 70 to 80 ciliary processes, and the pars plana, which is the posterior flat 4 mm of the CB (thus, for a vitrectomy, usually enter 3.5 mm posterior to the limbus to avoid the ciliary processes). The CB forms the aqueous, vitreous MPS, affects outflow, forms and supports the zonules, is responsible for accommodation, and is the attachment for the anterior vitreous base.

- Ciliary processes have a double epithelium. The outer, pigmented, cuboidal layer of cells is a continuation of the RPE and is contiguous with the posterior (inner) iris epithelium. The inner, nonpigmented, columnar layer is a contination of the neurosensory retina and is the site of aqueous production (*apigmented* = aqueous). The blood–aqueous barrier is formed by tight junctions of the inner epithelium and the nonfenestrated iris vessels.
- Three ciliary muscles:

  - Longitudinal (meridional): attaches SS/TM to the ora serrata (thus, miotics may cause RD). Contracture opens the TM and increases outflow and decreases uveoscleral outflow (thus, pilocarpine and Xalatan counteract each other).
  - Circular (sphincteric): contraction reduces the diameter of the ciliary ring and thus relaxes zonular tension (accommodation).
  - Oblique (radial): lies between the longitudinal and circular muscles. Contraction increases uveoscleral outflow and shallows the AC by pulling the lens diaphragm forward (thus increased risk of angle closure with miotics).
- Vasculature: major arterial circle is poorly defined and is more vascular in the anterior ciliary body (more hyphemas in the anterior chamber). It is formed from the two long posterior ciliary arteries and seven anterior ciliary arteries (two from each rectus muscle except the LR; thus, there is a risk of anterior segment ischemia with multiple muscle surgery).

AQUEOUS FLUID The aqueous provides a clear medium and nourishment (more glucose in the posterior chamber, more lactate in AC, acidic pH of 7.2, and decreased protein but 15× more ascorbate than serum) and maintains IOP (to prevent pthisis). Volume is about 200–300 μL and is produced at 2–3 μL/minute; thus, there is a complete turnover every 100 minutes.

- Produced by active transport (Na^+, Cl^-, HCO_3^- pumped across basal cell surface, and H_2O follows), ultrafiltration (H_2O and soluble products), and diffusion (lipid solubles pass via osmosis).
- Glaucoma is caused by outflow obstruction, not hypersecretion, as would be needed to increase production 8× to get IOP to 40 mmHg. Production decreases with age, surgery, and inflammation. Measure production with fluorophotometry.

OPTIC NERVE See Chapter 8. The optic disk is a vertical oval and is smaller in Caucasian versus African-American patients. Rim thickness normally follows the ISNT rule: **i**nferior rim broadest, then **s**uperior, followed by **n**asal and **t**emporal. This creates an optic cup that is normally a horizontal oval (becomes more vertical in glaucoma, which does not follow the ISNT rule, and inferior and superior nerve fiber layer axons are preferentially lost). The lamina cribrosa is stacked fenestrated collagen (type IV) and laminin plates, with larger openings and thinner walls superiorly and inferiorly (possibly less supportive and more easily damaged).

DEFINITION AND PATHOGENESIS OF GLAUCOMA Optic neuropathy characterized by nerve head cupping with associated loss of visual field. Diagnosis is typically made if two of three conditions are present: increased

IOP, ON cupping (11% of normals have a cup to disk ratio > 0.5), or VF defect. Visual function tests show decreased magnocellular function (M-type ganglion cells) as the body "sacrifices" peripheral fibers first. Neuronal cell death (ganglion axon loss) is the end result of glaucoma despite disputed mechanism (mechanical, vascular, etc.). Pathology shows retinal atrophy of ganglion cell and nerve fiber layers (has an intact inner nuclear layer as opposed to ischemic retinopathy, which shows dropout of retinal inner third). Etiology may be from

- Ischemia: fluorescein angiogram shows hypoperfusion in glaucoma.
- Mechanical: axonal compression with decreased axoplasmic flow.
- Apoptosis: programmed cell death with no inflammatory response or trace of the original cell. Theories of apoptosis include excessive glutamate that excessively binds to the ganglion cell and opens calcium channels, leading to cell death (also found in high concentration in the vitreous of glaucoma patients).
  - Neuroprotection: IOP reduction is the only proven form of neuroprotection. Calcium channel blockers may benefit the 10% of normal tension glaucoma (NTG) patients who progress despite maximum treatment. In animal models, Alphagan may preserve ganglion cells after crush injury to the ON.

EPIDEMIOLOGY Glaucoma is the second leading cause of blindness in the United States (first among African-Americans). Types of glaucoma in the United States: POAG (80%), secondary open-angle glaucoma (3%), angle closure (5%), congenital (< 1%), and glaucoma suspects (11%). Prevalence: Caucasians (1%), African-Americans (5%). Fifty percent of patients are undiagnosed, and 50% have IOP < 22 mmHg on first visit. About 4% of Caucasian patients and 8% of African-American patients are blind in both eyes (OU) from glaucoma, defined as VA < 20/200 in the better eye or VF < 20 degrees by Goldmann III4e.

Signs and Symptoms

BLOOD IN SCHLEMM'S CANAL ON GONIOSCOPY (See red line just posterior to the pigmented posterior TM.) Caused by increased EVP (Sturge-Weber syndrome, arteriovenous fistula, carotid–cavernous sinus fistula, pressure from large gonioscopy prism such as Goldmann, superior vena cava obstruction), hypotony, and thyroid eye disease.

CASE PRESENTATIONS Glaucoma in a young myopic athletic male: pigment dispersion syndrome (PDS). Elderly white female (or Asian patient) hyperope with cataract and high eye pressure: relative pupillary block (RPB). Glaucoma in an elderly Norweigan male with hairy ears: pseudoexfoliative glaucoma (PXG).

HYPOTONY Resulting from either decreased aqueous production (pthisis, beta-blockers, carbonic anhydrase inhibitors, postoperative, ocular ischemic syndrome, etc.) or increased outflow (rhegmatogenous retinal detachment, cyclodialysis cleft, wound leak, filtering bleb, etc.).

INFERIOR ANGLE PECULARITIES Most metabolically active, most open, most pigmented (posterior TM more active than anterior), and has the most iris processes.

IRIDODONESIS (excessive iris movement) Seen with zonular dialysis, lens dislocation, trauma, pseudoexfoliation syndrome (PXS), and myopia.

IRIS PIGMENT ABNORMALITY Seen with iris nevus, Fuchs' HIC, glaucomatocyclitic crisis, hemangioma, neurofibroma, and siderosis or chalcosis.

IRREGULAR ANGLE NARROWING Seen with subacute angle closure or RPB, lens dislocation, iris cysts, and PAS (angle narrowing at 12 o'clock is normal).

IRREGULAR ANGLE WIDENING Seen with angle recession, lens dislocation, and cyclodialysis.

IRREGULAR IRIS Seen with lens dislocation, iris cyst or tumor, and segmental atrophy (HZV, surgical trauma, or previous episodes of acute glaucoma).

"LYTIC" GLAUCOMAS All involve macrophages that ingest a product and obstruct the TM, such as phacolytic (high-molecular-weight lens protein), melanolytic (pigment breakdown from melanoma), and hemolytic glaucoma (red blood cells [RBCs]).

PIGMENT SPRINKLING Seen with PDS, PXS, melanoma, iris or CB cysts, uveitis, trauma, and IOLs.

SAMPAOLESIS'S LINE (pigment deposition along Schwalbe's ring or peripheral cornea) Seen classically with PXS, PDS, and other pigment sprinkling syndromes.

SCLERAL SPUR CHARACTERISTICS Visible (angle open), hidden (uveal meshwork commonly seen nasally, narrow angle, angle closure or synechia, inflammatory precipitates or exudates commonly seen inferiorly), prominent, and white (torn uveal meshwork, torn ciliary muscle, cyclodialysis cleft).

TM PIGMENTATION Increases with age and seen with PDS ("black crayon" appearance), PXS ("brown sugar" appearance), uveitis, trauma (including post-LPI or surgery), hyphema (pigment "balls" inferiorly), melanoma, and Sampaolesis's line.

Exam and Imaging

EXAM, ANTERIOR CHAMBER EVALUATION Van Herick grading measures peripheral AC depth compared with corneal thickness at the temporal limbus, with a slit lamp beam slightly off-center. If AC depth is equivalent to corneal thickness, then the angle is likely to be open (usually equivalent to Shaffer grade IV); if AC depth is one-quarter cornea thickness, then the angle is most likely occludable (grade II and consider a LPI). Risks of a persistent shallow chamber include increased AC inflammation, increased fibrin, and PAS (can form within 7 to 10 days).

EXAM, GONIOSCOPY Gonio prisms are needed to see into the angle because of total internal reflection. May give either a direct view (e.g., Koeppe) or an indirect view, which gives an inverted image of the opposite angle (e.g., Zeiss, Posner, Sussman, and Goldmann).

- Iris contour and width: open 45 degrees, narrow 10–20 degrees (hyperopes). Can also grade as 1+ convex (normal), 3+ convex (hyperopia, angle closure, or RPB), flat (myopia, aphakia, pseudophakia, or plateau iris), or concave (pigment dispersion, cyclitic membrane, PAS in aphakia, or pseudophakia).
- Ciliary band (anterior face of ciliary body): look for widened ciliary body, indicating angle recession with broken iris processes.
- Scleral spur: an extension of the sclera where the longitudinal ciliary muscle inserts. The angle is open if the spur is visible. May be pathologically dehisced with trauma, called a cyclodialysis cleft, seen as a white band or "fish mouth" behind the scleral spur (looking at the white sclera into the suprachoroidal space); may have hypotony and a retrodisplaced iris root.
- Corneoscleral TM: from scleral spur to Schwalbe's ring, posterior three fifths more pigmented and active; look for synechiae (uveal meshwork).
- Angle blood vessels: normal vessels include circumferential loops of the major arterial arcade up to the scleral spur (if cross, scleral spur is most likely abnormal) and short vertical vessels from the anterior ciliary or radial vessel from the iris. Abnormal vessels include vertical vessels that cross the scleral spur and arborize over the TM. Neovascularization shows a flat table-top iris surface and fibrovascular membrane with a red hue, from aqueous VEGF draining through the TM.

EXAM, GONIOSCOPY GRADING SYSTEMS

- Becker goniogram: two concentric circles are drawn, representing Schwalbe's ring and the scleral spur; angle pathology can be illustrated easily on the diagram.
- Shaffer: most commonly used grading system; grades the angle of iris insertion with the plane of TM: grade IV, wide-open 45 degree angle, CB is seen, closure not possible; grade III, open angle up to 35 degrees, scleral spur is seen; grade II, 20 degree angle, only TM is seen and angle closure is possible; grade I, 10 degree angle, only Schwalbe's ring or bare TM is seen and closure is probable; and grade 0, the angle is closed. Iris insertion is graded A–D, from posterior to anterior. In reality, most people use a modified Shaffer system.
- Scheie: grade I–IV, opposite of Shaffer grading system (grade IV is closed, and grade I is open to the scleral spur).
- Spaeth: four variables. 1. Iris insertion: A (anterior insertion, equal to Shaffer grade D), B, C, D (equal to Shaffer grade A), or E (posterior insertion, angle recession). 2. Estimated angle degree from 0 to 50%. 3. Iris configuration graded Q, R, or S (Queer = concave, as in reverse pupillary block; Regular = flat; or Steep = 3+ convex). 4. TM pigmentation graded from 0 to 4+. For example, D30R is normal.

IMAGING Stereo photographs are able to provide reliable documentation of glaucomatous optic neuropathy.

- GDx: a scanning laser polarimeter that estimates retinal nerve fiber layer thickness through measurement of a polarized laser light passing through the naturally birefringent nerve fiber layer and cornea. The orderly arrangement of microtubules within the axons and the arcuate bundles of nerve fibers separated by Müller's cells creates birefringence and thus polarizes light in phase and retards light that is out of phase.
  - The GDx machine plots the NFL retardation along two rings 10 degrees apart around the ON. The graphical printout divides the nerve into four quadrants and averages 1500 points in each quadrant (excluding NFL overlying retinal blood vessels). Colors indicate NFL thickness, and red-orange warm colors represent more retardation and thus a thicker NFL (usually superior and inferior); the cool blue colors indicate less retardation and a thinner NFL.
  - One problem is confounding birefringence from the corneal stroma and lens. Corneal polarization is usually 20 degrees down and nasal, which is adjusted for by the GDx machine. However, some people have different corneal orientation and thus may have false negative reading, with usually a nasal or temporally shifted red colors.

- Optical coherence tomography (OCT) and retinal thickness analyzer (RTA) are able to image the optic nerve with high resolution. They are analogous to an ultrasound but use light instead of sound, and may be used as adjuncts for glaucoma diagnosis.

INTRAOCULAR PRESSURE (IOP) SCREENING IOP screening has very low sensitivity and specificity for POAG. Mean pressure is 16 mmHg and is nongaussian and skewed toward higher IOPs.

- Schiotz: tests ocular rigidity. High rigidity gives a falsely high IOP, as seen with high hyperopia, long-standing glaucoma, age-related macular degeneration, and vasoconstrictors. Low rigidity gives a falsely low IOP, as seen with high myopia, miotics, RD or any ocular surgery, intravitreal gas, and thyroid disease. Problems include increased IOP from the instrument indentation. The principle behind the Schiotz test assumes that all eyes respond in the same way.
- Goldmann applanation: based on the Imbert-Fick principle ($P_{pressure} = F_{force} / A_{area}$) and is equivalent to the force required to overcome the resistance of the capillary action of tears and flatten a 3.06 mm^2 area of cornea (the area of the applanation tip; could have been 2–4 mm^2, but 3.06 allows the scale reading in grams $\times$ 10 = IOP). Biprism splits image, allowing Vernier acuity to estimate IOP. Astigmatism (4 D = 1 mmHg) has average horizontal and vertical readings.
  - IOP is overestimated by thick semicircles and corneas (except corneal edema underestimates) and globe pressue (squeezing, thyroid restrictive >6 mmHg increase in upgaze). A significant percentage of ocular hypertension (OHT) patients have thick corneas.
  - IOP is underestimated by thin corneas (e.g., following PRK) or fluid under a LASIK flap.
- Perkins: applanation like Goldmann.
- Tonopen: applanation and indentation; overestimates low IOP, underestimates high IOP. Similar to MacKay-Marg tonometry.
- Others: manometry only true measure of IOP. Pneumotonometer is least affected by corneal thinning (good after refractive surgery). Noncontact air-jet is unreliable with glaucoma. Tonography measures facility by Schiotz over 4 minutes.

OPTIC NERVE EVALUATION ON assessment is the most important factor in glaucoma diagnosis; it is objective, unlike VF testing.

- Most important diagnostic signs: vertical elongation of cup (in only 10% of normals; usually horizontal) or asymmetric cupping (difference in cup to disk ratio < 0.2 is seen in only 1% of normal individuals), rim notching or thinning, disk hemorrhage, and no rim pallor.
  - Axonal loss: with modest damage, usually NFL loss is at the inferotemporal rim (leading site of most damage; thus, a superior

nasal step or arcuate VF defect is the most common specific VF finding). With moderate damage, the temporal rim may show prominent loss, and advanced damage may leave only a remnant of the nasal rim. No axons cross the horizontal midline; thus, glaucomatous defects respect the horizontal visual field.
  - Drance hemorrhage (splinter hemorrhage of the NFL on or near the disk): most frequently seen with NTG and is a strong risk factor for progression of glaucoma (4–5× increased risk of VF loss when present; glaucoma progresses in 71% of patients vs. 33% without hemorrhage; POAG patients are 14× more likely to progress during the year after hemorrhage diagnosed than are patients without Drance hemorrhage). Prevalent in one third of NTG patients, one tenth of POAG, and one hundredth of normals (usually from posterior vitreous detachment, diabetes, hypertension, papillitis, or AION). Prevalence increases with severity of glaucoma but decreases with very advanced disease. Usually inferotemporal location and transient (average resolution in 10 weeks) but recurrent in two thirds of patients. Mechanism: microinfarcts, microvenous occlusion, and mechanical rupture.
- Less specific signs: peripapillary atrophy (PPA), baring of a circumlinear disk vessel, angulated vessel at disk margin (bayoneting), laminar dots of the cribriform plate, focal arteriolar narrowing in severely damaged eyes, overpass phenomenon, NFL defects, acquired ON pit, and saucerization (difficult to distinguish where the cup starts and the rim ends).
  - Cupping: not as important as the health of the neural rim. Can lose up to 50% of axons before clinical glaucomatous changes are seen. Sixty-six percent of normal patients have a C:D <0.3, and only 6% of normal patients are >0.5 (this latter group is disproportionately referred to ophthalmology). C:D ratio is larger in African-American patients. Cupping may be reversible in children, increases with age, and is larger when seen in stereo.
  - PPA: beta zone atrophy is more prevalent in glaucoma and shows marked RPE and choriocapillaris atrophy closer to the disk (present in only 20% of normal patients); alpha zone atrophy is seen in almost all normal eyes and shows irregular hypo- or hyperpigmentation.
  - Nerve fiber layer analysis: best seen with high magnification, high illumination, and a red-free filter. Light is normally reflected by the NFL and RPE; however, red-free light eliminates the RPE reflection and allows better NFL visualization. Often see a grainy appearance from Müller cell processes. Brighter and whiter reflection indicates a thicker NFL obscuring the underlying vessels. A

NFL defect may precede a glaucomatous VF defect; may see diffuse atrophy versus wedge-shaped defect.

- Other presentations: young patients with high IOP may show diffuse cupping with regular thinning. Focal glaucoma, usually in females with vasospastic risk factors (migraine, Raynaud's phenomenon, etc.), may show very localized rim loss usually inferiorly. Senile sclerotic glaucoma is often seen in older patients with hypertension or ischemic coronary artery disease and may show marked PPA, sloped cup, and pale rim (saucerization).

PERIMETRY, NORMAL AND ABNORMAL VISUAL FIELDS The visual field can be pictured as "a hill of vision in a sea of darkness."

- Normal VF: 50 to 60 degrees superiorly, 60 degrees nasally, 70 to 75 degrees inferiorly, and 90 to 100 degrees temporally. The normal blind spot is 15 degrees temporal to fixation and is 6 degrees wide × 8 degrees high. The temporal VF does not necessarily respect the horizontal meridian.
- Glaucomatous VF defects: represent nerve fiber bundle defects. The ganglion cell layer and glaucomatous damage respect the horizontal meridian (vs. chiasm and posterior defects, which respect the vertical midline; thus, if VF defect respects the vertical midline, consider neuroimaging). Ninety percent of early glaucomatous damage is in the central 30 degrees.
    - Arcuate defect: within 10 to 20 degrees of fixation; most common and earliest finding in glaucoma.
        - Bjerrum's scotoma: complete arc from blind spot to the horizontal meridian
        - Seidel's scotoma: proximal small comma-like arcuate scotoma off the blind spot
        - Central island: superior and inferior Bjerrum's scotoma
    - Nasal step: relative depression of a horizontal hemifield; may be generalized nasal or binasal depression
    - Paracentral scotoma: <10 degrees of fixation; for example, a Derringer scotoma connects a paracentral scotoma with the blind spot.
    - Temporal wedge: from the blind spot extending temporally, wedge shape pointing toward blind spot; represents nasal disk loss (uncommon).
    - Altitudinal defect: advanced glaucoma

PERIMETRY, MEASUREMENT A decibel is a relative log unit of scale. By convention, the brightest light generated by the perimeter machine is 0 dB; thus, a light that is 1 log order of magnitude dimmer than the brightest light is 10 dB.

- Frequency-doubling technology (FDT): beneficial in glaucoma diagnosis, as it differentiates selective magnocellular axon loss based on testing modulation. Looks at temporal modulation, spatial frequency, and contrast sensitivity.
- Goldmann perimetry: kinetic perimetry (stimulus size and intensity are constant and moved in the field until seen). The stimuli used to plot an isopter are identified by a roman numeral, a number, and a letter.
  - Stimulus size is noted by roman numerals I ($0.25\,mm^2$), II ($1\,mm^2$), III ($4\,mm^2$), IV ($16\,mm^2$), and V ($64\,mm^2$). Thus, each size increment equals a 2× increase in diameter and a 4× increase in area.
  - Stimulus intensity is noted by a number from 1 to 4 and a letter from *a* to *e*. A change of one number represents a 5 dB (0.5 log unit) change in intensity, and each letter represents a 1 dB (0.1 log unit) change in intensity. Thus, 4e = 1000 apostilbs (brightest); each number below 4 indicates 5 dB decrease, and each letter before *e* is a 1 dB decrease.
- Humphrey visual field (HVF): automated threshold (stimulus seen and missed 50% of the time, suprathreshold 95% chance that stimulus is seen). When reading the printout, ensure correct patient and prescription, then look at gray scale, glaucoma hemifield test (GHT), and global indices. Next, look at the pattern deviation, and check that three nonedge points >5 dB and one is at least 10 dB.
  - Full threshold: seen stimulus is presented 4 dB dimmer until not seen (infrathreshold), then brightened by 2 dB until seen (suprathreshold), then bracketed, crossing the threshold point twice in 2 dB increments.
  - FASTPAC: uses 3 dB increments and only single bracketing to find "threshold." Good for quick screening test but not best for following glaucomatous VF loss. Is up to 40% faster for normal patients, although short-term fluctuation increases up to 25%, and focal loss can be underestimated in glaucoma.
  - SITA (Swedish interactive thresholding algorithm): uses continuous modeling of the hill of vision to limit test time.
  - Reliability parameters:
    - Fixation loss: stimuli presented in blind spot. Low test reliability if >33%.
    - False-positive error: VF machine generates a noise without a stimulus presented. Low reliability if >20%, usually with an alert, nervous patient.
    - False-negative error: after retinal sensitivity at a location is established, a brighter stimulus is presented that should be seen if the patient is attentive. Low reliability if >20%, usually in a drowsy patient.
  - Global indices:

- Mean defect (M): represents how far "the island of vision has sunk into the sea of darkness." The lower the value, the higher the decrease in sensitivity.
- Glaucoma hemifield test (GHT): mathematical model that compares the superior VF to the mirror image of points in the inferior VF; highly predictive of glaucomatous VF loss.
- Pattern standard deviation (PSD) and corrected PSD (CPSD): the lower the number, the higher the decrease in sensitivity in a localized manner. CPSD is not available with SITA. A low PSD indicates localized decreased sensitivity. If both PSD and CPSD are low, then there is a significant decreased VF, and most likely glaucoma is present. This index factors out any generalized reduction and looks at how regular or irregular is the shape of the "island of vision."

○ Artifactual defects:
- Lens rim defect: superior edge defect
- Cloverleaf pattern: advanced glaucoma or inattention; patient loses concentration, and the four paracentral areas that are mapped the most show deeper scotomas.
- Generalized field depression: caused by cataract, miotic therapy, and inappropriate optical correction
- The myope not wearing a contact lens has an enlarged blind spot that is moved out when viewing through the HVF lens versus the aphakic patient's blind spot, which is minimized and moved in.

○ Short-wavelength automatic perimetry (SWAP): blue-yellow perimetry to identify early magnocellular (M cell) loss. (M cells are not damaged earlier in glaucoma, but there is less redundancy with the M cell system; thus, may identify damage from a single axon). May identify VF defect 3 years earlier than with HVF perimetry. High false-positive rate.

Infantile and Pediatric Glaucoma

CONGENITAL GLAUCOMA, PRIMARY TRABECULODYSGENESIS 50 to 70% of cases of pediatric glaucoma are congenital, with a 1:12,500 incidence (increased with inbreeding). Two thirds of patients are male, two thirds of cases are bilateral. Defect is on chromosome 2, autosomal recessive, with increased gene frequency in patients of Middle Eastern ancestry (may have an X-linked variant, but do not confuse with X-linked megalocornea).

- Two main symptoms: tearing and photophobia. Two main signs: corneal edema and buphthalmos (occurs only if age <3 years; the neonate cornea is normally 10 mm, 11 mm by 1 year). Also

blepharospasm, increased IOP, Haab's striae (horizontal Descemet's membrane breaks that extend to the limbus). Patient may also have poor vision from progressive myopia due to globe enlargement.
- Pathogenesis: "fetal angle configuration," with a high insertion of the iris root; reported Barkan's membrane, although a membrane is rarely seen covering the TM.
- Treatment: a surgical disease, but treat IOP first with topical medication; when cornea clears, surgically open TM with goniotomy (90% curative for one to three surgeries) or trabeculotomy if the cornea is cloudy. May use Diamox, but generally avoid topical carbonic anhydrase inhibitors, Alphagan, and Xalatan in infants.
- Poor visual prognosis if myopia, anisometropic amblyopia, strabismus, irregular astigmatism (from Haab's striae), corneal edema, cornea >14 mm, and optic neuropathy. Amblyopia is the leading long-term cause of vision loss.

JUVENILE OPEN-ANGLE GLAUCOMA (JOAG) Autosomal dominant, chromosome 1q21–q31 GLC1A gene defect coding for myocilin (formerly TM induced glucocorticoid response [TIGR]) protein. Similar gene defect also present in 3 to 5% of POAG patients and in steroid-response glaucoma (increased TM GAG). Age of onset >3 years; thus, no risk for buphthalmos. JOAG has very high IOP and aggressive course.

SECONDARY GLAUCOMAS FROM CONGENITAL ANOMALIES

- Aniridia: 50 to 75% secondary ACG from peripheral iris stump obstructing TM, bilateral. Associated with nystagmus, foveal hypoplasia, ON hypoplasia, corneal pannus, and anterior polar cataract. From PAX 6 gene defect, most are autosomal dominant, but if sporadic, then there is a 20% incidence of Wilms' tumor (nephroblastoma).
- Axenfeld-Rieger syndrome: 50% of patients have glaucoma from trabecular dysgenesis and PAS. It is an autosomal dominant, bilateral neural crest abnormality with iridocorneal adhesions; also associated with maxillary hypoplasia, dental abnormalities, hypospadias, and inguinal or, more specifically, umbilical hernias.
- Lowe's oculocerebrorenal syndrome: 67% risk of glaucoma. It is an X-linked recessive disorder characterized by bilateral cataracts, renal rickets, and aminoaciduria.
- NF I: 50% unilateral glaucoma if upper-lid plexiform neurofibroma is present.
- Peters' anomaly: 50% glaucoma from anterior segment dysgenesis with lens attached to cornea, along with the absence of Descemet's membrane and endothelium. May be autosomal dominant, recessive, or sporadic.

- Sturge-Weber syndrome: 33% glaucoma if lid or conjunctiva is involved with the hemangioma; patients may have late-onset glaucoma from increased EVP and blocked aqueous outflow.
- Rubella: trabeculodysgenesis usually from in utero infection in the third trimester (TM forms in the third trimester vs. rubella cataract, which is usually from infection in the second trimester, when the lens forms; thus, they are not seen together). Patients may also have cardiac abnormalities, salt and pepper retinopathy. Responds well to goniotomy, even with adults.
- Others: PHPV, microphthalmia, nanophthalmos, traumatic, uveitic, and ectropion uveae

Primary Open-Angle Glaucoma

Primary open-angle glaucoma (POAG), which represents 80% of glaucoma cases in the United States, is an acquired, chronic, bilateral disease that is often characterized by asymmetric ON damage. It is diagnosed by the appearance of the disk and VF abnormality, with open angles and no secondary cause. Genetic mutation is seen in some patients at chromosome 3q21–24 gene GLC1C (probably is late-onset variant of autosomal dominant hereditary glaucoma). Etiology is probably from decreased outflow (increased GAG in the TM and loss of trabecular beam endothelial cells).

- Diagnosis is done by ruling out angle closure or secondary causes. Usually two of three conditions are present: characteristic ON appearance, glaucomatous VF defect, and increased IOP. May use water provocative test: 1 liter H_2O increases IOP >8 mmHg.
- Six major risk factors: weaker association with hypertension, coronary artery disease, migraine, or other vasospasm disorder.
  - Age: better predictor of glaucoma than IOP (Collaborative Glaucoma Study).
  - Diabetes: 2–3× more prevalent.
  - Elevated IOP: if IOP is 20–25 mmHg, 7% have ON or VF damage; 26–30 mmHg, the risk of glaucoma is 12%; >30 mmHg, the risk is 28%. The yearly risk of VF loss if IOP is 21–30 mmHg is 1%; if >30 mmHg, the risk is 10%.
  - Heredity: 25% of POAG patients have a positive family history. There is a 10% risk of POAG if a first-degree relative is affected (especially a sibling).
  - Myopia: 3× POAG risk if greater than −6 D. Glaucoma diagnosis may be confounded by myopic signs: PPA, tilted or oval disk, and scleral crescent.
  - Race: African-American patients have higher IOP, larger C:D ratio, and greater glaucoma prevalence, with earlier onset and 8× increased risk of blindness from glaucoma.

- Treatment: often begin with a topical beta-blocker or prostaglandin agonist, then add other medications as needed. Topical alpha agonists (Alphagan or Iopidine) have similar efficacy as beta-blockers but have more side effects (allergy, respiratory issues in children, etc.). Most drops are equivocal (timolol is the most studied; Ocupress has intrinsic sympathomimetic activity and is thus better in treating hyperlipidemia and nocturnal hypotension but is only a partial agonist). Adding a topical carbonic anhydrase inhibitor (e.g., dorzolamide) to timolol will decrease IOP about 2–3 mmHg. May also use ALT early in treatment course. For medication or laser treatment failures, consider trabeculectomy.
  - Collaborative Initial Glaucoma Treatment Study (CIGTS): an ongoing, randomized, controlled clinical trial evaluating initial medical treatment versus trabulectomy, and has thus far found no difference in glaucoma progression between the two groups.

NORMAL TENSION GLAUCOMA (NTG) Characterized by ON cupping and VF loss with normal IOP. VF defects tend to be steeper, deeper, and closer to fixation and more commonly have disk hemorrhage, which is a predictor of VF deterioration. Some patients have chromosome 2cen-q13 defect in GLC1B gene and also etiology from vascular factors.

- Differential diagnosis: burned out POAG, SOAG, shock optic neuropathy (hypotensive episode, anemia), AION, myopic disk, other optic neuropathies (think of especially in younger patients, or if rim pallor, central VF loss or color deficits are present). Consider work-up with CBC and ESR to rule out anemia and giant cell arteritis or temporal arteritis (GCA).
- Collaborative Normal Tension Study Group (CNTSG): a multicenter, controlled clinical trial that randomized normal tension glaucoma patients into treatment (medications, laser, or surgery) versus observation groups. Thirty-five percent of untreated eyes worsened within 3 years (the other 65% eventually showed some slow progression); 7% of treated eyes worsened. The CNTSG is the first conclusive study that showed decreasing IOP by 30% prevents vision loss (aim for IOP <15 mmHg), but 9% of patients progress even despite a very low IOP.

OCULAR HYPERTENSION (OHT) Characterized by IOP >21 mmHg, with an open angle, no ON or VF defect. Only 1% of patients per year develop VF loss or diagnosis of true glaucoma.

- Ocular Hypertension Treatment Study (OHTS): an ongoing, multicenter, controlled clinical evaluation of medical treatment for OHT, which has thus far shown that subjects who received topical glaucoma medication experienced conversion to glaucoma at less than half the rate of subjects who were monitored without treatment.

Secondary Open-Angle Glaucomas

APHAKIC OR POSTKERATOPLASTY Glaucoma may develop from angle distortion or anatomic change or from PAS (especially postkeratoplasty), alpha-chymotrypsin, or zonule fragments (post-ICCE).

ELEVATED EPISCLERAL VENOUS PRESSURE (EVP) From venous obstruction (thyroid orbitopathy, superior vena cava syndrome, orbital tumors, cavernous sinus thrombosis), arteriovenous fistula (carotid–cavernous sinus fistula, Sturge-Weber syndrome), or idiopathic. Signs and symptoms: dilated and tortuous episcleral vessels, chemosis, proptosis, orbital bruit or pulsation, blood in Schlemm's canal.

FUCHS' ENDOTHELIAL DYSTROPHY 10 to 15% of Fuchs' patients develop glaucoma; autosomal dominant disorder characterized by collagen deposition on Descemet's membrane with bilateral corneal guttae, usually in late adulthood female patients.

GHOST CELL GLAUCOMA Vitreous hemorrhage usually following trauma, vitrectomy, or cataract extraction, with disruption of the anterior hyaloid face. The degenerated, tan, rigid, spherical RBCs clog the TM; may see Heinz bodies (hemoglobin congealed on the inside of the RBC cell membrane) on pathology. May need vitrectomy.

HEMOLYTIC GLAUCOMA TM obstructed by macrophages that have ingested RBCs after hyphema (usually traumatic: look for lens subluxation or phacodonesis). Old hemorrhage may also cause hemosiderotic glaucoma, or siderosis from hemoglobin iron may produce TM endothelial cell dysfunction.

MELANOMALYTIC GLAUCOMA Macrophages with melanin pigment from melanoma block the TM. Tumors may also seed or directly extend into the angle.

PHACOLYTIC GLAUCOMA Mature or hypermature cataract leaks high molecular weight proteins through an intact capsule; the proteins are then ingested by macrophages and clog the TM. Usually characterized by abrupt onset, with a red painful eye with AC flare and precipitates of white flocculent material, in the setting of a mature cataract. Control the inflammation and glaucoma, then remove lens.

PHACOTOXIC OR LENS PARTICLE GLAUCOMA Disrupted lens capsule (postoperative, YAG laser capsulotomy, trauma, etc.) in which the retained cortex and lens particles obstruct the TM. Characterized by delayed onset; may see white fluffy cortical material in AC and some inflammation, with an open angle on gonioscopy. Control IOP and inflammation; surgery may be needed. (Compare with phacoanaphylaxis, which is zonal granulomatous uveitis from disrupted lens capsule and usually has hypotony, not glaucoma.)

PIGMENT DISPERSION SYNDROME (PDS), PIGMENT DISPERSION GLAUCOMA (PDG) Autosomal dominant, chromosome 7q35–q36 defect of iris pigment epithelium, causing an iris that is too large for the eye. The iris has redundant folds and posterior bowing, with friction on the zonules, causing the release of pigment and signs of the syndrome. Profile: young, white, middle-aged, myopic male. Twenty-five to 45% of PDS patients develop pigmentary glaucoma from pigment granules that clog the TM and damage the TM endothelium. The increased AC IOP pushes the iris posterior, causing a reverse pupillary block.

- Signs and symptoms: Krukenberg spindle (vertical layering of pigment on the corneal endothelium), midperipheral iris TID, peripheral concave iris ("queer" iris configuration with wide 45 degree open angle), 360 degree heavily pigmented TM (almost black), Sampaolesis's line, and Scheie's stripe (posterior lens pigment settles where the anterior hyaloid face meets the posterior capsule). May see aliquots of aqueous enter the AC with blink or lid squeeze.
- Treat with miotics, ALT, and traditional glaucoma therapy. Can follow TID as a marker for progression, and exercise may provoke dispersion. The reverse pupillary block needs very peripheral small PI that creates a "black hole" effect as aqueous rushes into the posterior chamber (PC), unlike the large peripheral iridectomy needed for narrow angle, in which aqueous and pigment rush out of the PC.

POST-TRAUMATIC GLAUCOMA May have immediate IOP rise from TM contusion or disruption, hyphema, massive choroidal hemorrhage, alkali chemical burn (initial IOP rise from scleral shrinkage and prostaglandin release; may have intermediate IOP increase from inflammation or late IOP elevation from TM damage or PAS). Delayed glaucoma from angle recession (decreased aqueous filtration, lifelong glaucoma risk), PAS, lens-induced (phacolytic, subluxation with pupillary block), ghost cell, closure of cyclodialysis cleft, epithelial downgrowth, or retained foreign body.

- Seven rings of tissue that may be injured with anterior segment trauma (plus cataract):
  - Pupil margin tears
  - Iris root tear: iridodialyisis
  - CB muscle tear: angle recession
  - TM tears
  - Scleral spur tear: cyclodialysis cleft
  - Zonular dialysis
  - Ora serrata or vitreous base: dialysis

- Angle recession, contusion angle deformity: tear in the face of CB seen as a widened CB band (cleavage created between the circular and longitudinal ciliary muscles). Typically has a deep AC with iris retroplacement, and may be accompanied by irido- or cyclodialysis. Also has posterior rotation of the ciliary processes: a line drawn through the scleral spur parallel to the visual axis usually bisects the first ciliary process, but in angle recession, the line would pass anterior to the ciliary processes. Angle recession does not cause glaucoma but indicates trauma to the TM; thus, patients have a lifetime risk of developing glaucoma. POAG is also a risk factor for development of angle recession glaucoma, and angle recession is treated like POAG when it develops.
- Hyphema: glaucoma risk is greatest following rebleeding (average 4 days after traumatic hyphema from clot lysis and retraction) from either RBCs and fibrin that obstruct the TM or a pupillary clot that may cause a RPB. Hyphema glaucoma risk: large hyphema, initial hypotony, African-American race, aspirin use, and sickle cell hemoglobinopathy.
- Iridodialysis: tear in root of iris; may need to be sutured in place if large, obstructing visual axis, or causing monocular diplopia.
- Cyclodialysis: disinsertion of longitudinal ciliary muscle from scleral spur; see white, bare sclera underneath. Usually has hypotony from aqueous flow into suprachoroidal space, but may have sudden increased IOP if it closes spontaneously. May need to be sutured or closed with cryotherapy if it is causing chronic hypotony.
- Descemetization: migration of Descemet's membrane over TM after surgery or trauma. Presents like apparent POAG, as the membrane is opaque.
- Epithelial ingrowth: devastating postoperative or post-traumatic complication from surface epithelium that proliferates into the eye. As it grows over the corneal endothelium, it causes segmental corneal edema, then progresses onto the TM, obstructing outflow. Epithelium induces underlying trabecular stoma to proliferate and thus changes the TM into fibrous tissue. Iris whitens with argon laser.
- Fibrous ingrowth: not as severe as epithelial ingrowth.

PSEUDOEXFOLIATION SYNDROME (PXS) OR PSEUDOEXFOLIATIVE GLAUCOMA (PXG) Most common SOAG; 70% of PXS patients develop glaucoma (50% have bilateral glaucoma, often with labile IOP). A bilateral disease that presents unilaterally, it causes a BM-like fibrillogranular white material to be deposited throughout the anterior segment and also systemically. Glaucoma develops as the material blocks the TM or is ingested by macrophages that block the TM. The disease always occurs in the elderly, with the highest incidence in Navajo Native Americans (38% incidence) and Scandinavians.

- Signs: target or bull's-eye lesion on the anterior lens capsule, "dandruff" on the pupillary margin, poor dilation, peripupillary TID, nuclear cataract, zonular dehiscence (phacodonesis, subluxation, increased vitreous loss with cataract extraction), pigment dispersion with patchy "brown sugar" colored TM and Sampaolesi's line.
- Pathology: eosinophilic "iron filings" and "sawtoothing" of iris pigment epithelium.
- PXG has a good response to ALT. Not cured by cataract extraction and remember poor zonular integrity with CE. Associated with increased incidence of chronic angle closure. Some call PXS "exfoliation" syndrome, however this is really "glassblower's cataract."

SCHWARTZ SYNDROME Rare, mild, uveitic glaucoma from RRD (often chronic, low-lying RD), with degenerated photoreceptor outer segments that pass forward through disrupted anterior hyaloid face and obstruct the TM. Not responsive to steroids.

STEROID-INDUCED GLAUCOMA Five percent of normal patients within 2 to 3 weeks after starting steroids develop increased IOP that almost always returns to baseline when stopped. Risks include POAG, first-degree relative of POAG, diabetes, myopia, and nonfluorinated steroids. Increased IOP develops from decreased facility of outflow from steroid-induced increased GAG in the TM extracellular matrix.

- Chromosome 1q defect found in the myocilin gene, as in JOAG. Some patients with the gene defect are steroid–responders, whereas others are not because of polymorphism (gene expressed differently in different individuals), and other genes regulate its expression.

UVEITIC GLAUCOMA Usually characterized by decreased IOP from aqueous production suppression and increased uveoscleral outflow. However, several uveitic syndromes are associated with increased IOP, notably herpetic uveitis and the following:

- Fuchs' HIC: unilateral, chronic, mild anterior uveitis with stellate KP; patients are usually 30 to 40 years old. Associated with hypochromia and cataract.
- Posner-Schlossman syndrome (glaucomatocyclitic crisis): characterized by unilateral, recurrent, mild anterior uveitis in young adults, with marked IOP elevations from idiopathic trabeculitis.
- Grant's syndrome: bilateral trabecular precipitates in patients that may progress to full uveitis; treat with steroids.
- Uveitis-glaucoma-hyphema syndrome (UGH): classic triad, but all parts may or may not be present. Usually from poorly positioned IOL (classically, AC IOL "tickles" the TM); may need lens exchange.

Primary Angle-Closure Glaucoma

PRIMARY ANGLE-CLOSURE GLAUCOMA (PACG) WITH PUPILLARY BLOCK (needs LPI) Characterized by shallow AC that further narrows the angle by increased IOP in the PC, pushing the peripheral iris into the angle obstructing the TM. Risks: age (decreased AC depth), Asian and Eskimo patients, females, hyperopia, and family history. Prototypical patient: middle-aged Asian female hyperope.

- Acute symptoms: severe pain, redness, blurred vision, nausea, vomiting, bradycardia, and diaphoresis. Subacute symptoms: vague, dull ache behind eye or unexplained headaches, slightly blurred vision, and colored halos (microcystic edema).
- Signs: IOP usually 40–60 mmHg, ciliary flush, microcystic epithelial corneal edema (vs. stromal edema seen with hypotony), shallow AC, cell and flare, irregular oval sluggish mid-dilated pupil (4–6 mm is critical diameter), sector iris atrophy, and glaukomflecken (infarcted anterior lens capsule epithelium); may see ON edema or central retinal vein occlusion (CRVO).
- Diagnosis: gonioscopy shows closed angle (or if corneal edema obstructs the view, the most important diagnostic clue is gonioscopy of the fellow eye, showing a narrow angle). Provocative tests include mydriasis (0.5% tropicamide), which causes IOP rise >8 mmHg (like water provocative test for POAG), and induced angle closure in dark room or prone position. Usually AC is peripherally shallow (van Herick AC depth < ¼ corneal thickness), but if it is centrally shallow, consider phacomorphic, posterior-pushing mechanism or aqueous misdirection. Rule out SOAG, perform gonioscopy, look for NVI, undilated check for CRVO, PDR, RD, and evaluate ON in both eyes.
- Precipitating factors: dim illumination (usually as mid-dilated pupil is coming down from full dilation), emotional stress, near work, anticholinergics (including antihistamines), adrenergics, and miotics
- Treatment for acute IOP rise:
    - Aqueous suppressants: beta-blocker every 5 minutes (2 doses), alpha-agonist every 5 minutes (2 doses), carbonic anhydrase inhibitor every 5 minutes (2 doses), and Diamox 500 mg IV or PO (not Sequels)
    - Hyperosmotics: Mannitol 1–2 g/kg IV 20% solution over 20 to 30 minutes, glycerin 1.0–1.5 g/kg PO on ice to clear cornea edema
    - After IOP <40 mmHg, then pilocarpine 2% every 5 minutes (three doses) to stiffen the iris (prevent anterior bowing), increase TM outflow, and set up for LPI. Do not use pilocarpine with inflammatory glaucoma, neovascular glaucoma (NVG), or if severe synechial angle closure. Miotics may cause paradoxical rise of IOP because of decreased uveoscleral outflow.

  - Keep patient supine, and perform repeated compression of central cornea (ocular "CPR" to force aqueous out of the eye). Consider a retrobulbar block to control pain and nausea.
  - A LPI is definitive treatment, followed with prophylactic LPI in the fellow eye (50 to 75% ACG risk to fellow eye).
- Chronic ACG: presents like POAG (may or may not be symptomatic; often painless, gradual), but has creeping, small PAS. Causes 70% of glaucoma in China. Associated with hyperopia, cataract progression (especially if myope with progressive cataract), increased age, and PXS. Needs LPI; pilocarpine can increase pupillary block. Chronic angle-closure glaucoma CACG develops in an eye with previous POAG (also known as combined-mechanism glaucoma).

PLATEAU IRIS (primary ACG without pupillary block) Needs peripheral iridoplasty primarily, but always perform a peripheral iridotomy first in order to eliminate any RPB (cannot confirm diagnosis of plateau iris without patent LPI). Anteriorly displaced ciliary body pushes peripheral iris forward, occludes angle, and increases IOP. M = F; patient usually 40 years old and myopic. Plateau iris is characterized by a flat iris plane, with deep central AC, and the "sine wave" sign on gonioscopy. Dilation can increase occlusion.

- Plateau iris configuration: anatomic predisposition but no glaucoma; do LPI.
- Plateau iris syndrome: ACG despite LPI; thus, needs peripheral iridoplasty or pilocarpine to pull peripheral iris out of angle.
- Pseudoplateau iris: iris cyst that pushes iris forward.

Secondary Angle-Closure Glaucoma

SECONDARY ACG WITH PUPILLARY BLOCK Needs LPI.

- Ectopia lentis: from anteriorly displaced lens. Do not use miotics at first (because they pull the lens–iris diaphragm anterior); give a mydriatic/cycloplegic, place patient supine to let lens settle back, then give a miotic and do LPI.
- Iris bombé: 360 degrees of posterior synechiae seen with severe or chronic intraocular inflammation.
- Phacomorphic glaucoma: enlarged, intumescent and cataractous lens causes pupillary block and secondary angle-closure glaucoma (maybe even in the setting of a patent PI). Presents with red painful eye, shallow AC despite LPI, and closed angle on gonioscopy. Treat by lowering IOP, then do LPI if cataract extraction is not expedient.

SECONDARY ACG WITHOUT PUPILLARY BLOCK May need peripheral iridoplasty.

- Anterior "pulling" mechanism: many causes, including epithelial downgrowth.
  - Inflammation: PAS from trauma, uveitis, untreated RPB, or flat chamber
  - Iridocorneal endothelial (ICE) syndrome: 50% of ICE patients develop glaucoma; acquired unilateral syndrome of abnormal corneal endothelial cells that become epithelial-like and migrate over the angle and iris. Disease spectrum encompasses Chandler's syndrome, with only corneal edema, and Cogan-Reese syndrome (iris nevus syndrome), characterized by pigmented iris nodules (stroma "pinched up" by cellular membrane), and essential iris atrophy from cellular membrane that contracts over the iris stroma, causing progressive iris atrophy, ectropion uvea, and stretch or melting iris holes. Yellow-colored PAS are pathognomic. ALT is ineffective; may try filtering surgery, but internal failure is common; often need an aqueous shunt. Profile: middle-aged 40-year-old female without family history or systemic disease. See also Chapter 3.
  - Neovascular glaucoma (NVG): anterior segment angiogenesis usually stimulated by VEGF released from hypoxic retina. Etiologies include PDR (50%), ischemic CRVO (up to 60% of cases get NVG; also known as "90-day glaucoma"), ocular ischemic syndrome, chronic RD, uveitis, melanoma, and RB (50%). Treat associated inflammation with steroids; use atropine to stabilize the blood–aqueous barrier and topical glaucoma medications as needed. If proliferative retinopathy is present, perform PRP. Trabeculectomy has a high failure rate; thus, typically use antimetabolites or implant a glaucoma filtering device.
  - Posterior polymorphous membrane dystrophy (PPMD): 15% incidence of glaucoma; autosomal dominant bilateral endothelial abnormality with endothelialization of angle, iris atrophy, and corectopia like ICE. PAS tend to close angle. Vesicles may be seen on Descemet's membrane with large dark areas on specular microscopy (ICE has dark areas within cells). See also Chapter 3.
- Posterior "pushing" mechanism: usually myopic shift, diffusely shallow AC, and poor response to LPI. If bilateral, consider possibility of drug reaction causing choroidal swelling with forward ciliary body rotation that pushes the lens–iris diaphragm forward and secondarily closes the angle.
  - Aqueous misdirection, ciliary block, "malignant" glaucoma: increased IOP from misdirected aqueous flow into the vitreous cavity that increases the vitreous volume, pushing the lens–iris

diaphragm forward and secondarily closing the angle. Usually occurs post-operatively (especially after trabeculectomy).

- Risk: ACG, nanophthalmos (increased choroidal effusions), intumescent lens, exfoliation, and history of aqueous misdirection
- Treat early before IOP >25 mmHg with aqueous suppressant medications and atropine (cycloplegic causes posterior displacement of the lens). May need to disrupt anterior hyaloid face (i.e., with YAG laser), and may need vitrectomy. Avoid miotics (cholinergics), as they exacerbate the block and increase inflammation.

- Contracting retrolental tissue: seen with retinopathy of prematurity or PHPV.
- CRVO: forward lens displacement from increased vitreous volume and fluid transudation.
- Uveal effusion syndrome, nanophthalmos: small eye (axial length <20 mm) and thus shallow AC plus uveal effusions that cause an anterior shift in the lens–iris diaphragm, causing ACG. Patients have abnormal and thickened sclera. Avoid intraocular surgery if possible. Dictum: "Beware the phakic patient with aphakic spectacles."
- Others: posterior uveitis such as VKH, scleral buckle (5% have shallow AC; vortex vein occlusion may cause ciliary body congestion and forward rotation), heavy PRP (CB swelling with forward rotation; treat with cycloplegics, steroids, iridoplasty), tumor, and choroidal hemorrhage or effusion.

BLIND, PAINFUL EYE WITH END-STAGE GLAUCOMA Treat with topical cycloplegic and steroid for comfort (may use aqueous suppressants for comfort but not necessarily for IOP control). Consider evisceration.

Surgery

ARGON LASER TRABECULOPLASTY (ALT) Laser with gonioprism used to place burns at the junction of the anterior and posterior TM to contract the tissue under the burn and to stretch open the spaces between the laser spots. Increases TM outflow (does not "punch holes" in the TM) and also "tickles" the TM endothelium to increase metabolic activity.

- Most useful for the "three P's"—**p**seudoexfoliation, **p**igmentary glaucoma, **P**OAG. Phakic, older patients as well as patients with more pigmented TM are more responsive. Typically use after patients have failed 2–3 drops; usually buys 6 months to 2 years before surgery is needed.

- Laser lenses include Goldmann three mirror (59 degrees), Thorpe four mirror (62 degrees), and Ritch trabeculoplasty lens (59 degrees, 64 degrees, and 17 D button). Laser settings: 0.1 second, 50 μm, and 400–1000 mW to make a tiny bubble or see blanching. Usually treat inferior 180 degrees and maybe treat the other 180 degrees if good effect. Postoperatively treat with alpha-agonist and steroid drop for 7 days.
- Check IOP in 6 to 8 weeks to assess efficacy. Eighty percent of POAG patients have 30% IOP decrease persisting to 1 year, decreasing to 50% at 5 years.
  - Glaucoma Laser Trial (GLT): a multicenter, randomized clinical trial designed to assess the efficacy and safety of starting treatment for POAG with ALT versus timolol 0.5% bid. ALT patients' IOP was 1–2 mmHg lower at 2 years, but 50% of patients required addition of medications. In the Glaucoma Laser Trial Follow-up Study (GLTFS), the ALT treated eyes required fewer medications, had 1.2 mmHg lower IOP, improved VF, and more stable and less variable IOP. It concluded that treatment with ALT was at least as efficacious as initial treatment with topical medication.
  - Advanced Glaucoma Intervention Study (AGIS): a multicenter, randomized clinical trial evaluating two treatment sequences in medically uncontrolled open-angle glaucoma. Many conclusions were drawn, including confirmation of increased risk of cataract formation following trabeculectomy, identification of risk factors for failure of ALT and trabeculectomy, and differential response to surgical treatment between black and white patients. African-American patients with advanced glaucoma benefited from ALT prior to trabeculectomy, which was not the case for Caucasian patients.
- Complications: if laser is placed in the posterior TM, may have tentlike PAS, IOP spike, inflammation, or pain (long posterior ciliary arteries at 3 and 9 o'clock). Do not perform ALT in eyes with active inflammation.

CYCLODESTRUCTIVE PROCEDURES End-stage glaucoma may use cyclocryotherapy (very painful and inflammatory) or the preferred cyclophotocoagulation (CPC) with the diode or YAG laser (case of sympathetic ophthalmia reported). Diode laser CPC: use "G probe," 810 nm wavelength, 16 to 18 applications, 1 to 2 seconds, 1.5–2.5 W. The diode has 71% scleral transmission and greater melanin absorption than YAG laser; about 50% of patients need retreatment.

GONIOTOMY Knife or needle tip swept into angle for congenital glaucoma. Just scratch angle; should not see blood or feel grit. There is a 70% success rate.

LASER IRIDOPLASTY OR GONIOPLASTY Large burns in the midperipheral iris used to pull iris root out of the TM for plateau iris syndrome, narrow angles, nanophthalmos, or other posterior-pushing ACG. Typical settings: argon laser 200–500 μm, 0.2 to 0.5 second, 300 mW, 24 spots total.

LASER PERIPHERAL IRIDOTOMY (LPI) Used to bypass RPB. Use pilocarpine preoperatively to tighten iris. Lenses may have a magnification button such as Abraham lens (66 D button) or Wise lens (103 D, more magnification and thus less laser energy required).

- Usually place LPI superonasal. May use argon or YAG lasers, and many clinicians begin with argon laser to photocoagulate (suggested settings: 50 μm, 500 mW, 0.1 second applied in a cloverleaf pattern) followed by YAG laser (2–5 mJ); often will see gush of fluid out of posterior chamber. If iris is bleeding, apply gentle pressure on the lens. Patency is not guaranteed by transillumination defects (best if the anterior lens capsule is seen).
- Postoperatively, usually treat with an alpha-agonist and steroid for 1 week. Dilate 1 to 2 weeks after treatment to break any posterior synechiae. Complications include IOP spike, inflammation, and lens opacity (caution in young phakic patients; may not even require direct damage).

SHUNTS Tube placed into the AC or PC that shunts fluid to a bleb, which is kept patent by a reservoir plate. May be valveless like Baerveldt and Molteno drainage devices (free flowing; thus, increased risk of early hypotony; can stent tube with suture, which can be removed after 6 weeks when plate is fibrosed), or may have pressure-sensitive valves like Ahmed and Krupin devices.

SUTURE LYSIS May use Hoskins or other lens to stabilize the eye and blanch the conjunctival vessels. Red laser is better if subconjunctival hemorrhage is present, as in the immediate postoperative period; otherwise, green laser is standard, usually at 50 μm, 600 mW.

TRABECULECTOMY The goal is to preserve vision when maximal tolerated medical therapy (MTMT) is insufficient to control VF loss. The procedure is 80 to 90% effective in Caucasian POAG patients over 65 years old to maintain IOP <21 mmHg. May be full thickness (not commonly used now; has thin cystic overhanging blebs, low IOP, and flat AC) or partial thickness, guarded (thicker blebs). Partial thickness trabeculectomies may be limbal-based (high, easily visible blebs) or fornix-based (diffuse, poorly defined blebs).

- Preoperative treatment: stop echothiophate 3 weeks prior, stop NSAIDs 2 weeks prior, and stop oral carbonic anhydrase inhibitors

1 day before surgery (may cause postoperative hypotony). Inspect the conjunctiva, and document a recent automated VF.

- Technique: usually superotemporal location (inferior associated with increased endophthalmitis). Limbal-based technique: incise conjunctiva 8–10 mm posterior to limbus, and dissect down to bare sclera. Judicious use of cautery (prevent chemotactic, fibroblast proliferation, but prevent charring), and dissect forward to the limbus. Apply antimetabolite if desired on a sponge for 3 to 5 minutes before the eye is entered. Create a partial-thickness conjunctival flap, then enter the AC. Use a punch (e.g., Kelly Descemet's punch) to remove tissue above the TM at Schwalbe's line. Create a PI, then suture the flap (as many as are needed to create a nearly watertight closure). Send tissue from repeat trabeculectomies for pathology to rule out epithelial ingrowth.
- Postoperative treatment: steroids are key to prevent episcleral fibrosis. Patency requires flow: if there is no flow, the flap will fibrose within 2 to 3 weeks or 2 to 3 months if antimetabolite is used. Keep open by laser suture lysis, digital pressure massage (finger on lower eyelid, applying gentle pressure for 20 seconds on and 20 seconds off). Also use topical antibiotics; may use cycloplegics (deepens the AC, stabilizes blood–ocular barrier, and offers ciliary spasm relief).

TRABECULECTOMY WITH ANTIMETABOLITES Indications for use (and risk factors for bleb failure): age <65, uveitis, neovascularization, previous ocular surgery (failed trabeculectomy, aphakia, pseudophakia), non-Caucasion (especially African-American patients). Avoid in high myopes (thin sclera with possible buckling and choroidal folds).

- 5-fluorouracil (5-FU): antifibroblastic cell-cycle specific; may cause corneal epithelial toxicity. Fluorouracil Filtering Surgery Study (FFSS): a randomized, controlled clinical trial comparing the success rate of standard glaucoma filtering surgery with and without adjunctive 5-FU treatment. 5-FU was beneficial after previous failed filtering surgery and in aphakic/pseudophakic eyes.
- Mitomycin C: antibiotic from *Streptomyces caespitosus*, DNA alkylating agent; not cell-cycle specific, may cause intraocular toxicity.

TRABECULECTOMY POSTOPERATIVE COMPLICATIONS

- Bleb-associated endophthalmitis: early onset, most commonly from staphylococcal species; late-onset, *S. pneumoniae* is the primary organism, also *Hemophilus influenza.* Increased risk with thin wall bleb, inferior location, and antimetabolite use.
- Bleb failure: leading cause is episcleral fibrosis; may also be from internal ostomy obstruction by iris, vitreous, or lens. Risk factors for failure: aphakia, uveitis, iris NV, young patient, African-American patients, and previous ocular surgery. Try needling if there is a failed

high, thick, elevated, encapsulated bleb. Subconjunctival 5-FU injection within the first 2 weeks postoperative may prevent scarring. Repeat trabeculectomy for scarred, flat bleb.

- Bleb leak: causes mild discomfort, tearing, blurred VA with shallow AC, low IOP, and low or flat bleb that is usually Seidel positive. Risks: high, thin, ischemic bleb usually after full-thickness filtering or antifibrotic use. Treat with pressure patch, aqueous suppressants, and BSCL; hold steroids, and consider compression suture. If severe AC reaction or hypopyon, suspect endophthalmitis.
- Choroidal (suprachoroidal) hemorrhage: flat AC, normal or increased IOP; fundus shows dark choroidal effusions that may be seen on ultrasound. Usually onset in early postoperative period, with a dull headache on affected side exacerbated by head lowering or Valsalva maneuver. May cause AC shallowing with no relief with PI, and can be observed if limited to moderate size. Treat with steroids, cycloplegics, analgesics, and aqueous suppressants. If necessary, may drain choroidals, but it is usually better to wait or, if necessary, to reform the AC with viscoelastic and let the hemorrhage resolve.
- Corneal dellen: corneal drying and thinning from adjacent high bleb; treat with lubrication.
- Hypotony: may cause corneal edema, shallow AC, ciliary body detachment, maculopathy, or ocular discomfort.

TABLE 4–1

Differential Diagnosis of Shallow Anterior Chamber after Filtering Surgery

IOP (mmHg)	Bleb	Problem	Treatment
<10	Elevated	Excessive filtration	Conservative; elevate head of bed, avoid Valsalva and ocular pressure
<10	Flat	1. Conjunctival leak 2. Ciliochoroidal detachment (may have cyclodialysis cleft) 3. RD	BSCL, resuture, or reoperate
Normal or elevated	Flat	1. Aqueous misdirection 2. Suprachoroidal effusion or hemorrhage 3. Pupillary block 4. Obstruction of internal ostomy	1. Vitrectomy or YAG laser the anterior hyaloid face 2. Observation 3. PI

- Hypotony maculopathy: especially prevalent with antimetabolite use, primary procedure, and in young myopes (more elastic sclera). Attempt to slow filtration with a pressure patch, BSCL, or blood patch, or reform AC with viscoelastic. If present >3 months, may cause permanent macular changes.
- Choroidal effusion/detachment: decreased IOP; see large choroidal effusions. Maximal on postoperative day 5; can usually observe without treatment.
- Flat AC (Table 4–1): if lens–cornea touch, immediate intervention is required to prevent corneal decompensation and cataract. If iris–cornea touch, can observe for a short time.
  - Grade 1: peripheral iris touch; usually resolves spontaneously.
  - Grade 2: pupil margin touch; reform the AC with BSS or viscoelastic via paracentesis, and treat increased IOP.
  - Grade 3: flat chamber, lens touch, emergency; must reform the AC (30 gauge needle at slit lamp).
- Malignant glaucoma, aqueous misdirection syndrome: treat with cycloplegic and possible vitrectomy; see earlier discussion.
- Pupillary block: flat AC, normal or increased IOP, and normal fundus without choroidal effusions.
- Tenon's cyst: vascular localized bleb with abrupt transition from conjunctiva to bleb, often with increased IOP. Usually just observe.

TRABECULOTOMY For congenital glaucoma with cloudy cornea. Forked knife or suture placed into Schlemm's canal that is then rotated or pulled, tearing canal opening in the AC; should see blood.

CHAPTER 5

Uveal Tract and Ocular Inflammation

Iris

IRIS ANATOMY (FIG. 5–1) Dimensions: 12 mm diameter, 37.5 mm circumference (length of Schlemm's canal); root of iris 0.18 mm thick, midstroma 0.5 mm; thickest at collarette. Radial vessels run from the major arterial circle at the root from two long posterior ciliary arteries and seven anterior ciliary arteries, with a minor circle under the collarette. Surface anatomy from outside in: peripheral crypts, ciliary iris, collarette, Fuchs' crypts, and pupil. Anterior iris has melanocytes, fibroblasts, and capillaries (increased with rubeosis or pseudorubeosis from iritis). Stroma is composed of collagen, GAG ground substance, channels, and clump cells (macrophages). Stromal pigmentation (neural crest origin) gives iris color, and resident melanocytes are postmitotic and not reactive like the RPE (thus the patency of PI). The iris is an extension of the choroid, which is attached to the sclera only at the vortex vein ostia (the cause of the cloverleaf pattern seen with choroidal effusions) and at the scleral spur.

- The iris dilator and sphincter muscles arise from the IPE. The dilator has sympathetic innervation that also stimulates pigmentation (thus, congenital Horner's syndrome has light-colored irides). The sphincter muscle has cholinergic innervation. Fuchs' and Michel's spurs connect the sphincter and dilator muscles; thus, when the iris contricts, it stretches the dilator muscle and vice versa. The iris constrictor shortens by 80% (unusual for a muscle) and thus needs crypts to allow for increased movement.
- Iris pigment epithelium (IPE): bilayer of anterior nonpigmented epithelium and posterior pigmented cells are in an apical-to-apical arrangement (like the ciliary body). Iris cysts form if the apical junction breaks down. Poor iris dilation is seen in patients with PXS from basement membrane material deposited into the muscle. Histopathologically, lacy vacuolization represents glycogen deposits seen in diabetic patients.

IRIS COLOBOMA Usually inferonasal.

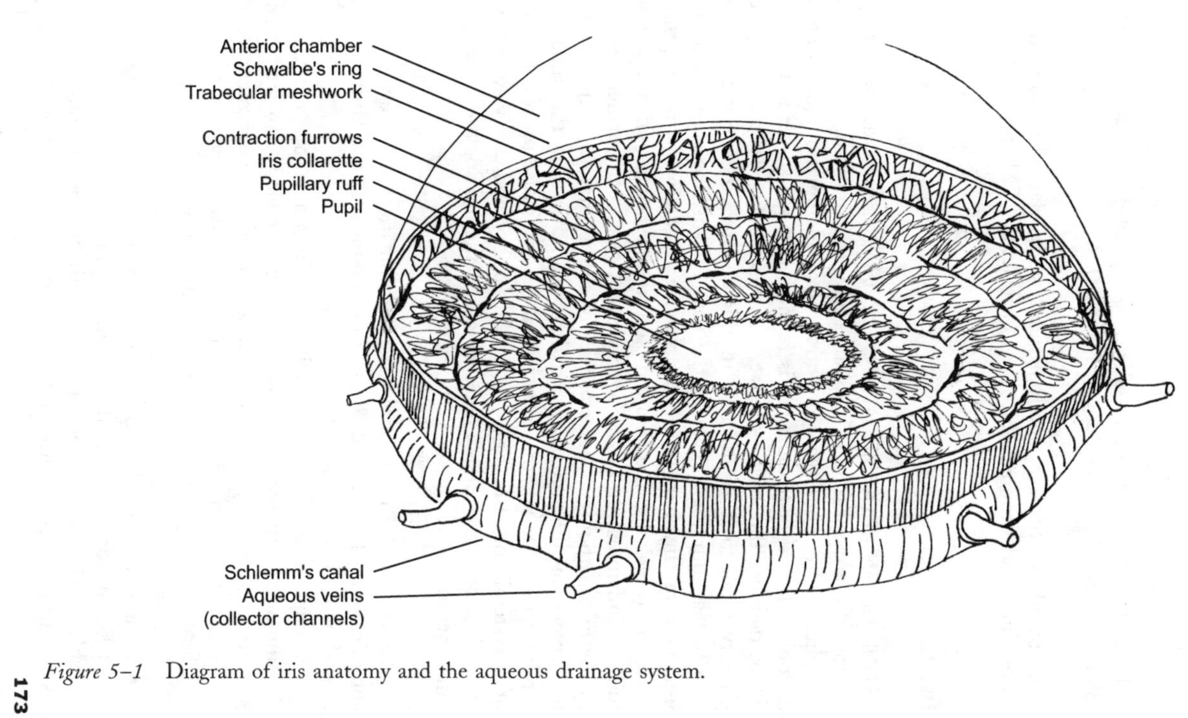

Figure 5–1 Diagram of iris anatomy and the aqueous drainage system.

IRIS MELANOMA Concern for melanoma if pigmented iris lesion is >2 mm. Increased risk of metastatic cancer increases with age, increased IOP, tumor in angle, extraocular extension, and prior surgery, but not the type of cells seen on pathology. There is a 5% risk of metastatic cancer at 10 years.

IRIDODIALYSIS Tear in root of iris; distinguish from coloboma (which is inferonasal and has the sphincter involved).

IRIDOSCHISIS Seen in elderly patients, with bilateral inferior iris stomal "shredding" and atrophy, which may obstruct the TM and cause glaucoma.

Uveitis

DEFINITION AND CLASSIFICATION *Uveitis* is broadly defined as inflammation of the uveal tract (iris, ciliary body, and choroid). The definition is complicated by other types of intraocular inflammation (e.g., infections, endophthalmitis, or toxoplasmosis retinitis that spills over to the choroid). Thus, defining the uveitic diseases involves careful classification as to the primary tissue that is affected. In this chapter, the uveitic diseases are classified as anterior (involving the iris and anterior segment primarily), intermediate (involving the pars plana and anterior vitreous primarily), posterior (involving the choroid and retina primarily), and panuveitis (diffuse inflammation of ocular tissues). Uveitis can further be classified by the histopathologic characteristics of granulomatous or nongranulomatous types of inflammation. Further delineation of the inflammation can be made as to whether it is a local ocular disease process only or part of a systemic disease. Thus, a careful history and a review of systems are important first steps in elucidating the etiology of the patient's inflammation.

GOALS OF THERAPY Suppress the inflammation and prevent secondary complications. Ten percent of cases of blindness in the United States are caused by uveitis complications.

- Complete elimination of all active inflammation and cells: most important therapeutic goal, because allowing chronic, even low grade (1 + cells), uveitis eventually produces permanent structural damage, such as chronic macular edema with cyst or macular hole formation, cyclitic membrane formation with hypotony, and ON damage.
- Limitation of total steroid used: long-term use of corticosteroids has a 100% incidence of significant undesirable side effects.

Tables 5–1 and 5–2 present diagnostic uveitis laboratory tests, and associations between uveitis and human leukocyte antigens (HLA).

TABLE 5–1

Selected Diagnostic Uveitis Laboratory Tests

Laboratory Test	Indication and Comments
ACE level	Elevated in two thirds of patients with active sarcoidosis
ANA	Family of antinuclear antibodies that are elevated in collagen-vascular diseases, particularly SLE and RA
C-ANCA	Cytoplasmic staining pattern of IgG autoantibodies against PMN antigen; 90% sensitive and specific for Wegener's granulomatosis
P-ANCA	Perinuclear staining pattern of IgG autoantibodies against PMN antigen; positive with microscopic PAN and Churg-Strauss syndrome, and also positive occasionally in Wegener's granulomatosis and crescentic glomerulonephritis
CBC	Elevated white cell count with infection or leukemia; eosinophilia with systemic toxocariasis, atopy, or Churg-Strauss syndrome; lymphopenia with SLE and HIV
ESR/CRP/C-25	Nonspecific inflammation and immune system activation
Hepatitis B surface antigen	Positive in 40% of PAN
Herpes virus antibodies	Because the prevalence of seropositivity is so high in the general population, a positive titer is virtually meaningless; however, a negative titer all but eliminates herpes from consideration; in contrast, antigen sampling with PCR amplification from an intraocular specimen is very specific
HIV tests	Antibodies against HIV are detected by ELISA and confirmed by Western blot test; in addition, T-lymphocyte levels are decreased in HIV infection, notably with a decreased ratio of CD4+ (T-helper) relative to CD8+ (T-suppressor) cells
Lyme serologies	ELISA immunoassay followed by confirmatory Western blot test for *Borrelia burgdorferi*; may be false-negative if early in the infection; false-positive result may be seen with syphilis or collagen vascular disorders
Lysozyme levels	Tend to parallel ACE levels, but may be a more sensitive indicator of active pulmonary saroidosis
Raj immune complexes	Circulating IgG
Rheumatoid factor (RF)	Class of autoantibodies (usually IgM) against the Fc fragment of IgG; seropositivity is nonspecific and may occur in a number of collagen vascular disorders, but 80% of patients with RA are RF positive

(*Continued*)

TABLE 5–1 (*Continued*)

Laboratory Test	Indication and Comments
Syphilis serologies	Antitreponemal tests (FTA-ABS and MHA-TP) are nearly 100% sensitive and specific regardless of infection stage, remain positive for life, and thus are the best screening tests for prior exposure; the nontreponemal tests (VDRL and RPR) detect antilipoidal Ab produced during active treponemal infection and reflect disease activity and thus may be used to gauge response to therapy; however, they may also have false-negative rates up to 30% in latent secondary syphilis and false-positive results in autoimmune disease and other spirochete infections (e.g., Lyme disease); both indirect and direct tests may be false-negative in patients with AIDS
Toxoplasma antibodies	Elevated ELISA IgM and IgG titers are always significant; IgM may remain elevated up to a year after infection; Sabin-Feldman dye test is the most sensitive and specific but availability is limited
Urine analysis	Proteinemia, hematuria or casts in Wegener's granulomatosis or SLE

Signs and Symptoms and Clinical Presentations of Uveitis

ACCOMMODATIVE DEFICIENCY Sympathetic ophthalmia

ACUTE UVEITIS Behçet's syndrome, VKH, toxoplasmosis, and acute multifocal placoid pigment epitheliopathy (AMPPE)

AFRICAN-AMERICAN PATIENTS Sarcoid and SLE have higher prevalence in African-American patients

AGE <20 YEARS Juvenile rheumatoid arthritis (JRA), toxoplasmosis, toxocariasis, and masquerade (RB, leukemia, JXG)

AGE 20 TO 60 YEARS Most uveitis occurs in this age group, including HLA-B27, sarcoid, Fuchs' heterochromic iridocyclitis (HIC), VKH, and SLE

AGE >60 YEARS Serpiginous choroidopathy, birdshot retinochoroidopathy, ARN, and masquerade (large cell lymphoma, uveal melanoma, metastatic CA, paraneoplastic)

AMBLYOPIA Toxoplasmosis or toxocariasis, causing a macular lesion

TABLE 5–2
Uveitis and Human Leukocyte Antigen (HLA) Associations

HLA	Disease Association
HLA Class I Antigens	
A1	Sarcoidosis
A11	Sympathetic ophthalmia
A29	Birdshot retinochoroidopathy (highest HLA disease association known)
B8	Uveitis in African-American patients, atopic disease
B27	Anterior uveitis, Reiter's syndrome, psoriatic arthropathy, inflammatory bowel disease, Whipple's disease, ankylosing spondylitis
B51, B12	Behçet's syndrome
HLA Class II Antigens	
DR1	RA
DR2, DR3	SLE
DR4	VKH, RA
DR8	JRA
DRw53	VKH

Note: HLA are gene products derived from the major histocompatability complex (located on chromosome 6q). HLA Class I antigens (A, B, and C subtypes) are present on almost every cell and mediate antigen presentation to cytotoxic T cells (CD8+). HLA Class II antigens (DR, DP, and DQ subtypes) are present on B cells and macrophages and mediate antigen presentation to helper T cells (CD4+). The HLA-DR region appears to exert its effect on autoantibodies.

APHTHOUS ORAL ULCERS Behçet's syndrome, mucocutaneous lymph node syndrome (MCLNS), OCP, SJS, SLE, HSV, Reiter's syndrome, ulcerative colitis, and Crohn's disease

ARTERIOLAR VASCULITIS PAN, SLE, ARN, Behçet's syndrome, and idiopathic. Less common than venulitis.

ARTHRALGIAS/ARTHRITIS Ankylosing spondylitis, JRA, Behçet's syndrome, sarcoidosis, Reiter's syndrome, SLE, relapsing polychondritis, Wegener's granulomatosis, inflammatory bowel disease (ulcerative colitis, Crohn's disease, Whipple's disease), RA, syphilis, brucellosis, psoriatic, Lyme disease, sporotrichosis, and gonococcal

ASIAN/MIDDLE EASTERN ANCESTRY Behçet's syndrome and VKH are more prevalent in these patients

ASTHMA/WHEEZE Systemic toxocara, tuberculosis, ascariasis, aspergillosis, Churg-Strauss syndrome, and sarcoidosis

BAND KERATOPATHY JRA, sarcoidosis, multiple myeloma, and chronic uveitis in children

BILATERAL CN VII PALSY Lyme disease and sarcoidosis

CASE HISTORIES AND WORK-UP

- Child with red, inflamed eye: many possible etiologies of inflammation, but always rule out RB.
- Child with recurrent or chronic iridocyclitis may have hypopyon, often white-appearing eye: get ANA (on two substrates; usually positive), RF (usually negative), and HLA-B8 to rule out JRA.
- Choroiditis with exudative retinal detachment and a history of episodic tinnitus: get fluorescein angiogram and audiometry, spinal tap, and MRI scanning of the brain to rule out VKH.
- Elderly female with new onset "vitritis," partially steroid sensitive: get vitreal biopsy for culture, cytology, and cytokines to rule out intraocular lymphoma or infection.
- Female with pars planitis and a history of episodic paresthesias: get MRI scanning of brain and spinal tap to rule out multiple sclerosis.
- Granulomatous uveitis: consider chest x-ray, serum ACE, serum lysozyme, serum calcium, liver function enzymes and bilirubin, intradermal skin tests, upper body gallium scan, and chest CT scan to rule out sarcoidosis or tuberculosis.
- Multifocal choroiditis, primarily posterior pole in a 35-year-old male: check HLA-A29, ERG to rule out birdshot choroiditis.
- Patient with erythema nodosum, alopecia, vitiligo, poliosis: likely VKH.
- Recurrent uveitis with a history of episodic diarrhea, possibly with mucus or blood in the stool: get gastroenterologist consultation with endoscopy and biopsy to rule out inflammatory bowel disease.
- Recurrent uveitis with a history of low back stiffness upon awakening: get HLA-B27 and lumbosacral spine films to rule out ankylosing spondylitis.
- Retinal vasculitis and a history of recurrent aphthous ulcers and pretibial skin lesions: consider biopsy of the skin lesions, HLA-B51, and HLA-B27 to rule out Behçet's syndrome.
- Retinal vasculitis with a history of subacute sinusitis: consider chest x-ray, sinus films, urine analysis, and serum ANCA to rule out Wegener's granulomatosis.
- Retinochoroiditis adjacent to a pigmented chorioretinal scar: get antitoxoplasma IgG and IgM antibodies to rule out toxoplasmosis.

- Unilateral iridocyclitis with fine white KP and a lighter iris in the affected eye: evaluate the lens, IOP, and gonioscopy to rule out Fuchs' HIC.

CHILDHOOD ANTERIOR UVEITIS JRA, ankylosing spondylitis, Behçet's syndrome, sarcoid, trauma, Fuchs' HIC, HSV, and tuberculosis

CHILDHOOD INTERMEDIATE UVEITIS Pars planitis

CHILDHOOD PANUVEITIS Pars planitis, sarcoidosis, VKH, and masquerade (leukemia, retinoblastoma)

CHILDHOOD POSTERIOR UVEITIS Toxoplasmosis and toxocariasis

CHOROIDITIS, CHORIORETINITIS, RETINAL PIGMENT EPITHELIITIS VKH, serpiginous choroidopathy, sympathetic ophthalmia, multifocal chorioretinitis and panuveitis (MCP), septic multifocal choroiditis, punctate inner choroidopathy, uveal effusion, sarcoidosis, syphilis, tuberculosis, candidiasis, ocular histoplasmosis syndrome (OHS), birdshot retinochoroidopathy, acute retinal pigment epitheliitis (ARPE), AMPPE, unilateral "wipe-out" syndrome of Gass (diffuse unilateral subacute neuroretinitis [DUSN], toxocariasis), and CMV inclusion

CHRONIC UVEITIS JRA, birdshot retinochoroidopathy, serpiginous choroidopathy, tuberculosis, *Propionibacterium acnes* infection, lymphoma, sympathetic ophthalmia, sarcoidosis, and MCP

COUGH OR PULMONARY INVOLVEMENT OHS, sarcoidosis, tuberculosis, coccidiomycosis, Wegener's granulomatosis, *Pneumocystis carinii*, malignancy, Churg-Strauss syndrome, and aspergillosis

DIARRHEA Inflammatory bowel disease (Crohn's disease, ulcerative colitis, Whipple's disease), Cogan's syndrome, AIDS or AIDS-related complex, amoeba, mucormycosis, giardiasis, ascariasis, and schistosomiasis

EAR, AUDITORY, OR VESTIBULAR SYMPTOMS Relapsing polychondritis, Wegener's granulomatosis, Cogan's syndrome, VKH, sarcoidosis, syphilis, GCA, and Eales' disease

EPIDIDYMITIS PAN and Behçet's syndrome

FEMALE PREPONDERANCE JRA, AMPPE, acute zonal occult outer retinopathy (AZOOR, 90% are female), birdshot retinochoroidopathy (vitiliginous chorioretinitis), multiple evanescent white-dot syndrome

(MEWDS, 80%), punctate inner choroidopathy (PIC, 70%), subretinal fibrosis and uveitis syndrome (SFU, 100%), sarcoidosis, VKH (60%), acute macular neuroretinopathy (AMN, 95%), acute idiopathic blind spot enlargement syndrome (AIBSE, 85%), and MCP (75%)

FEVER Reiter's syndrome, Behçet's syndrome, PAN, GCA, colitis, AIDS-related complex/AIDS, Whipple's disease, HZV, tuberculosis, brucellosis, leptospirosis, Lyme disease, candidiasis, coccidiomycosis, amoeba, mucormycosis, Cogan's syndrome, serum sickness, trypanosomiasis, and VKH

FLU OR MONONUCLEOSIS-LIKE Histoplasmosis, leptospirosis, toxoplasmosis, CMV, AMPPE, ARPE, MEWDS, and ascariasis

GENITAL SORES OR ULCERS Reiter's syndrome, Behçet's syndrome, syphilis, and OCP

GEOGRAPHY Coccidiomycosis (U.S. Southwest desert), histoplasmosis (Mississippi River valley), Lyme disease (everywhere in the United States, especially the Northeast), and cysticercosis (Central and South America)

GLAUCOMA Posner-Schlossman syndrome (glaucomatocyclitic crisis), HSV, HZV, Fuchs' HIC, JRA, sarcoidosis, intraocular lymphoma, VKH, sympathetic ophthalmia, Behçet's syndrome, toxoplasmosis, rubella iridocyclitis, and any severe chronic iridocyclitis. However, uveitis usually has lower IOP.

HEADACHE OR MENINGITIS VKH, sarcoidosis, Behçet's syndrome, cryptococcus, HSV, histoplasmosis, leptospirosis, sympathetic ophthalmia, toxoplasmosis, tuberculosis, Lyme disease, HZV, brucellosis, intraocular lymphoma, uveal effusion, Whipple's disease, Churg-Strauss syndrome, PAN, and giardiasis

"HEALTHY" PATIENTS DUSN, pars planitis, HSV, OHS, toxoplasmosis, toxocariasis, traumatic, Fuchs' HIC, birdshot retinochoroidopathy, sympathetic ophthalmia, MEWDS, AMPPE, ARPE, MCP, serpiginous choroidopathy

HEMATURIA PAN, SLE, and Wegener's granulomatosis

HEPATOSPLENOMEGALY CMV, toxocariasis, toxoplasmosis, leptospirosis, AIDS, brucellosis, and sarcoidosis

IRIS NODULES Sarcoidosis, tuberculosis, syphilis, herpetic retinitis, and leprosy

JAUNDICE Brucellosis, schistosomiasis, leptospirosis, and CMV

MALE PREPONDERANCE HLA-B27 and Eales' disease

MASQUERADES OF UVEITIS Congenital (PHPV, myopia), metabolic (amyloid, cholesterolosis, asteroid), vascular (Coats' disease, CRVO, systemic hypertension), trauma (IOFB, RD, ghost cell, phacolytic, anterior segment ischemia), neoplastic (intraocular lymphoma, leukemia, retinoblastoma, MM, systemic lymphoma), and infectious disease (endophthalmitis)

MEDICATIONS Sulfa, pamidronate disodium (inhibits bone resorption in osteoporosis), rifabutin (treatment for *Mycobacterium avium*), and cidofovir (treatment for CMV)

NEPHRITIS Vasculitis (PAN, Wegener's granulomatosis, etc.), Behçet's syndrome, tuberculosis, sarcoidosis, toxoplasmosis, Cogan's syndrome, cryoglobulinemia, and tubulointerstitial nephritis–uveitis (TINU) syndrome

NEURITIS, CRANIAL Syphilis, Lyme disease, sarcoidosis, subacute sclerosing panencephalitis, and Churg-Strauss syndrome

NEURITIS, PERIPHERAL Lyme disease, leprosy, HZV, sarcoidosis, multiple sclerosis, and Behçet's syndrome

NIGHT SWEATS Tuberculosis, coccidiomycosis, and sarcoidosis

PERIPAPILLARY CHOROIDITIS Tuberculosis (Jensen's disease), toxoplasmosis, and toxocariasis

PHARYNGITIS, TONSILLITIS Sarcoidosis, viral infection, candidiasis, AIDS-related complex/AIDS, Whipple's disease, and gonococcal

PNEUMONIA, PNEUMONITIS CMV, AIDS-related complex/AIDS, sarcoidosis, Wegener's granulomatosis, SLE, Whipple's disease, coccidiomycosis, aspergillosis, and sporotrichosis

POOR HANDWASHING Toxoplasmosis toxocariasis

POSTERIOR INFLAMMATION Toxoplasmosis (18%), idiopathic vasculitis (18%), idiopathic choroiditis (18%), OHS (10%), toxocariasis (7%), CMV retinitis (6%), idiopathic retinitis (6%), serpiginous choroidopathy, AMPPE, ARN, birdshot retinochoroidopathy, leukemia, intraocular lymphoma, candidiasis, tuberculosis, and SLE

PROSTATITIS, CYSTITIS Whipple's disease, Reiter's syndrome, ankylosing spondylitis, and gonococcal

PSYCHOSIS VKH, sarcoidosis, Behçet's syndrome, SLE, and steroids

"QUIET EYE" JRA, pars planitis, Fuchs' HIC, Behçet's syndrome, sarcoidosis, syphilis, toxocariasis, IOFB, CMV retinitis, masquerade syndromes, and most posterior uveitic diseases

RAW MEAT Toxoplasmosis and cysticercosis

RECENT EYE SURGERY Endophthalmitis, lens-induced, sympathetic ophthalmia, and iritis from anterior segment ischemia after strabismus surgery

RETINAL ARTERIAL OBSTRUCTION FROM INFLAMMATION Collagen vascular diseases and vasculitis (PAN, SLE, GCA, Wegener's granulomatosis, Behçet's syndrome), toxoplasmosis, and Lyme disease

RETINAL PERIPHLEBITIS Tuberculosis, Eales' disease, syphilis, sarcoidosis, and multiple sclerosis

RETINAL VASCULITIS Infectious (DUSN, HZV, syphilis, toxoplasmosis, CMV, ARN, larval embolization), immune (idiopathic, Eales' disease, Behçet's syndrome, Kawasaki disease, PAN, GCA, Wegener's granulomatosis, pars planitis, sarcoidosis, primary Sjögren's syndrome, multiple sclerosis, SLE, Takayasu's disease, Berger's disease (thromboangiitis obliterans), and vascular causes (hemoglobinopathies, severe systemic hypertension, hyperviscosity syndrome, diabetes mellitus)

RETINAL "WIPEOUT" Bilateral acute retinal necrosis (BARN), Behçet's syndrome, PAN, and DUSN

RPE DETACHMENT VKH, sympathetic ophthalmia, intraocular lymphoma, and leukemia

RPE DROPOUT Birdshot retinochoroidopathy, SFU, MEWDS, ARN, Behçet's syndrome, DUSN, and PAN

RPE HYPERPLASIA RP, syphilis, PIC, ARPE, VKH, and AMPPE

SADDLE NOSE Syphilis (congenital), Wegener's granulomatosis, and relapsing polychondritis

SCLERITIS, DIFFUSE Vasculitis (RA, Wegener's granulomatosis, SLE, PAN, relapsing polychondritis, Takayasu's disease), syphilis, HSV, HZV,

Reiter's syndrome, VKH, toxoplasmosis, tuberculosis, inflammatory bowel disease, Behçet's syndrome, sarcoidosis, leprosy, mumps, and masquerade (melanoma)

SCLERITIS, SECTORAL Tuberculosis, gout, and syphilis

SECTORAL IRIS ATROPHY HSV, HZV, previous attacks of angle closure glaucoma, and Fuchs' HIC

"SICK ANIMAL" EXPOSURE Brucellosis and trichinosis

SINUSITIS Wegener's granulomatosis, sarcoidosis, Whipple's disease, Churg-Strauss syndrome, relapsing polychondritis, and mucormycosis

SKIN NODULES Behçet's syndrome, ulcerative colitis, histoplasmosis, sarcoidosis, Crohn's disease, AMPPE, leprosy, and onchocerciasis

SKIN RASH Behçet's syndrome, syphilis, Lyme disease (erythema chronicum migrans), rubella, rubeola, Reiter's syndrome (keratoderma blennorrhagicum), leprosy, toxoplasmosis, SLE, ulcerative colitis, sarcoidosis, SJS, mucocutaneous lymph node syndrome, psoriatic, giardiasis, loiasis, schistosomiasis, and HZV

"SPILLOVER" IRIDOCYCLITIS Pars planitis, VKH, toxoplasmosis, toxocariasis, candidiasis, and herpetic retinitis

SPLENDORE-HEPLIN PHENOMENON Histopathologic finding of a IgM, IgA, and IgG reaction with eosinophils in a ring around a parasite

SUBRETINAL FIBROSIS SFU, ICSR, age-related macular degeneration (AMD), large nevi, melanoma, serpiginous choroidopathy, sarcoidosis, and OHS

SUBRETINAL NEOVASCULARIZATION (CNVM) OHS, toxoplasmosis, Behçet's syndrome, birdshot retinochoroidopathy, sarcoidosis, choroiditis, toxocariasis, VKH, rubella, serpiginous choroidopathy, and coccidiomycosis

"SUNSET GLOW" FUNDUS VKH and syphilis

SYNECHIAE JRA, syphilis, VKH, Behçet's syndrome, Reiter's syndrome, psoriasis, sarcoidosis, pars planitis, HZV, ankylosing spondylitis, and SFU

UNPASTEURIZED MILK Tuberculosis and brucellosis

UNPROTECTED SEX HIV, HSV, CMV, and syphilis

URETHRAL DISCHARGE Reiter's syndrome, chlamydia, syphilis, HSV, and gonococcal

VASCULITIS, CEREBRAL AMPPE, Behçet's syndrome, HSV, syphilis, and Lyme disease

VIRAL ETIOLOGY OF RETINAL DISEASE AMPPE, MEWDS, and Leber's stellate neuroretinitis

WHITE-DOT SYNDROMES THAT ARE UNILATERAL MEWDS and DUSN

WHITE-DOT SYNDROMES WITH GOOD PROGNOSIS AMPPE, ARPE, PIC, and MEWDS

WHITE-DOT SYNDROMES WITH GUARDED PROGNOSIS (may have CNVM or chronic course) Birdshot retinochoroidopathy, DUSN, MCP, and serpiginous choroidopathy

WHITE-DOT SYNDROME WITH POOR PROGNOSIS SFU

WHITE-DOT SYNDROMES IN YOUNG PATIENTS AMPPE, MEWDS, ARPE, MCP, and DUSN

WHITE-DOT SYNDROME MASQUERADES Sarcoid, B-cell lymphoma, sympathetic ophthalmia, and VKH

CAUCASIAN PATIENTS HLA-B27 and multiple sclerosis

Anterior Uveitis Diagnosis and Work-Up

General: Anterior uveitis accounts for 28% of all cases of uveitis.

- Signs and symptoms: acute pain, blurred vision, photophobia, red eye with ciliary flush (except JRA), hypotony (if increased IOP, consider HSV), AC cell, KP (granulomatous type has mutton-fat KP, epithelioid or giant cells, and Arlt's triangle on inferior cornea secondary to convection currents), which may spill into anterior vitreous, hypopyon (if in a quiet eye, consider masquerade), iris atrophy, and Koeppe or Busacca iris nodules. Chronic iridocyclitis: lymphocytes and plasma cells (Russell's bodies), isolated or part of ankylosing spondylitis, psoriatic arthritis, inflammatory bowel disease, Fuchs' HIC, JRA, phacoanaphylaxis, and sarcoidosis.
- Basic work-up: order MHA-TP or FTA, CBC, electrolytes, and chest x-ray, then add other tests as suspicion warrants.

ANTERIOR UVEITIS, GRANULOMATOUS WITH LOCAL OCULAR DISEASE

- Trauma
- Infectious: chronic anaerobic endophthalmitis, HSV, HZV, onchocerciasis, and schistosomiasis
- Autoimmune: sympathetic ophthalmia, lens-induced (phacoanaphylactic), and Fuchs' HIC. Consider HLA-A11, S-Ag, vitreous culture, and look for Dalen-Fuchs nodules.
- Masquerade: juvenile xanthogranuloma

ANTERIOR UVEITIS, GRANULOMATOUS WITH SYSTEMIC DISEASE

- Infectious: syphilis, tuberculosis, toxoplasmosis, leprosy, brucellosis, and helminthic. Consider PPD, VDRL, FTA-Abs, eosinophil count, and Cowdry-A test.
- Autoimmune: sarcoidosis and VKH. Consider ACE, calcium, anergy, chest x-ray, conjunctival biopsy, gallium scan, poliosis, vitiligo, and hearing exam.
- Masquerade: intraocular lymphoma and leukemia

ANTERIOR UVEITIS, NONGRANULOMATOUS WITH LOCAL DISEASE

- Trauma: surgical or nonsurgical, UGH syndrome, graft versus host disease, and polypropylene reaction
- Infectious: HSV, HZV, and *Staphylococcus aureus*
- Autoimmune: Fuchs' HIC, lens-induced (phacogenic), glaucomatocyclitic crisis, and idiopathic
- Masquerade: juvenile xanthogranuloma, tumor, and pigment dispersion syndrome

ANTERIOR UVEITIS, NONGRANULOMATOUS WITH SYSTEMIC DISEASE

- Infectious: syphilis, HSV, HZV, Lyme disease, leptospirosis, amoeba, and giardiasis. Consider VDRL, FTA-Abs, anergy panel, stool for amoeba, Lyme serology, and corneal sensitivity.
- Autoimmune with joint involvement: JRA, HLA-B27, ankylosing spondylitis, psoriatic, inflammatory bowel disease, Reiter's syndrome, and Sjögren's syndrome. Consider sacroiliac x-rays, ANA for JRA, RF, ESR, uric acid, VDRL, FTA-Abs (MHA-TP), HLA-B27, ear biopsy, Schirmer's testing, and salivary biopsy.
- Autoimmune with vasculitis: Behçet's syndrome, PAN, relapsing polychondritis, serum sickness, mucocutaneous lymph node syndrome, and rarely RA. Consider CRP, ESR, cryoglobulins, C3, C4, CH50, circulating immune complexes (CIC), skin biopsy, eosinophils, ANA, RF, ANCA, chest x-ray, tuberculosis skin, urinanalysis, properdin factor B, serum lysozyme, and 1-acid glycoprotein.

Anterior Uveitis Diseases

BRUCELLOSIS Acquired from undercooked animal meat, causing an acute febrile illness with possible iridocyclitis; treat with tetracycline.

FUCHS' HETEROCHROMIC IRIDOCYCLITIS (HIC) (9% of anterior uveitis) Unilateral mild iritis with heterochromia from stromal thinning (darker irides become lighter and vice versa), diffuse fine stellate KP, PSC cataract, glaucoma (15%), and rubeosis or vessels crossing the TM that may lead to hyphema. Associated with chorioretinal scars (toxoplasmosis with possible reaction to previous infection).

HALLERMANN-STREIFF SYNDROME Characterized by skin disease, alopecia, short stature, congenital cataract, glaucoma (PAS and posterior synechiae), and severe granulomatous uveitis, with onset usually at about age 20.

HERPES SIMPLEX VIRUS (HSV) (6%) Keratouveitis often with increased IOP from trabeculitis.

HLA-B27 RELATED (11%) Most common identifiable cause of acute anterior uveitis.

- Anklyosing spondylitis, 5% of cases of acute anterior uveitis: acute, recurrent, usually unilateral uveitis with fibrinous AC reaction, typically in males with low back pain from spondyloarthritis (x-ray the sacroiliac joints) or pauciarticular arthritis; 5% of patients have aortitis that may lead to aortic insufficiency. Average age of onset is 9 years. Uveitis may be prodrome for systemic disease. Ninety-five percent of cases are HLA-B27 positive.
- Reiter's syndrome: classic triad of bilateral papillary conjunctivitis, nongonococcal urethritis, and arthritis (mnemonic: can't see, can't pee, can't climb a tree). Often have a conjunctival mucopurulent discharge, corneal punctuate epithelial erosions (PEE), and punctate SEI or infiltrate, and may have uveitis, keratoderma blennorrhagicum (red, scaly rash on palms and soles), and circinate balanitis. Age of onset: 16 to 40 years; 75 to 95% of cases are HLA-B27 positive. May result from immunologic reaction to infectious antigen (*Chlaymdia, Yersinia, Campylobacter, Shigella,* etc.).
- Psoriasis: 10% of patients have iritis but only if joints are involved (20% of psoriatic patients).
- Inflammatory bowel disease (ulcerative colitis, Crohn's disease, Whipple's disease): mild iritis that coincides with bowel symptoms; 75% of cases are B27 positive.

IDIOPATHIC (43%) No work-up needed if it is first episode, mild, and unilateral.

JUVENILE RHEUMATOID ARTHRITIS (JRA) (10%) Chronic synovitis with extraarticular manifestations such as chronic iridocyclitis. Typically involes white eye and is bilateral and nongranulomatous; associated with cataract (60%), glaucoma (22%), and band keratopathy (50%). JRA is usually seen in females (80%), 4 to 6 years old; 80% of patients who are ANA positive develop anterior uveitis. If untreated, JRA will lead to decreased VA within 2 years. Ocular symptoms may persist into adulthood even though joint symptoms resolve.

- Four types:
  - Type 1: most common iritis; pauciarticular (four or fewer joints involved), early onset (25 to 40% of JRA), large joint disease. Ninety-five percent of patients who are ANA positive and RF negative have uveitis.
    - Chronic iridocyclitis of young girls: same as type 1 but no joint involvement
  - Type 2: boys with pauciarticular B27+
  - Type 3: polyarticular (40% of JRA)
  - Type 4: severe systemic JRA, Still's disease
- Treat iritis initially with hourly steroids and cycloplegic if case is mild or with atropine if severe. Consider steroid ointment at bedtime (qhs), NSAID, and immunosuppressives. Must eliminate all cell (is a very "sticky" inflammation) and treat cell, not flare. Once quiet, usually see patients every 3 months if ANA positive or yearly if negative; follow slit lamp exam to rule out posterior synechiae.

MASQUERADES OF ANTERIOR UVEITIS Intraocular lymphoma, leukemia, postoperative endophthalmitis (consider vitreous biopsy or tap), RB, chronic RD, retained IOFB, and melanoma

MEDICATIONS Cobalt (tattoos), oral contraceptives, quinidine, sulfa, Xalatan, topical beta-blockers, diethylcarbamazine (treatment for loiasis), MMC, cidofovir (for CMV retinitis), rifabutin (prophylaxis against *Mycobacterium avium* complex in AIDS patients; may cause severe uveitis with hypopyon when used with clarithromycin or fluconazole).

OCULAR OR ANTERIOR SEGMENT ISCHEMIA Scleral buckle procedure, multiple muscle surgery, carotid disease (chronic inflammation with few KP, poorly reactive pupil), and GCA. Treat with steroids, cycloplegics.

ONCHOCERCIASIS *Onchocerca volvulus* microfiliarial death in eye incites inflammatory response.

OTHER VIRAL CAUSES OF UVEITIS HZV (40% of patients develop uveitis), CMV, HIV, and influenza

PANUVEITIS Behçet's syndrome, sympathetic ophthalmia, sarcoidosis, VKH, syphilis, and tuberculosis

PHACOANTIGENIC UVEITIS, PHACOANYPHYLACTIC Lens proteins leak through ruptured capsule, causing zonal granulomatous inflammation, usually following trauma or surgery; 3 to 7% coincidence with sympathetic ophthalmia. Treat by cataract extraction.

POSNER-SCHLOSSMAN SYNDROME Glaucomocyclitic crisis: iritis, increased IOP, and corneal edema

POSTSURGICAL May be normal inflammation, lens-induced, or infectious

POSTERIOR UVEITIS SPILLOVER Candidiasis, toxoplasmosis, or toxocariasis

SCHWARTZ SYNDROME Acute anterior uveitis from chronic RRD

Intermediate Uveitis Diagnosis and Work-Up

General: Intermediate uveitis comprises 15% of all cases of uveitis. Patients typically present asymptomatic with a white eye or with floaters and blurred vision from vitreous cells. Patients also may have mild anterior segment inflammation, retinal vessel sheathing, pars plana snowbanking, inferior retinal "snowballs," CME, cotton-wool spots, PSC cataract, vitreous hemorrhage, or RD.

INTERMEDIATE GRANULOMATOUS UVEITIS WITH LOCAL DISEASE
- Infectious: toxocariasis (consider *Toxocara* titer)
- Autoimmune: pars planitis (consider ESR)
- Masquerade: IOFB (consider ultrasound)

INTERMEDIATE GRANULOMATOUS UVEITIS WITH SYSTEMIC DISEASE
- Infectious: Lyme disease
- Autoimmune: sarcoidosis and multiple sclerosis

INTERMEDIATE NONGRANULOMATOUS UVEITIS WITH LOCAL DISEASE
- Autoimmune: Fuchs' HIC, pars planitis, and idiopathic senile vitritis (look for heterochromia, TID, and angle vessels)
- Masquerade: ophthalmia nodosa (tarantula hair) and familial exudative vitreoretinopathy

INTERMEDIATE NONGRANULOMATOUS UVEITIS WITH SYSTEMIC DISEASE
- Infectious: Lyme disease (consider Lyme titers and western blot)

- Autoimmune: multiple sclerosis (consider MRI, neurologic exam)
- Masquerade: amyloid

Intermediate Uveitis Diseases

PARS PLANITIS Forty-five percent of intermediate uveitis is caused by pars planitis. It is usually seen in children and young adults, with uveitis of unknown etiology that is bilateral in 75% of cases. Patients may be asymptomatic or have floaters or decreased VA, usually from CME. They may also have band keratopathy, low-grade AC cell with endothelial dusting, numerous vitreous cells, "snowbanking" (white aggregates composed of glial elements and fibrovascular tissue), cyclitic membrane, disk edema with diffuse leakage on FA and staining, and peripheral retinal NV (poorer prognosis). There is a smoldering course without exacerbations in 59% of cases, with exacerbations in 31%, and a benign self-limited course in 10%. Associated with cataract (42%), chronic CME (28%), and RD (5%).

- Most cases are idiopathic but may be autoimmune or familial. HLA-DR2 in 67% of cases; also found in 50 to 70% of multiple sclerosis patients versus 20 to 25% of normal controls. There is a 20% 5-year incidence of multiple sclerosis.
- No treatment (do not treat every AC cell). Treat CME with steroids or carbonic anhydrase inhibitors. May laser or cryotherapy the pars plana membrane, especially if there is NV. Rule out secondary causes.

CHRONIC CYCLITIS Same as pars planitis but without exudate; work-up with CXR, ACE, and FTA-Abs.

IDIOPATHIC AGE-RELATED VITRITIS Age of onset: 60 to 70 years. Consider large cell lymphoma (needs diagnostic vitrectomy and DNA PCR), Whipple's disease, syphilis, pars planitis, tuberculosis, and sarcoidosis. Steroids are ineffective.

LYME DISEASE Spirochete *Borrelia burgdorferi* carried by *Ixodes dammini* tick found on rodents, deer, birds, cats, and dogs, usually in early summer to midautumn. Causes up to 3% of cases of intermediate uveitis.

- Three stages:
  - Stage 1: erythema chronicum migrans, follicular conjunctivitis, headache, malaise, myalgia, arthralgias, and fever
  - Stage 2: follows in 1 to 4 months with neurologic (in 30 to 40% of cases; usually CN VII palsy, encephalitis, or meningitis), musculoskeletal (arthritis, tendonitis), cardiac (myocarditis, heart block), and ophthalmic symptoms (keratitis, iritis, intermediate uveitis, vitritis, panophthalmitis, or optic neuritis)

  - Stage 3: >5 months; shows chronic atrophic skin changes, keratitis, chronic meningitis, chronic arthritis, and respiratory distress.
- Diagnose with enzyme-linked immunosorbent assay (ELISA) IgM and IgG (negative in early stage 1) and immunofluorescent antibody titers; beware of false (+) FTA-Abs.
- Treat with tetracycline, erythromycin, penicillin, or intravenous ceftriaxone or penicillin if there is CNS involvement.

OTHERS Fuchs' HIC (27%), sarcoidosis (14%), multiple sclerosis (5%), toxoplasmosis, toxocariasis, and tuberculosis

Posterior Uveitis Diagnosis and Work-Up

General: Posterior uveitis represents 38% of all cases of uveitis. Patients usually present with decreased VA and may have pain, floaters, metamorphopsia, and systemic symptoms. There are many etiologies, but the most common are toxoplasmosis (18%), idiopathic vasculitis (18%), idiopathic choroiditis (10%), multifocal choroiditis from tuberculosis or syphilis, histoplasmosis (10%), and toxocariasis (7%).

POSTERIOR GRANULOMATOUS UVEITIS WITH LOCAL DISEASE

- Infectious: toxoplasmosis, OHS, BARN (HZV, HSV-2), and toxocariasis
- Autoimmune: sympathetic ophthalmia and pars planitis (consider ultrasound, FA)
- Masquerade: intraocular lymphoma

POSTERIOR GRANULOMATOUS UVEITIS WITH SYSTEMIC DISEASE

- Infectious: CMV, tuberculosis, syphilis, toxoplasmosis, brucellosis, coccidiomycosis, helminthic, ascariasis, onchocerciasis, microfilaria, cysticercosis, and schistosomiasis (consider tuberculosis, VDRL, FTA-Abs, chest x-ray, *Toxocara* titer, histoplasmosis or coccidio skin test, and eosinophils)
- Autoimmune: sarcoidosis and VKH (consider ACE, calcium, chest x-ray, gallium scan, anergy, and conjunctival biopsy; look for poliosis, vitiligo, and hearing problems)
- Masquerade: fungal endophthalmitis (candidiasis, sporotrichosis, aspergillus) and amyloid

POSTERIOR NONGRANULOMATOUS UVEITIS LOCAL OCULAR DISEASE

- Trauma: radiation vasculitis
- Infectious: CMV, HZV (BARN), DUSN, ophthalmomyiasis, and rubella (consider eosinophils, serum glutamic-oxaloacetic transaminase [SGOT], lactate dehydrogenase [LDH], FA, and HIV)

- Autoimmune: MEWDS, AMPPE, punctate inner choroidopathy, subretinal fibrosis and uveitis syndrome, birdshot retinochoroidopathy, acute retinal pigment epitheliitis, MCP, serpiginous choroidopathy, and posterior scleritis (consider FA, ERG, electro-olfactogram [EOG], hepatitis B virus surface antigen, HLA-A29, vitiligo, Epstein-Barr virus [EBV] titers with ELISA assay and IgM)
- Masquerade: retinitis pigmentosa, amyloid, and tumors

POSTERIOR NONGRANULOMATOUS UVEITIS WITH SYSTEMIC DISEASE

- Infectious: syphilis, HSV, HZV, Lyme disease, CMV, trypanosomiasis, rubella, measles, Whipple's disease, *Acanthamoeba*, and giardiasis
- Autoimmune vasculitis: Behçet's syndrome, SLE, relapsing polychondritis, Crohn's disease, Wegener's granulomatosis, PAN, scleroderma, dermatomyositis, cryoglobulinemia, Sjögren's syndrome, Eales' disease, and multiple sclerosis (consider ANA, RF, cryoglobulins, ESR, ANCA, CIC, tuberculosis, spinal tap, SPEP, hepatitis B surface antigen, chest x-ray, sinus, l-acid-glycoprotein, and properdin factor B)
- Masquerade: intraocular lymphoma, endogenous endophthalmitis, familial exudative vitreoretinopathy, and leukemia (consider CBC)

Posterior Uveitis Diseases

ACUTE MACULAR NEURORETINOPATHY (AMN) Rare bilateral white-dot syndrome that affects young healthy adults with posterior pole middle and outer retinal lesions.

ACUTE MULTIFOCAL PLACOID PIGMENT EPITHELIOPATHY (AMPPE) Acute illness that is postviral in one third of patients, usually seen in young females (average age: 25) who present with a headache and variably decreased VA; bilateral (maybe weeks later). Exam shows multiple deep, large (1 DD) white placoid RPE lesions in the posterior pole and vitreous cells in 50%. On FA, blocks early from obliterative choroidal vasculitis and stains late (hyperfluorescent). The early multifocal hypofluorescence looks like hypertensive Elschnig's choroidal infarctions. Has full recovery; 80% are 20/40 or better, but may leave permanent RPE disturbance. No treatment necessary (rarely has CNVM, CME, cerebral vasculitis, or pleocytosis).

ACUTE RETINAL PIGMENT EPITHELIITIS (ARPE), KRILL'S DISEASE Usually seen in young adults with decreased VA and gray macular spots with yellow-white halos, which resolve in 6 to 12 weeks.

ACUTE ZONAL OCCULT OUTER RETINOPATHY (AZOOR) Very rare white-dot syndrome of young women with damage of outer retinal layers without noticeable fundus changes but with progressive VF loss, photopsias, and central distortion. FA shows confluent hyperfluorescence with granularity. Has ERG changes.

BIRDSHOT RETINOCHOROIDOPATHY, VITILIGINOUS CHORIORETINITIS Seen in older (average age: 51) women with bilateral decreased VA, floaters, photopsias, and nyctalopia. Exam shows numerous vitreous cells and cream-colored depigmented large (1000 μm) lesions throughout the fundus. CME present in 50% with disk staining. Typically a chronic course, with late disk pallor and vessel attenuation. HLA-A29.2 is positive in 96% of cases (highest known HLA-associated disease; normal population is 7% positive). Thought to be a response to retinal S antigen (arrestin). May treat CME with steroids.

DIFFUSE UNILATERAL SUBACUTE NEURORETINITIS (DUSN) Nematode migration under retina often from parasite carried by raccoons.

EALES' DISEASE Rare, idiopathic, bilateral occlusive peripheral retinal vasculitis (possible allergy to tuberculoprotein) affecting 20- to 40-year-old males in India and the Middle East. Presents with floaters or blurring, retinal nonperfusion, NV, vitreous hemorrhage (VH), vessel sheathing, and tortuosity; often have branch retinal vein occlusion (BRVO), and occasionally have vestibulo-auditory symptoms. No specific therapy; 54% end with VA 20/20–20/50.

MULTIFOCAL CHORIORETINITIS AND PANUVEITIS (MCP) Older age, bilateral white-dot syndrome with marked AC and vitreous cell, multiple 50–200 μm lesions (smaller than AMPPE) in the posterior pole (more punched out and discrete than birdshot retinochoroidopathy) that block early and stain late. Chronic course with CME, CNVM (present in 45% of cases, the major cause of vision loss). The second eye may not be involved until years later. Treat with steroids or cyclosporine, but expect poor visual prognosis.

MULTIPLE EVANESCENT WHITE-DOT SYNDROME (MEWDS) Young (average age: 28) myopic women (75%) without viral prodrome but with good VA, unilateral shimmering photopsias, and paracentral scotomas or enlarged blind spot. Exam shows multiple 100–200 μm punctate perifoveal lesions with macular granularity and possibly a few vitreous cells. "Wreath" sign seen on FA with lesions that hyperfluoresce early and stain late (also late disk staining). Good prognosis; self-limited course lasts 7 weeks; no therapy.

PUNCTATE INNER CHOROIDOPATHY (PIC) May be a subgroup of MCP (similar HLA association) in young myopic females without vitreous cells but with small dots in the posterior pole. Benign course, less recurrence than MCP.

SERPIGINOUS CHOROIDOPATHY Seen in middle-aged (40 to 50 years old) Caucasian patients with bilateral chronic chorioretinitis starting at the ON and extending through the posterior pole (predilection for the macula) with vitreous cells. Lesions wax and wane, lasting months, then regress, leaving overlying RPE loss, and new lesions form at border of old lesions. FA blocks early and stains late with pathognomonic hyperfluorescent "brushfire border." Indolent course; steroids 1 mg/kg have not proven beneficial, and immunosuppressives do not work well. Twenty-five percent of cases have CNVM.

SUBRETINAL FIBROSIS AND UVEITIS SYNDROME (SFU) Very rare, chronic, bilateral disease of young healthy, female, usually African-American patients with multifocal choroiditis that progresses to subretinal plaques, with profound vision loss and poor visual prognosis.

TOXOPLASMOSIS Protozoan *Toxoplasma gondii* infection with moderate to severe vitritis and focal white necrotizing retinitis. Typically retinitis reactivates next to an old pigmented scar. Fifty percent of cases have "mutton-fat" granulomatous KP and AC cell. Subnormal ERG; may develop retinal NV or CNVM. Usually due to reactivation of congenitally acquired toxoplasmic cysts latent in retina that were acquired early in pregnancy, often with bilateral retinochoroiditis with macular predilection. May cause 30 to 50% of posterior uveitis. Very common in developing countries, and decreases cataract surgical success rate there by 20%.

- Organism is highly prevalent in North America. Obligate intracellular parasite in cats (the definitive host) that shed oocysts in their feces. Cysts may remain viable for up to 1 year. Humans are intermediate host, usually from ingestion of oocysts in contaminated food (especially raw meat) or soil (such as cat litter), resulting in human infection with predilection for the retina and other CNS structures.
    - Congenital: transplacental, excavated macular scar, hydrocephaly, seizures, cerebral calcifications, jaundice, and hepatosplenomegaly
    - Acquired: only 10 to 20% are symptomatic with febrile illness. In AIDS patients, is usually newly acquired, and 30 to 50% have toxoplasmic encephalitis; thus, order CT.
- Diagnose clinically, plus order serum antibodies (any titer is signficiant in the presence of a fundus lesion). Also may use Sabin-Feldman dye test. Associated with Fuchs' HIC.
- Many cases resolve and do not need treatment. However, in general, treat the active infection if it is within the arcades or peripapillary, large (>1 DD) lesion, or has severe vitritis. Do not treat during pregnancy. Mepron (Atovarone) may be available for monotherapy

and is active against cysts, but typically use triple therapy (cannot rid cysts):

- Pyrimethamine: 150 mg load, then 25 mg qid for 6 weeks. Check CBC weekly for bone marrow suppression.
- Sulfadiazine: 4 g load, then 1 g qid for 6 weeks. May use Bactrim as substitute.
- Folinic acid: 5 mg po qid. Leucovorin rescue to prevent megaloblastic anemia, as the protozoan cannot import folate and thus makes its own.
- If macula-threatening, add clindamycin 300 mg qid (watch for pseudomembranous colitis) and prednisone 80–100 mg (avoid depot injection).

WHIPPLE'S RETINITIS Systemic malabsorption syndrome caused by *Tropheryma whippelii* (corynebacterium), seen in 40- to 70-year-old patients with anterior or posterior uveitis. May have vitreous cells, pars plana exudates, cotton wool spots (CWS), retinal vasculitis, papilledema, nystagmus, gaze palsy, external ophthalmoplegia, dementia, ataxia, and arthritis. Diagnose with jejunal biopsy, vitreous biopsy to see periodic acid Schiff stained macrophages. Differential diagnosis: large cell lymphoma and sarcoidosis. Treat with tetracycline or penicillin.

Panuveitis/Diffuse Uveitis

General: Panuveitis and diffuse uveitis represent 18% of all cases of uveitis and have the signs and symptoms of any of the previously mentioned uveitic diseases. Technically, panuveitis is an inflammation that involves three noncontiguous ocular tissues.

PANUVEITIS, GRANULOMATOUS WITH LOCAL OCULAR DISEASE

- Infectious: toxoplasmosis, toxocariasis, ARN/BARN, and ophthalmomyiasis (consider toxocara ELISA, toxoplasma serology)
- Autoimmune: sympathetic ophthalmia, pars planitis, birdshot retinochoroidopathy, phacoantigenic, Fuchs' HIC, and masquerade (consider history of injury, vitiligo, fluorescein angiography, and ultrasound)
- Masquerade: intraocular lymphoma (consider thick smear, VDRL, FTA-Abs, toxoplasmosis, other agents, rubella, cytomegalovirus, herpes simplex [TORCH], jejunal biopsy, toxoplasma titers, Lyme serology, HIV ELISA, and measles titer)

PANUVEITIS, GRANULOMATOUS WITH SYSTEMIC DISEASE

- Infectious: HSV, tuberculosis, toxoplasmosis, helminthic, coccidiomycosis, sporotrichosis, brucellosis, cryptococcal, and Kawasaki disease

(consider tuberculosis skin test, chest x-ray, *Toxocara* titer, *Toxoplasma* titer, eosinophils, *Brucella* serology, and vitreous biopsy for fungal cultures)
- Autoimmune: sarcoidosis, VKH, and amyloid (consider ACE, calcium, chest x-ray, gallium scan, anergy, conjunctival biopsy, exam for poliosis, vitiligo, and hearing problems)
- Masquerade: candidiasis

PANUVEITIS, NONGRANULOMATOUS WITH LOCAL DISEASE
- Infectious: ARN/BARN, endophthalmitis from surgery, injury, and endogenous (consider AC to vitreous cultures, CH50, and CIC)
- Autoimmune: birdshot retinochoroidopathy, MCP, subretinal fibrosis and panuveitis, Fuchs'HIC, pars planitis, idiopathic senile vitritis, and lens-induced uveitis (consider HLA–A29, S antigen, brain CT, and EBV titers)
- Masquerade: intraocular lymphoma and leukemia (consider x-ray for IOFB)

PANUVEITIS, NONGRANULOMATOUS WITH SYSTEMIC DISEASE
- Infectious: tuberculosis, syphilis, Lyme disease, HSV-2, brucellosis, and giardiasis (consider VDRL, FTA-Abs, anergy panel, Lyme serology, chest x-ray, tuberculosis skin test, and giardia in stool)
- Autoimmune: PAN and Behçet's syndrome (consider eosinophils, CIC, C3, C4, RF, ANA, ESR, ANCA, serum lysozyme, 1-acid glycoprotein, and properdin factor B)
- Masquerade: intraocular lymphoma and leukemia (consider CBC)

IDIOPATHIC Most cases (45%) are of an unknown cause, with negative work-up.

BEHÇET'S Causes 10% of panuveitis from an occlusive vasculitis secondary to immune complex deposition. Usually presents in third decade. Leading cause of acquired blindness in Japan and Turkey, with an immunologic predisposition along the old Silk Road trading routes. Associated with HLA B51, the same region that codes for immune response, circulating immune complexes, and neutrophil diapodesis.
- 20% of patients present first to an ophthalmologist, often with explosive bilateral nonsimultaneous panuveitis; usually acute, but may be chronic, may have an evanescent, shifting hypopyon. May also present with a white-eye and posterior vasculitis (no isolated vitritis). Retinal veins are affected more than arteries, and the primary posterior presentation is BRVO from venous engorgement. "Cut-off" sign from obliterative vasculitis. Characterized by hemorrhage/exudate, papilledema, and frosted branch angiitis. English walnuts may precipitate inflammation.

- Chronic relapsing course over 10 years that waxes and wanes. Chronic disease shows decreased anterior attacks, more retinal pathology; may look RP-like, with narrow, sheathed vessels and severe chorioretinal atrophy with RPE alterations. May have capillary dropout, macular ischemia, and NV.
- Four major diagnostic criteria:
  - Aphthous oral ulcers (98%): especially hard palate and uvula
  - Genital ulcers
  - Erythema nodosum (70%): tender, raised skin lesions
  - Uveitis
- Minor criteria: arthritis (52%; seen especially in Japan, usually the knee joint), epididymitis, intestinal involvement, vascular occlusions (8%; "angio-Behçet's"; also aneurysms, thrombus, and thrombophlebitis in 10% of cases), neurologic complications (10% have CN palsies, psychiatric disorders, vertigo, or hearing loss similar to VKH). Also cutaneous hypersensitivity (pathergy), developing a lesion with skin prick (ask about previous blood draws, shaving lesions). Acneiform lesions (58%; may be complicated by steroid use).
- Differentiate from other posterior uveitis: sarcoidosis (more free to behave as it will, less explosive, indolent), venulitis (not as occlusive), and viral retinitis (larger, progressive coalescence of retinal whitening)
- Treatment: immunosuppression with systemic steroids initially, then steroid sparing agents (e.g., Cytoxan, chlorambucil, cyclosporin). Consider PRP for NV.

SARCOIDOSIS Cause of 21% of panuveitis. Autoimmune, noncaseating, multisystem granulomatous inflammation that is a type 4 hypersensitivity (T cell reaction). Ocular disease may precede the systemic disease up to 7 years, and course usually runs 2 to 10 years. Thirty percent of patients with systemic disease have ocular involvement, with uveitis, lacrimal infiltration, conjunctival nodules, interstitial keratitis, or erythema nodosum.

- Usually presents with iridocyclitis, mutton-fat KP, Koeppe (margin) and Busacca (stromal) iris nodules, or cataract. Characterized by dense synechia with possible glaucoma from iris bombé pupillary block, PAS, or TM damage (11 to 23%). Intermediate uveitis with large epithelioid cells in the anterior vitreous, snowbanking and "snowballs" usually 360 degrees, unlike pars planitis. Posterior uveitis is less frequent but has perivenous sheathing ("candle-wax drippings"), retinitis, CME, retinal NV, choroiditis, and granulomas of the choroid or ON.
- Primarily affects Caucasians worldwide, but more prevalent in African-American patients in the United States. F > M; 20 to 50 years old. Younger patients usually have acute unilateral disease versus older patients with bilateral chronic disease. Rare in children who may only have rash, arthritis, and uveitis.

- Work-up: consider serum ACE, lysozyme, CXR, skin testing, gallium scan, tissue biopsy if lacrimal involved or granuloma of the skin or conjunctiva, or broncho-alveolar lavage.
- Treat with prednisone 80–100 mg qd and PF 1% every 1 hour; taper oral dose with response to 10–20 mg over 3 to 4 weeks. Cyclosporine for steroid-sparing agent.

SYMPATHETIC OPHTHALMIA (SO) Rare but classic chronic, bilateral, granulomatous panuveitis from immune reaction to the injured (exciting) eye, causing the fellow (sympathizing) eye to also become inflamed anywhere from 10 days to 50 years later. Estimated incidence of 0.2% of eyes postinjury, 0.007 to 0.7% postcataract extraction, 1.4% of uveitis. Sixty-five percent occur within 2 weeks to 2 months, 80% occur within 3 months, and 90% within 1 year.

- Hippocrates noted injury in one eye led to disease in fellow eye. Mackenzie (1840) described first case series. Fuchs (1905) elucidated etiology. Highest incidence reported during U.S. Civil War in 1860s, then few cases in World War I and II; none in Korean or Vietnam wars.
- Immune reaction against self-antigen (possible retinal S or uveal antigen). Peripheral lymphocytes reacting against melanin may account for the vitiligo and poliosis that are often seen. Anterior chamber associated immune deviation (ACAID) causes AC antigen suppression. There is a reported decreased SO incidence after glaucoma filtering surgery. Associated with HLA-A11.
- Presents with insidious pain and photophobia in both eyes, with decreased VA and early loss of accommodation from cyclitis. Granulomatous iridocyclitis with large mutton-fat KP, extensive PAS, nodular thickened iris, and choroid. Dalen-Fuchs nodules are cream-colored choroidal lesions that are sub-RPE excrescences of Bruch's membrane composed of T cells, 60–700 μm, in the midperiphery. The choroiditis spares the choriocapillaris and the retina (unlike VKH); thus, not likely to have serous RD. Patients may also have cataract, rubeosis, glaucoma, and papillitis. May look like VKH, with poliosis, vitiligo, and meningeal signs, but with an ocular trauma history. FA shows irregular choroidal filling, multiple leakage, and early hypo- and later hyperfluorescence.
- Differential diagnosis: VKH, phacoantigenic (SO has up to a 25% coincidence with lens-induced uveitis from traumatic etiology), syphilis, and sarcoidosis
- Treatable with lifelong immunosuppression with steroids and cyclosporin. Sixty-five percent of patients retain 20/60 vision or better. Prevent SO following trauma by enucleating a blind, painful eye within 2 weeks.

SYPHILIS Sexually transmitted chronic, systemic infection caused by the spirochete *Treponema pallidum*, and is the cause of 1 to 3% of all uveitis.

Is a uveitis that can be cured, it is considered the "great masquerader." May be acquired or congenital if mother was in primary or secondary stage of infection. Risk increased in AIDS patients.

- Screen patients with treponemal tests FTA-Abs or MHA-TP. The nontreponemal tests, VDRL and RPR, detect antilipoidal Ab produced during active treponemal infection and may be normal after treatment or in tertiary disease; also may be falsely negative with RA, SLE. Ocular involvement implies neurosyphilis; thus, do lumbar puncture, and check CSF VDRL.
- Four potential stages:
  - Primary: incubation period of 3 weeks, followed by skin or mucous membrane chancre from 8 days to 6 weeks after infection with regional lymphadenopathy. Painless chancre heals within a few weeks. If congenital, may cause bilateral acute interstital keratitis with stromal vessels and later ghost vessels, keratouveitis, retinitis with salt and pepper fundus, RPE degeneration, and optic atrophy (looks like RP).
  - Secondary: if untreated, the spirochetemic stage follows within a few weeks or months after disappearance of the primary chancre, with fever, malaise, headache, generalized lymph node enlargement, arthralgias, and rash. Also may have conjunctivitis, keratitis, uveitis (granulomatous or not, can look like anything) with iris nodules. Usually not posterior, but may have focal or multifocal choroiditis, exudates around disk and arterioles, arteritis, extensive RPE hypertrophy, and papillitis neuroretinitis. Secondary stage subsides, even without antibiotic therapy, and the infection becomes latent.
  - Latent: untreated patients with historic or serologic evidence for syphilis but with no clinical manifestations have latent syphilis. Secondary syphilitic relapses may develop during this state of latency. Most patients stay latent.
  - Tertiary (neurosyphilis): 30% of untreated cases will progress to the tertiary stage, with syphilitic inflammatory lesions of the heart, aorta, brain, kidney, bone, eye, or skin. Ocular findings include Argyll-Robertson pupils with blurred vision, chorioretinitis (bilateral in 50%), vitreous haze, flame hemorrhages, chorioretinal atrophy, periarterial sheathing, diffuse neuroretinitis, IK, and punctate keratitis.
- Treat with IV penicillin 12–24 million units/day for 10 days, then Benzathine penicillin G 2.4 million units IM for 3 weeks plus topical steroids for ocular inflammation. Watch for Jarisch-Herxheimer reaction (increased inflammation and exudate with treatment from death of treponemes). Check CSF every 6 months until cells, protein, and VDRL normalize.

TUBERCULOSIS Aerobic bacillus with predilection for highly oxygenated tissues (lung apex and choroid) that may cause uveitis from direct infection or hypersensitivity reaction (type IV). At-risk populations: health care workers, endemic areas, indigent or immunocompromised patients. May present as a granulomatous iridocyclitis, vitritis, choroiditis with yellow-white choroidal nodules, retinal periphlebitis, vascular occlusions, or papillitis. Check PPD (confounded by bacille Calmette-Guérin [BCG] vaccine and atypical *Mycobacterium* infections), CXR, and possibly aqueous PCR. May give a Schlaegel trial: isoniazid (INH) for 2 weeks. Treat active tuberculosis with INH, rifampin, and pyrazinamide.

VOGT-KOYANAGI-HARADA DISEASE (VKH), UVEOMENINGEOENCEPHALITIS Cause of 18% of panuveitis, usually with severe bilateral granulomatous inflammation with bilateral serous RD, iridocyclitis, choroidal thickening, disk edema, meningeal irritation, poliosis, and vitiligo. Vogt described the first case (1906), Harada added retinal findings (1926), and Koyanagi described neurologic characteristics (1929).

- Almost always presents in pigmented races, especially Asian and Native American. Sixty percent of patients are female, usually 20 to 50 years old. Rarely affects children or Caucasians. Higher incidence in Japan than in Japanese immigrants in the United States. Etiology is likely from sensitivity to melanin, as evidenced by vitiligo, poliosis, iris depigmentation with recurrent anterior attacks, "sunset glow" fundus with chronic posterior inflammation as the body depigments, high-frequency hearing loss (cochlea contains melanin), and neurologic symptoms (melanin in the CNS meninges). Asians have more recurrent anterior uveitis than Westerners, who have more posterior signs and symptoms.
- Diagnosis: clinical findings, may have positive HLA-DR4, Dw53 in 75% of cases. Ultrasound shows diffuse low choroidal reflectivity (usually increased with posterior scleritis).
- Three stages:
  - Prodromal stage: few days of headache, nausea, tinnitis, dysacusis or hearing loss, and orbital pain.
  - Uveitic or ophthalmic stage: rapid onset with bilateral posterior uveitis, choroidal fullness, retinal edema, papillitis, multifocal choroidal inflammation, and SRF accumulation with serous RD; may have ACG from annular choroidal effusion.
  - Convalescent stage: Dalen-Fuchs nodules are present with chorioretinal scarring. Sugiura sign is pathognomonic with perilimbal vitiligo from loss of basal melanosomes.
- Differential diagnosis: syphilis (may also have bilateral serous RD) and birdshot retinochoroidopathy (may have retinal lesions associated with vitiligo)

- Treat with immunosuppression: usually steroids first, then other agents such as cyclosporine (T-cell mediated disease); typically flares less than 1 year.

Surgery

CATARACT SURGERY IN UVEITIC PATIENTS Usually wait until the eye is quiet for at least 6 months. Surgery is often complicated by small pupils and rebound uveitis. In general, avoid IOLs in JRA and VKH. Consider sulcus placement of IOL to prevent posterior synechiae to the anterior capsule. Often need aggressive immunosuppression with corticosteroids (oral, periocular, or topical) prior to and following cataract surgery.

CHAPTER 6

Lens

Anatomy and Physiology

EMBRYOLOGY Derived from surface ectoderm, with inward sequestration instead of desquamation of aging cells. Majority of lens development occurs at 3 to 8 weeks in utero.

- At the 4 mm stage, the optic vesicle that is apposed to the surface ectoderm initiates the formation of the lens placode. A single layer of columnar cells is seen as the fovea lentis (lens pit) and invaginates concomitantly with the optic vesicle conversion to a double-layered optic cup. The lens vesicle separates from the cornea at the 9 mm stage, with basal cell membranes external and apices facing the lumen.
- The lens capsule forms at the 10 mm stage, as does the tunica vasculosa lentis, which fully encompasses the lens by the 40 mm stage. The posterior vascular capsule begins from the hyaloid artery anteriorly to join with the choroidal vein, then proceeds to join the long ciliary artery to form the anterior vascular capsule (pupillary membrane).
- The posterior cells of the lens vesicle elongate to obliterate the lumen by 16 mm (forming the primary lens fibers, later known as the embryonic nucleus). Anterior vesicle cells remain as the lens epithelium and at 25 mm begin to proliferate at the germinative zone, then differentiate at the equatorial transitional zone and are added internally as secondary lens fibers. Secondary fibers never reach both the anterior and posterior poles, and thus form the anterior upright Y suture and posterior inverted Y (the Y sutures enclose the fetal nucleus). Later adult fibers form more complex stellate sutures.

ANATOMY (Fig. 6–1) Elongated adult lens fibers have a basal process posterior beneath the capsule and an apical process anterior beneath the epithelium. The nucleus assumes a more anterior position as the fibers internalize, producing the lens bow. Fibers denucleate, lose organelles, and form complex interdigitations with other fibers; the lens cortex contains the most recently created fibers. Anterior radius of curvature is about 10 mm, and the posterior surface curvature is 6 mm.

- Capsule: the basement membrane of the lens epithelial cells. Composed of type IV collagen with heparin sulfate, it is thinnest at the posterior pole (2–9 μm) and thickest paraequatorial (12–21 μm).

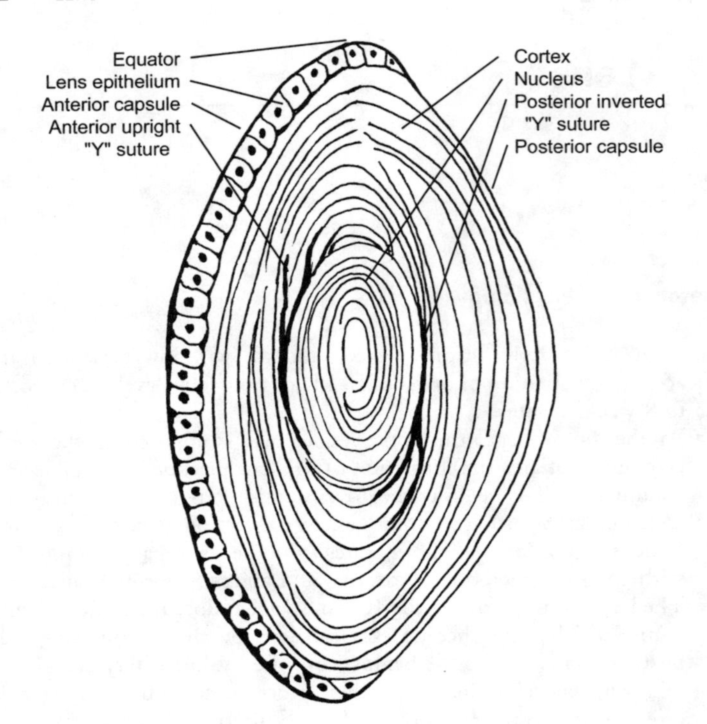

Figure 6–1 Anatomy of the adult lens in cross section.

- Lens epithelium: an anterior cuboidal monolayer. The equatorial cells form lens cell "fibers" by inward sequestration throughout life (older cells are in the nucleus). Arranged in lamellae, the fibers meet at the Y sutures.
- Lens proteins: 33% of the lens is protein that is either water soluble or insoluble. Water-soluble crystallines are labeled alpha (30%), beta (55%), and gamma (15%), derived from two unrelated protein superfamilies (alpha proteins are the most highly conserved). Water-insoluble proteins are characterized as urea soluble or insoluble; they increase with age and are responsible for cataract genesis.

PHYSIOLOGY Nearly all of the lens metabolic needs are supplied by glucose that is converted into adenosine triphosphate (ATP) from glycolysis. Most energy is derived from anaerobic glycolysis (70–90%), and to a lesser extent, from the hexose monophosphate shunt, the sorbitol pathway, and the tricarboxylic acid (TCA) cycle. The lens has limited immune sequestration (not complete but diminished access to immune system). It receives passive nutrition from the aqueous. Accommodation is from zonular relaxation, allowing the central anterior lens to bulge.

- Hardening of the lens, not loss of ciliary muscle tone, causes presbyopia.
- In diabetes, the lens converts excess glucose into sorbitol, which is not transported out; as sorbitol collects, it causes lens hydration and myopic shift.

OPTICAL PROPERTIES Progressive increase of refractive index, from 1.38 in the periphery to 1.50 at the center. The lens is transparent because lens cells lack nuclei. It has homogeneous cytoplasm, with ordered crystalline proteins and fibers ordered in a paracrystalline array. It has minimal extracellular space and is avascular.

ZONULES Comprising the tertiary vitreous, zonules arise from the pars plana and are composed of elastic fibrillin.

Signs and Symptoms

ECTOPIA LENTIS May be from trauma, inherited as autosomal dominant or autosomal recessive, or secondary to systemic disease, such as Marfan syndrome ("sun rise" dislocation), Weill-Marchesani syndrome (dislocates anterior into the AC), homocystinuria ("sun set" luxation), hyperlysinemia, sulfite oxidase deficiency, aniridia (20% incidence), megalocornea, Kniest syndrome, coloboma (absence of zonules; may be part of the CHARGE association), PHPV, tertiary syphilis (always do work-up for syphilis), and Ehlers-Danlos syndrome. Classified as subluxation (partial loss of zonular support), luxation (total loss of zonular support), or dislocation (lens out of place). In general, avoid surgery if possible.

GLAUKOMFLECKEN White epithelial and anterior cortical opacities that represent focal anterior lens epithelium necrosis following acute glaucoma.

RETAINED NUCLEI IN LENS Asssociated with rubella (epithelial cell migration into lens), microphthalmia, dermal aplasia, and sclerocornea (MIDAS) syndrome, Leigh syndrome, trisomy 13, Lowe's syndrome, and Down syndrome.

UNILATEAL MATURE CATARACT May be normal variant, but rule out underlying chronic RD, trauma, or tumor.

Congenital and Genetic Disease

CATARACT, CONGENITAL OR INFANTILE Present at birth (congenital) or during first year (infantile) in 1/2000 live births. One third of cases are associated with systemic disease, one third are inherited, and one third are from undetermined cause. Important to obtain a red reflex history, family history, full pediatric exam, date of onset, and associated signs and symptoms. Can characterize based on laterality (bilateral vs. unilateral) and by morphology of cataract.

CATARACT, LATERALITY Narrows the differential diagnosis.

- Bilateral: 60% idiopathic, 30% herditary (usually autosomal dominant), 10% from a metabolic or systemic disorder such as diabetes, galactosemia, Lowe's, Down, Alport's, or Marfan syndromes, Fabry's disease, trisomies 13–15, hypoglycemia, myotonic dystrophy, hypoparathyroidism, aniridia, anterior segment dysgenesis, corticosteroids, radiation, and TORCH, especially rubella. Work-up with TORCH titers, VDRL, RBC galactokinase level, urine for reducing substances, and calcium and phosphorus levels.
- Unilateral: 80% idiopathic, 10% traumatic (rule out NAT), 10% from local dysgenesis and not inherited such as PHPV, anterior segment dysgenesis, posterior lenticonus, anterior polar, posterior pole tumors, or rubella. Check TORCH titers.

CATARACT, MORPHOLOGY Lamellar is the most common.

- Cerulean: bluish, central, and not visually significant.
- Coronary: crownlike peripheral.
- Lamellar: most common congenital cataract (40%) from involvement of secondary lens fibers, zonular, with disk-shaped layers of opacification surrounding a clearer center. Bilateral, symmetrical, usually autosomal dominant, or sporadic cases usually from transient toxic influence (e.g., prenatal tetany).
- Membranous: traumatized lens resorbs proteins and forms dense white anterior membrane.
- Nuclear (pulverulent, Coppock cataract, cuneiform): opacification of embryonic nucleus (from disturbance in first 3 fetal months). May be bilateral (usually autosomal dominant) or unilateral, typically in a small eye.
- Persistent hyperplastic primary vitreous (PHPV): usually posterior cortical opacification that progresses to complete cataract that is unilateral and sporadic. Bilateral cases usually seen with chromosomal trisomies.
- Polar: subcapsular cortex and lens capsule opacity.
    - Anterior polar: small, bilateral, symmetric, nonprogressive; usually autosomal dominant but may be unilateral and sporadic. May be

associated with microphthalmos, PPMD, anterior lenticonus, and Peters' anomaly.
  - Posterior polar: more visual impairment than anterior, progressive, usually autosomal dominant and bilateral, but may be sporadic and unilateral. Associated with remnants of tunica vasculosa lentis, PHPV, and lentiglobus or lenticonus. May have capsular fragility during CE.
- Posterior lenticonus: sporadic, unilateral, polar.
- Posterior subcapsular: acquired, developmental. Usually associated with Down syndrome, steroid use, RP, or trauma if unilateral.
- Sutural: common fetal stellate cataract from opacified Y suture; bilateral, symmetric, and usually autosomal dominant, but not visually significant.
- Capsular: protrudes into the AC, unlike anterior polar cataract; usually not visually significant.

CATARACT, FROM ASSOCIATED SYSTEMIC OR SYNDROMIC CONDITIONS

- Aniridia: anterior and posterior lens opacities at birth and cortical, subcapsular, and lamellar opacities in 50 to 85% of cases within first two decades. Associated with poor zonular integrity and ectopia lentis.
- Galactosemia: autosomal recessive inability to convert galactose to glucose from an enzyme defect in galactose-1-phosphate uridyl transferase (most common), galactokinase, or UDP-galactose-4-epimerase. Classic "oil droplet" cataract in 75% of cases from accumulation of galactose and galactitol, with osmotic lens swelling; early cataract may be reversed with dietary changes. Patients also have mental retardation, malnutrition, hepatomegaly, and jaundice within a few weeks of birth. Galactosemia is fatal if not treated by elimination of milk from diet.
- Lowe's (oculocerebrorenal) syndrome: X-linked recessive disorder, with bilateral anterior lenticonus or micropunctate cortical cataracts with flat discoid lens and retained nuclei. Female carriers may have cortical lens opacities and aminoaciduria. Associated with glaucoma in 67% of cases from trabeculodysgenesis; also microphthalmia, nystagmus, strabismus, mental retardation, renal tubular acidosis (Fanconi syndrome), renal rickets, and hypotonia. CE is often difficult (total cataract).
- Myotonic dystrophy: autosomal dominant disorder, with "Christmas tree" polychromatic iridescent crystals in the lens cortex, that progresses to complete opacity. Associated with delayed relaxation of contracted muscles (patients cannot let go when they shake your hand), frontal balding in males, ptosis, and cardiac conduction defects.
- Peters' anomaly: may have adhesions between the lens and the cornea, with anterior polar or cortical cataract, microspherophakia, and anterior lens displacement.

- Rubella cataract: RNA togavirus infection in the first trimester, with cardiac defects, deafness, and mental retardation (Gregg's syndrome, rubella embryopathy). Usually bilateral (20% are unilateral). May have complete or pearly white nuclear opacifications in 15% of cases, with retention of live virus (no women of childbearing age should be in the OR during CE; may have postoperative inflammation from viral endophthalmitis) and retention of lens nuclei. May also have diffuse pigmentary retinopathy (salt and pepper fundus), microphthalmos, glaucoma, and corneal clouding.

CONGENITAL APHAKIA Primary lens plate fails to form; more commonly from secondary spontaneous resorption of lens.

ECTOPIA LENTIS FROM CONGENITAL CAUSES Trauma is the most common cause, but may be inherited as autosomal dominant (simple) or recessive (et pupillae) or secondary to systemic disease. In general, avoid surgery if possible.

- Ectopia lentis et pupillae: bilateral, progressive autosomal recessive displacement of the lens and pupil in opposite directions. Associated with axial myopia, RD, enlarged cornea, early cataract, and TID with poor dilation from hypoplastic iris sphincter muscle.
- Homocystinuria: autosomal recessive inborn error of methionine metabolism, most commonly from deficiency of beta-synthase, that converts homocysteine to cystathionine; 1:15,000 incidence. Seen in tall, blond, Marfan-like patients, except they have mental retardation and stiff joints. Patients are normal at birth, then develop seizures, osteoporosis, and progressive mental retardation in 50% of cases.
    - Lens dislocation occurs in 30% of affected infants and in 80% by age 15. Ectopia lentis is bilateral and symmetric from brittle cysteine-deficient zonular fibers. The lens displaces into the AC in 77% and posteriorly in 23% of cases (although classic answer is inferonasally on exams). Pathology shows periodic acid–Schiff (PAS) stained material on the zonules and on the surface of the ciliary epithelium.
    - Patients have increased serum and urine homocysteine (check sodium nitroprusside urinary test) and methionine. Increased homocysteine increases risk of thrombosis and small vessel disease (small strokes); patients are prone to thromboembolic events, especially during general anesthesia.
    - Fifty percent mortality by age 20. Treat with low-methionine (no meat) and high-cysteine diet, along with extra vitamin B_6. Patients need heparin and a beta-blocker.
- Hyperlysinemia: inborn error of lysine metabolism associated with mental retardation, muscular hypotony, and ectopia lentis, typically with Louisiana Cajun ancestry.

- Marfan syndrome: autosomal dominant (however, no family history in 15% of cases) gene defect of glycoprotein fibrillin 15, which is the major component of elastic tissue throughout the body, including zonules.
    - Seen in tall patients with arachnodactyly, normal intelligence, hyperextensible joints, chest wall abnormalities, and often a dilated aortic root (large vessel disease, unlike homocystinuria) and mitral valve prolapse.
    - Eighty percent of patients have ectopia lentis that is bilateral and symmetric, from stretched zonular fibers. Seventy-five percent have subluxation superotemporal (mnemonic: picture Abraham Lincoln, who was probably marfanoid, holding his arms up and out), often associated with cataract.
    - Patients also may have megalophthalmos (abnormal scleral fibrillin) with high axial myopia, enophthalmos (absence of retrobulbar fat), increased corneal diameter (13–14 mm), flat cornea (K 38–39 D), deep AC, glaucoma, poor dilation from hypoplasia of the iris dilator muscle, TID, increased vitreous loss with cataract extraction, a normal vitreous (unlike Stickler's syndrome), RD (usually can treat with just a buckle), staphyloma and Fuchs' spots, strabismus (in 20% of patients), and often amblyopia.
    - Treat with good optical correction (meticulous retinoscopy; cylinder is usually in the axis of lens dislocation), as patients can have good VA and will need reading aid. Treat cataract and glaucoma (may have RPB from microspherophakia) if needed, but may be hazardous and may need lensectomy using vitrectomy. Typically suture a large single-piece IOL, and trabeculectomy usually works well (because this is a connective tissue disorder). Prescribe a beta-blocker early to delay aortic aneurysm formation.
- Simple ectopia lentis: autosomal dominant; is likely the milder end of a spectrum with Marfan syndrome (less severe mutation in fibrillin 15 gene).
- Sulfite oxidase deficiency: autosomal recessive disorder of sulfur metabolism; associated with severe mental retardation, myoclonus, seizures, and ectopia lentis in 50% of cases.

LENS COLOBOMA May be primary and isolated or secondary from lack of ciliary body or zonular development, usually inferonasal. Also may be acquired from ciliary body tumors (especially medulloepithelioma).

LENTICONUS AND LENTIGLOBUS Localized cone-shaped (conus) or spherical deformation (globus) of the lens. Posterior location is more common and is usually seen in females, both unilateral and axial. Anterior lenticonus usually affects males and is bilateral; associated with Alport's syndrome. Retinoscopy shows a distorted and myopic reflex; may appear as oil droplet (do not confuse with oil droplet cataract of galactosemia).

- Alport's syndrome: hereditary hemorrhagic nephritis and sensorineural deafness from an X-linked (in 85% of cases) defect of type IV collagen (found in basement membranes) from mutation of the COL4A5 gene at Xq22. Ten to fifteen percent of patients have anterior lenticonus cataracts OU (early) and flecked retinopathy (late) from lens capsule and Bruch's membrane defects.

MICROSPHEROPHAKIA Small, spherical lens from faulty secondary lens fiber development. Patients are highly myopic; disorder may be isolated or seen with Weill-Marchesani syndrome (most common cause), congenital rubella, Peters' anomaly, and Marfan, Alport's, and Lowe's syndromes.

- Weill-Marchesani syndrome: autosomal recessive cause of microspherophakia (lens volume reduced by 25–40%), with lens equator visible through dilated pupil; often dislocates anteriorly or inferiorly (usually in second decade). Also has progressive lenticular myopia of 15–20 D, microcornea, and shallow AC.
  - Patients have "antimarfanoid" habitus with short stature, broad hands, stubby fingers, bradydactyly, reduced joint mobility, hearing defects, and normal intelligence.
  - Dominant spherophakia (McGavic type) has been reported as autosomal dominant Weill-Marchesani syndrome but is more like homocystinuria.
  - Lens can cause pupillary block angle-closure glaucoma that is aggravated by miotics. Thus, treat with cycloplegics to pull the lens–iris diaphragm posteriorly, then perform an LPI.

REMNANTS OF THE TUNICA VASCULOSA LENTIS

- Mittendorf's dot: remnant of a hyaloid corpuscle seen as a dense white spot inferonasal on posterior lens capsule where the hyaloid artery attached in utero.
- Epicapsular star: brown specks on the anterior lens capsule; also called "chicken tracks."
- Persistent pupillary membrane: fine filaments arising from the iris collarette to the anterior capsule.
- PHPV, retrolental fibroplasia, persistent fetal vasculature (PFV): unilateral eye maldevelopment with cataract, leukocoria, usually small eye in a full-term infant (distinguish from ROP). See Chapter 7.

Metabolic and Degenerative Disease

CATARACT, ACQUIRED, AGE-RELATED Most common cause of visual morbidity worldwide.

- Nuclear sclerosis: slowly progressive, bilateral impairment of distant vision more often than near vision. Often has a myopic shift ("second sight" for presbyopic patients), monocular diplopia from abrupt change in refractive index between the sclerotic nucleus and the cortex, or poor blue hue discrimination.
  - Older nuclear cells lose organelles and cell membranes, with increasing density and dehydration and accumulation of yellow urochrome pigment (possible photo-oxidation product). Pathology shows homogeneity of nucleus, with loss of cellular laminations and increased eosinophilia. When advanced, becomes brown (brunescent) or black (cataracta nigra).
  - Risk factors: older age, smoking, and lower socioeconomic status
- Cortical: soft cataract from changes in ionic composition that lead to cortex hydration and cuneiform opacities; often bilateral but asymmetric. Patients often complain of glare and monocular diplopia. On examination, may see cortical spokes, water clefts, or vacuoles from hydropic swelling of lens fibers; may have secondary cortical changes with crystal formation (cholesterol, calcium oxalate), dystrophic calcification, or even bone or fat formation. Risks include age, diabetes, UV light, and lower socioeconomic status.
  - Morgagnian globules: spherules of degenerated liquefied lens cortex protein (not cellular accumulation, like the fluid-filled bladder cells seen with PSC).
  - Mature cataract: intumescent and white total cortical opacity.
  - Morgagnian cataract: sclerotic nucleus sinks in a bag of liquefied cortex.
  - Hypermature cataract: cortical material leaks through capsule, leaving it wrinkled and shrunken (may have associated phacolytic glaucoma).
- Posterior subcapsular (PSC): axial cupuliform (saucer-shaped) opacities seen typically in younger patients that causes glare and poor photopic vision, especially with miosis, thus reducing near vision more than distant vision. Risk factors include age, diabetes, trauma, steroids, inflammation, ionizing radiation, UV light, and lower socioeconomic status. From posterior migration of lens epithelial cells that form aberrant swollen lens fibers (Wedl or bladder cells).
- Anterior subcapsular (ASC): local metaplasia of epithelial cells that synthesize collagenous plaque beneath the anterior capsule. Usually from an injury or irritant or associated with atopic dermatitis.

CATARACT, ACQUIRED, ASSOCIATED WITH OCULAR CONDITIONS Associated with many conditions, including uveitis, PXS, RP, essential iris atrophy, chronic hypotony, glaucoma, myopia, RD, and intraocular tumor (especially ciliary body melanoma).

Systemic and Vascular Disease

DIABETIC OR SUGAR CATARACT Classic diabetic "snowflake" cataract is bilateral, abrupt, progressive subcapsular lens changes in young patients with uncontrolled diabetes. Senescent cataract is also seen more frequently and earlier. In addition, patients may have earlier presbyopia, decreased amplitude of accommodation, and transient refractive changes (usually myopic) from increased aqueous glucose that enters the lens by diffusion and is converted by aldose reductase to sorbitol, which is not metabolized and causes influx of water and lens swelling.

HYPOCALCEMIA, TETANIC CATARACT Punctate iridescent cortical opacities, usually from idiopathic hypocalcemia or parathyroid removal.

ISCHEMIC CATARACT Anterior segment ischemia (carotid disease, multiple muscle surgeries, etc.) may cause rapidly progressive cataract (usually PSC). Also seen with Takayasu's arteritis (pulseless disease) and Buerger's disease (thromboangiitis obliterans).

OTHER SYSTEMIC CAUSES OF CATARACT Hypoparathyroidism, hypothyroidism, cretinism, aminoacidurias, and infantile hypoglycemia

WILSON'S DISEASE, HEPATOLENTICULAR DEGENERATION Autosomal recessive disorder of copper metabolism in which patients may have "sunflower" cataracts from cuprous oxide deposition on the anterior lens capsule and Kayser-Fleischer ring from deposition in Descemet's membrane.

Physical Disease

CHEMICAL AND ELECTRICAL INJURY Alkali injury is more likely to cause cataract because it penetrates the eye more easily than acid, increasing the aqueous pH and decreasing glucose and ascorbate. Electrical shock may cause protein coagulation and cataract, first seen as vacuoles.

DEPOSITION CATARACT FROM INTRAOCULAR FOREIGN BODY

- Chalcosis: copper foreign body may cause deposition in basement membranes (e.g., Descemet's or the anterior lens capsule), seen as the characteristic "sunflower" cataract (as in Wilson's disease) but usually not visually significant. If the foreign body is pure copper, patients often have a severe inflammatory reaction.
- Siderosis bulbi: from an iron IOFB or hemosiderosis with iron depostion in epithelial and endothelial cells (e.g., the TM, lens epithelium, iris, and retina). When advanced, may see complete cortical cataract.

DRUG-INDUCED CATARACT OR LENS CHANGES Many drugs are associated with cataract formation.

- Amiodarone: may cause stellate anterior axial pigment deposition.
- Corticosteroids: one third of patients on chronic dose of prednisone 10 mg/day develop cataract, usually PSC. Cataract may be reversible in children, and any route of steroid therapy (systemic, topical, subconjunctival, nasal sprays, etc.) may lead to cataract.
- Miotics and anticholinergics: especially seen with echothiophate iodide and demecarium bromide, primarily in adults (84% of patients have anterior subcapsular vacuoles). Twenty percent of patients after 55 months on pilocarpine develop vacuolar cataracts. Topical anticholinesterases are also associated with large iris cysts.
- Phenothiazines: cause pigmented deposits in the anterior lens epithelium; axial but usually not visually significant.
- Others: dinitrophenol (formerly used for weight control, as it uncouples oxidative phosphorylation), ergot poisoning, paradichlorobenzene, and Myleran.

RADIATION CATARACT Nearly all forms of radiation have been reported to cause lens changes.

- Ionizing radiation: may cause latent cataract up to 20 years later. Younger patients (more actively growing lens cells) are more susceptible. Cataract not typically seen from microwave radiation.
- Infrared radiation ("glassblower's cataract"): anterior capsular damage causes the capsule to delaminate and "peel off" (true exfoliation), and the outer lamella scrolls up on itself.
- Ultraviolet radiation: UVB increases cortical and PSC cataracts.
- Argon laser: blue light is absorbed by yellow sclerotic nucleus.

RESIDUAL CATARACT FOLLOWING CATARACT SURGERY

- Elschnig's pearls: proliferation of residual epithelium cells after cataract extraction form aberrant lens fibers (identical to bladder cells).
- Soemmering's ring: retention of peripheral ring of cortex after cataract extraction.

TRAUMATIC CATARACT Usually seen as a stellate or rosette-shaped axial opacity from blunt injury; may occur with even seemingly minor trauma (e.g., rubber-band snap to eye). Also look for Vossius' ring from pupillary margin pigment sticking to the anterior capsule following blunt injury. Check for phacodonesis, subluxation, or dislocation, indicative of zonular trauma. If the lens capsule is ruptured by the trauma, lens hydration and rapid opacification are typical. Perforating or penetrating injury may cause complete cataract or focal opacity. Also observe for phacoantigenic uveitis (phacoanaphylactic) if the capsule is open.

TRAUMATIC ECTOPIA LENTIS Most common cause of ectopia lentis. Lens trauma is also associated with retinal dialysis or tears, as the posterior capsule is attached to the anterior hyaloid face via Weigert's ligament, and thus may transmit the traumatic forces to the vitreous base.

Inflammatory and Immune Disease

ATOPIC DERMATITIS, ATOPIC CATARACTS Skin and lens share a common embryologic origin. Cataract is seen in 25% of patients with atopic dermatitis; patients are usually 20 to 30 years old with bilateral anterior subcapsular shieldlike plaques that tend to do poorly at surgery. Cataract also seen in ectodermal dysplasia (Rothmund's and Werner's syndromes) and acrodermatitis enteropathica.

PHACOANTIGENIC UVEITIS, PHACOANAPHYLAXIS Lens proteins leak through ruptured capsule, causing zonal granulomatous inflammation (histopathologic "zones" of inflammatory cells: PMN infiltrate first around the lens material, followed by epithelioid histiocytes, then finally a mononuclear infiltrate). Almost always seen following trauma or surgery (thus, a 3–7% coincidence with sympathetic ophthalmia). Treat by cataract extraction and anti-inflammatory medication.

UVEITIC CATARACT Usually PSC, seen with any chronic uveitis but especially with JRA (especially pauciarticular, RF negative, ANA positive) and Fuchs' heterochromic iridocyclitis (70% have cortical cataract, with favorable prognosis after CE).

Cataract Surgery

PREOPERATIVE

Determine visual disability: note functional complaints, record loss of BCVA, and do a complete eye exam. Particularly note physical exam factors that may complicate surgery or recovery, such as deep brow, presence of conjunctival filtering bleb, corneal guttae, shallow AC, poor dilation, presence of pseudoexfoliation or phacodonesis, and fundus pathology that needs treatment or that may limit visual recovery.

- Phacoemulsification after vitrectomy: may have zonular instability and little posterior support, with a "floppy" posterior capsule. If there is a need to convert to extracapsular cataract extraction (ECCE), expression is often difficult, and lens must be lifted out.
- Diabetic retinopathy: potential massive progressive of DR after surgery, especially with vitreous loss and increased risk of CME.

- Complete medical history: especially inquire about the use of anticoagulants (Coumadin, aspirin, Plavix, Ticlid, etc.) and anesthesia risks (coronary artery disease, emphysema, etc.).
- Determine surgical plan: A-scan, keratometry, presence of astigmatism, and refractive goal. Typically have an IOL available for the "bag," sulcus (0.5 D less power), and AC. Obtain and document informed consent.

PREPROCEDURE CHECKLIST On the day of surgery, at least mentally review these issues for each patient (mnemonic: ABC-ATLS-ABC).

- **A**ccurate patient and eye
- **B**ig pupil
- **C**heck consent and preop note
- **A**-scan review
- **T**able (set up the bed, wrist rest, etc.)
- **L**enses (ensure IOLs of proper power are available)
- **S**cope (ensure working order, and zero the X, Y, Z axes) and **s**upplies (ensure nursing has the instruments that you need)
- **A**nesthesia (retrobulbar, topical, etc.)
- **B**allottement of the globe if retrobulbar anesthesia used
- **C**leanse patient and surgeon (scrub)

EXTRACAPSULAR CATARACT EXTRACTION (ECCE) TECHNIQUE Many variations on surgical technique; goal is to get the cataract out as efficiently as possible with as few complications as possible.

- Administer retrobulbar anesthesia: may also use topical, sub-Tenon's, parabulbar, etc.
  - Technique: use 1:1 mixture of 2% lidocaine without epinephrine and 0.75% bupivacaine (and may use Wydase), 1.25 inch, 22 gauge needle. Ensure that the patient and surgeon are in a comfortable position. Have the patient's eyes in primary gaze, place finger on the inferior orbital rim about at the junction of the medial two-thirds of the eyelid and lateral one-third (approximately at the temporal limbus). Begin lateral to finger, and advance needle horizontally through the eyelid half the needle length with bevel up (may also pull down the lid and enter through the conjunctival fornix). Once past the globe equator, aim for the contralateral occiput, entering approximately 1 inch total length (never exceed 31 mm and never cross the midsagittal plane). Inject 4–5 cc, remove the needle, then apply external compression to the eye for several minutes of 20 seconds pressure and 10 seconds release. Beware of patients with deep-set eyes or long axial length.
  - Complications: retrobulbar hemorrhage (1–3%) with rapid orbital swelling, proptosis, globe immobility, elevated IOP, inability to separate the eyelids, massive ecchymosis of the lids and conjunctiva,

and decreased VA (optic neuropathy or CRAO); treat with lateral canthotomy/cantholysis, digital pressure to create orbital pulsations, and osmotic diuresis. Also common are globe perforation (1:1000) or direct CNS spread (1:350–1:500), seen as confusion, extraocular paresis or amaurosis in the contralateral eye, shivering, convulsions, nausea, vomiting, and significant changes in vital signs.

- Administer lid or facial nerve block, such as a modified van Lint injection at the lateral canthus.
- Adjust wrist rest, tape head, prep and drape patient, and place lid speculum.
  - The most important part of the preparation is use of povidone-iodine (Betadine) and a drop placed in the conjunctiva fornix (if patient is allergic to Betadine, use baby shampoo scrub and topical antibiotics).
  - The most important part of the draping is to drape the lashes out of the surgical field.
- Consider bridle suture if there is poor superior limbus exposure or deep socket: hold the SR with large forceps, and pass 5.0 silk on a blunt (e.g., BV) needle underneath the muscle, then attach suture to drape.
- Measure white to white with calipers.
- Do peritomy, using 0.12 forceps and blunt Westcott scissors.
- Use wet-field cautery to obtain scleral hemostasis.
- Groove perpendicularly with crescent blade, 1–2 mm posterior to the limbus, 11 mm chord length, one-half scleral thickness.
- Tunnel in a lamellar plane with crescent blade toward the limbus; keep blade flat against the globe, and advance until the blade tip is seen in the limbal vessels.
- Do paracentesis.
- Instill viscoelastic into AC.
- Enter AC with microkeratome through the central wound; keep level with iris plane to create triplanar wound.
- Perform capsulotomy with cystotome, can-opener versus capsulorrhexis.
- Hydrodissect and may hydrodelineate the lens with BSS.
- Rock the nucleus: push down toward 3 o'clock, then 9, 6, and finally 12 o'clock.
- Extend the wound with cresent blade or corneoscleral scissors to the left and right.
- Preplace safety sutures, using 10.0 nylon, at 10 and 2 o'clock.
- Express nucleus using lens loop superior to push down wound edge and use gentle pressure with muscle hook inferiorly at limbus.
- Tie the two safety sutures.
- Perform irrigation and aspiration with manual Simcoe cannula, engage cortex peripherally, pull to center, and aspirate.

- Place viscoelastic into bag.
- Place IOL, use McPherson's forceps to grasp lens oriented as a backwards "*S*." Place inferior haptic first, and use Sinskey-type hook to spin lens into bag.
- Apply Miochol to constrict pupil.
- Suture wound with 10.0 nylon; ensure watertight closure.
- Remove bridle suture; close conjuctiva with cautery or 8.0 Vicryl, and inject subconjunctival Decadron 8 mg and Ancef.
- Remove speculum and drapes, clean off Betadine, then place Maxitrol ointment, two eye pads, and Fox shield. Instruct patient not to bend, lift, strain, or cough.
- At 1 day postop, remove patch, begin steroid and antibiotic drops, and advise patient regarding activity restriction and shield or glasses over eye at all times.

INTRAOPERATIVE COMPLICATIONS

- Suprachoroidal hemorrhage: risk factors include chronic glaucoma, hypotony, older age, hypertension, and atherosclerosis. See loss of red reflex, experience posterior pressure, with risk of loss of intraocular contents. Immediately place finger over wound, and quickly suture wound closed, then consider sclerostomies.
- Vitreous loss: signs include sudden iris or lens bounce, change in pupil size or peaked pupil, decreased AC depth, decreased phacoemulsification power or inefficient aspiration, and posterior loss of lens particles. Stop phacoemulsification, but do not immediately remove phacoemulsification instruments; maintain AC with viscoelastic. If there is adequate compartmentalization with no mixture of vitreous and lens and rent is small, can continue slow phacoemulsification with low flow. However, phacoemulsification will not cut vitreous and increases risk of RD if vitreous is aspirated by phacoemulsification.
  - Risk of vitreous loss: zonular weakness (PXS, trauma, Marfan syndrome, etc.), small pupil, and previous vitrectomy.
  - Anterior vitrectomy: avoid hydration and traction of vitreous. Remove vitreous down to posterior capsule plane; may perform core vitrectomy. Consider pars plana vitrectomy, which offers greater vitreous cleanup: small peritomy; using 20 gauge microvitreoretinal (MVR) blade, enter at 3–4 mm posterior to limbus, then vitrectomy through pars plana with separate irrigation through paracentesis.

POSTOPERATIVE COMPLICATIONS

- Astigmatism: most likely caused by a tight suture following ECCE; may cut suture at steep axis after 6 weeks if >3 D of astigmatism.
- Corneal edema: usually temporary, but may be irreversible if there is significant endothelial cell loss (preexisting guttae or other corneal pathology or excessive phacoemulsification time). Also, historically,

Brown-McLean syndrome with peripheral corneal edema from flat AC may be seen following ICCE.

- Capsular block syndrome: typically occurs 1 to 2 weeks postop, with a clear space seen between the IOL and posterior capsule without capsular fibrosis that represents retained viscoelastic. May be treated with YAG laser capsulotomy. Also seen months or years later, with milky substance posterior to IOL and myopic shift, from hydration of retained cortex with fibrosis of anterior capsule to IOL; prevent fluid egress from the bag.
- Capsular centration syndrome, capsular phimosis: anterior capsule contraction with decreasing capsulorrhexis size that may cause IOL decentration.
- Cystoid macular edema: 50% incidence by FA after ICCE, 20% after ECCE, and much less after routine, uncomplicated, fast phacoemulsification. Usually occurs at 4 to 14 weeks postop. Risk factors include age, vitreous loss, AC IOL, diabetes, and microscope light toxicity. Edema mostly caused by inflammatory release of prostaglandins created from arachidonic acid derived from cell membranes. Treat with a topical NSAID and/or steroid (e.g., Volaren and PF 1% qid). Ninety percent of patients with a PC IOL recover >VA 20/40.
- Delirium: may be from anticholinergic toxicity, sensory deprivation, RD, fall, or stroke.
- Diabetic retinopathy progression: most important predictor of good postop VA in diabetic patients is the absence of preop DR. Ninety percent of nondiabetic patients are 20/40 or better after surgery versus only 60 to 70% of diabetic patients; one third of NPDR will progress in the operative eye postop.
- Epithelial or fibrous downgrowth: may cause segmental corneal edema after penetrating injury (trauma or surgery).
- Glaucoma: after CE, one third of patients have a mildly increased IOP, one third remain normal, and one third have a lower IOP. Glaucoma may develop from a very high early IOP spike, usually from retained viscoelastic or inflammation, or from long-term elevated IOP, usually from TM damage or steroid induced.
- IOL decentered or wrong power: explant by tilting IOL vertically, then cut horizontally with intraocular scissors, and pull out in two pieces. Best time to explant is within 7 days before significant fibrosis occurs.
- Posterior capsule opacification: incidence depends on IOL type, although usually <10%; needs YAG laser capsulotomy.

PEDIATRIC CATARACT EXTRACTION Consider surgery if opacity is >2 mm and in visual axis; a posterior opacity is more amblyogenic. Earlier surgery is better; operate for congenital cataract within 6 weeks of life. Critical period of visual development is in first few months; thus, bilateral visually significant cataracts can cause irreversible amblyopia and sensory nystagmus. Surgery for bilateral cataracts before age 2 months has better visual prognosis (80% of patients are 20/50 or better). Mean VA for congenital unilateral cataracts operated on within 2 months of age is 20/60; after 20 months, is 20/160.

- Surgery is usually lensectomy (often can just aspirate lens), primary capsulotomy, and anterior vitrectomy if patient is <5 years old. Expect strong Weigert's ligament; thus, avoid ICCE. Typically leave aphakic if patient is <2 years old; if older, place one piece PMMA or acrylic lens in the bag.
- Extended wear CL preferred over aphakic spectacles to reduce aniseikonia and astigmatism. Historically epikeratophakia was attempted. Remember that lifelong loss of accommodation is typical after CE; thus, prescribe bifocals.
- Pediatric postoperative complications: posterior capsule opacification (PCO) in 100% of patients, amblyopia, second membrane formation from proliferation of retained lens cells, glaucoma (5–30%), RD (5%), postoperative inflammation, CME rarely, and corneal decompensation, especially with Peters' anomaly.

PHACOEMULSIFICATION TECHNIQUE An ECCE technique that allows removal of the lens through a smaller incision—often without sutures and with topical anesthesia—with a lower complication rate. The phacoemulsification unit utilizes ultrasound energy to emulsify the lens nucleus in the eye. Diaphragm machines have slow but exponential rise in vacuum. Peristaltic machines use rollers to "milk" the fluid through the tubing and have a rapid stepwise rise in vacuum (e.g., Alcon Legacy). Venturi systems use gas flowing across a port to build a vacuum and show a rapid linear rise in pressure; also, the aspiration tip does not need to be occluded to build pressure (e.g., Storz Millennium).

VISCOELASTICS Complex molecules used to maintain intraocular spaces, provide protective coating, and assist surgical maneuvering.

- Cohesive (e.g., Healon, Provisc, Amvisc): sodium hyaluronidase, high molecular weight; adhere to themselves and are easy to remove.
- Dispersive (e.g., Viscoat, Ocucoat): low molecular weight; provide better coating of the endothelium.

YAG LASER CAPSULOTOMY Uses the photodisruptive power of the YAG laser to open the posterior capsule. Wait at least 6 weeks after CE; plate-type IOLs may decenter even years later. Treat with an alpha-agonist preprocedure, then defocus the laser posteriorly and apply the laser energy usually in a cruciate or circular pattern at 0.5–2.0 mJ. Has a 1% risk of RD; thus, perform DFE at 4 weeks.

Refractive Lens Surgery

CLEAR LENS EXTRACTION Often used for high myopia; some studies have shown up to a 17% long-term RD risk, but is likely much less.

IOL CALCULATION AFTER REFRACTIVE SURGERY Contact lens method is probably the most accurate, as it determines a corrected K value by overrefracting with a plano RGP. If the patient has a myopic shift with the overrefraction, convert the RGP base curve into diopters, and subract the myopic shift diopters to obtain the new K.

- Example: a post-LASIK patient's current spherical equivalent = +0.25. With overrefraction using a plano RGP and with a base curve of +35.0 D, the spherical equivalent changes to −2.00 D. Because of the myopic shift, the cornea must be weaker than the base curve of the CL by 2.25 D. Therefore, the new cornea K must be 32.75 (35.0 – 2.25).
- Keratometer and topographers are based on a net index of refraction = 4/3 ($n = 1.33$). However, because refractive surgery changes the shape of the anterior but not the posterior cornea, the 4/3 index is no longer valid. These instruments thus overestimate the power of the cornea by up to 14%.

PHAKIC IOL Early studies showed a high incidence of pupillary block glaucoma, especially in hyperopes, and usually prevented by two patent LPIs preoperatively. About 2% incidence of focal lens opacity and <1% incidence of visually significant cataract are seen within a few years of surgery.

CHAPTER 7

Retina and Vitreous

Anatomy and Physiology

EMBRYOLOGY The neuroectodermal monolayered optic vesicle invaginates to form a bilayered optic cup with inferior defect (choroidal fissure that closes at 7 weeks). Neural crest mesenchyme migrates through the choroidal fissure and develops into the hyaloid artery. Early on, the cavity of the optic vesicle is contiguous with the diencephalon via the optic canal, and the outermost layer nuclear zone (later the photoreceptors) have ciliated cells that are continuous with ependymal cells of the third ventricle.

- The retinal pigment epithelium (RPE) forms from the outer thinner layer of the optic cup, and the neural layer develops from the inner layer. The anterior one fifth of the inner layer remains as a monolayer along with the pigment layer, extending anteriorly as the ciliary body and posterior iris epithelium. The posterior four fifths of the inner layer proliferates into the outer nuclear and the inner marginal zones. The nuclear zone invades the marginal zone to form the inner and outer neuroblastic layers. The inner neuroblastic layer forms ganglia (first retinal cells to recognizably differentiate), amacrine, and Müller's cells. The outer neuroblastic layer gives rise to the horizontal, bipolar, and rod and cone cells by the eighth fetal month.
- Macula development begins just after midterm, with an increase in the number of ganglion cell nuclei that begin lateral displacement by 7 months, leaving a fovea centralis. The cones decrease in width and increase in density but are not fully developed until 3 to 4 months after birth.

VASCULATURE Retinal inner three fifths is supplied by branches from the central retinal artery (cilioretinal artery from choroidal circulation present in 20%) and the outer two fifths from choroidal circulation. Central retinal artery pressure = 80/40 mmHg. Retinal veins drain to the central retinal vein, and vortex veins drain to the superior ophthalmic vein, then into the cavernous sinus. Retinal vein at disk = 125 μm wide; 80% of the population has spontaneous venous pulsations.

- Choroid is vascularized by two posterior ciliary arteries, supplying the lateral and medial choroid. Thus, a vertical line through the disk is a watershed zone for choroidal infarction. Choroid is vascularized in inner half only.

- Blood–retinal barrier: formed by tight junctions of retinal blood vessels, RPE tight junctions; the internal limiting membrane (BM of Müller's cells) protects retina from vitreous.

VITREOUS Composed of hyaluronic acid (secreted mostly from nonpigmented pars plana epithelium) and thin collagen fibrils from hyalocytes. Volume about 4 mL (1 teaspoon). The strongest attachment of the vitreous framework is to the pars plana and around blood vessels and somewhat less around the macula.

- Berger's space is an area between the anterior vitreous (anterior hyaloid face) and the posterior lens capsule. Weigert's ligament (hyaloideocapsular ligament) is the firm attachment between the anterior hyaloid and the posterior lens capsule. The Weiss ring is the posterior vitreous detachment from the optic disk that floats in the prepapillary space of Mortegiani. Another anatomic space between the vitreous and the retina exists in the premacular bursa.
- In infancy, the primary vitreous is mesenchymal vascularized tissue from ectoderm, mesoderm, and neuroectoderm. The secondary adult vitreous is secreted by the retina and Müller's cells and thus is of neuroectodermal origin. Finally, the tertiary vitreous comprises the zonules derived from ciliary epithelium.
- With age (and accelerated in high myopes, postsurgical, hereditary vitreoretinopathies), liquefaction pockets develop within the vitreous cavity and vitreous fibrils conglutinate, causing floaters. Eventually the internal collapse of the vitreous structure may cause a posterior vitreous detachment (PVD).

RETINAL PERIPHERY The vitreous base inserts 2 mm onto the ora serrata anteriorly and posteriorly 4 mm onto the retina. The posterior base is the main origin of tears, as radial collagen fibers insert perpendicularly into the retina.

- Ora serrata: scalloped edge of approximately 48 dentate processes and ora bays.
- Enclosed ora bays: may give appearance of retinal hole; may tear at posterior margin after PVD.
- Meridional fold: ridgelike elevation of retina perpendicular to the ora in the meridian of ciliary processes, lies partly across the pars plana.
- Meridional complex: large dentate process, with occasional thinning posterior to the ridge; completely crosses pars plana.
- Cystic retinal tuft: white vitreoretinal mound; may cause up to 10% of RDs.
- Ora serrata pearls: small basement membrane material at the ora; not clinically significant, but may be confused for small RB in children. Present in 20% of autopsy eyes.

- White without pressure: posterior extension of vitreous base, especially temporally and in darkly pigmented and myopic patients; does not predispose to RD.

RETINA LAYERS (Fig. 7–1) At the posterior pole retina is 0.5 mm thick (choroid 0.4 mm and sclera 1 mm).

- Inner limiting membrane: BM of Müller's cells
- Nerve fiber layer: axons of ganglion cells; site of juvenile retinoschisis and flame hemorrhages.
- Ganglion cell layer: projects via the NFL to lateral geniculate and pretectal nuclei.

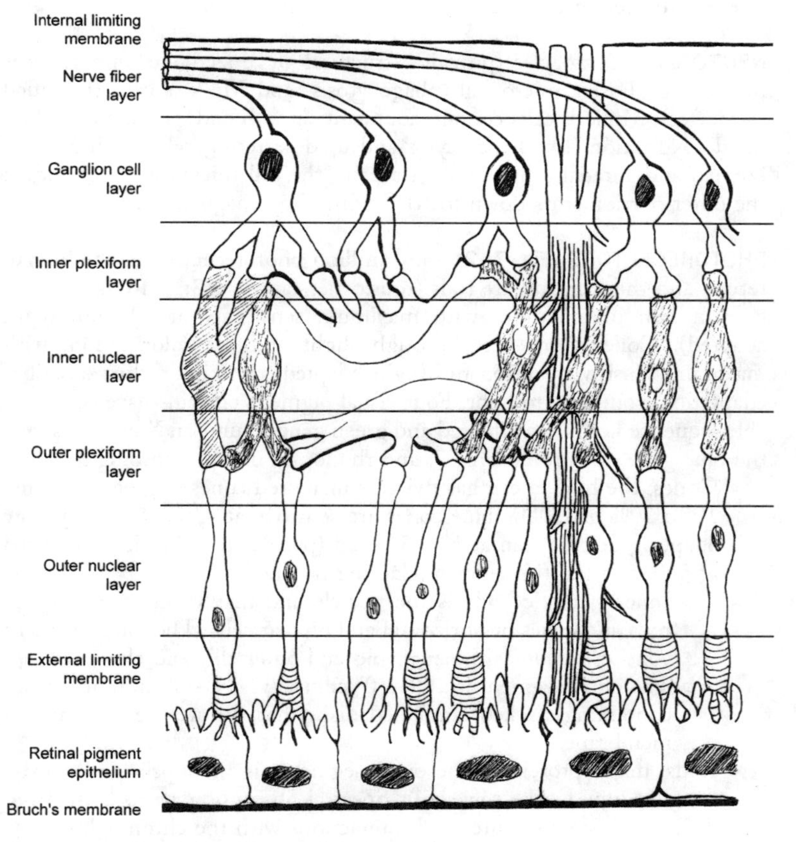

Figure 7–1 Simplified schema of the histologic layers of the retina and its cellular components.

- Inner plexiform layer: bipolar-ganglion cell and bipolar-amacrine cell synapses
- Inner nuclear layer: Müller, horizontal, bipolar, and amacrine cell bodies. Approximate limit of retinal circulation (outer retina supplied by the choroid).
- Middle limiting membrane (histological artifact)
- Outer plexiform layer: site of photoreceptor-bipolar and bipolar-horizontal cell synapses. Also site of CME (cystic spaces from the radiating fibers of Henle), cystoid degeneration, typical degenerative retinoschisis, and lipoprotein exudates.
- Outer nuclear layer: rod and cone nuclei
- Outer limiting membrane: not a true membrane, but the cell junction of photoreceptors.
- Photoreceptor layer: cell bodies of rods and cones

NEUROGLIA Astrocytes (provides structural and metabolic support, proliferates to gliosis), microglial (phagocytosis) and Müller's cells (modified astrocytes). Müller's cells contain abundant smooth endoplasmic reticulum for detoxification (like hepatocytes and lipid-secreting cells, such as meibomian and adrenal cells), and it traverses the full thickness of the retina; the outer portion scars down to RPE with photocoagulation.

PHOTORECEPTORS (Fig. 7–2) 130 million photoreceptors in the human retina, and the majority are rods (rods:cones ratio = 13:1). Rods function best in dim illumination, with maximum sensitivity at 504 nm (dark adapted). Cones work best in bright light and for color vision, with maximum sensitivity at 555 nm (light adapted). Purkinje's shift describes adaptation from dark to light. Four visual pigment proteins have considerable sequence homology: the red and green genes found on X chromosome, the blue gene on chromosome 7, and rhodopsin on chromosome 3.

- Cones: the human eye has twice as many red cones as green and only 10 to 20% blue. The blue cones are sensitive at 420–445 nm (yellow adapting field), green at 530–545 nm (purple adapting field), and red at 560–575 nm (blue-green adapting field).
    - Inner synaptic body is the pedicle and may connect with other rods and cones or horizontal and bipolar cells. The inner segment consists of conical inner myoid and outer ellipsoid elements.
    - The outer segment is a "9 + 0" cilium (vs. "9 + 2" in motile cilia) containing stacked laminated disks that are attached to the cell membrane.
- Rods: major protein in the outer segments is rhodopsin and consistency is liquid (like olive oil). Spectral absorption peaks arise from different opsin structures and interactions with the chromophore.
    - The inner synaptic body is the spherule connecting to two horizontal cells or one or more bipolar cells. The inner segment

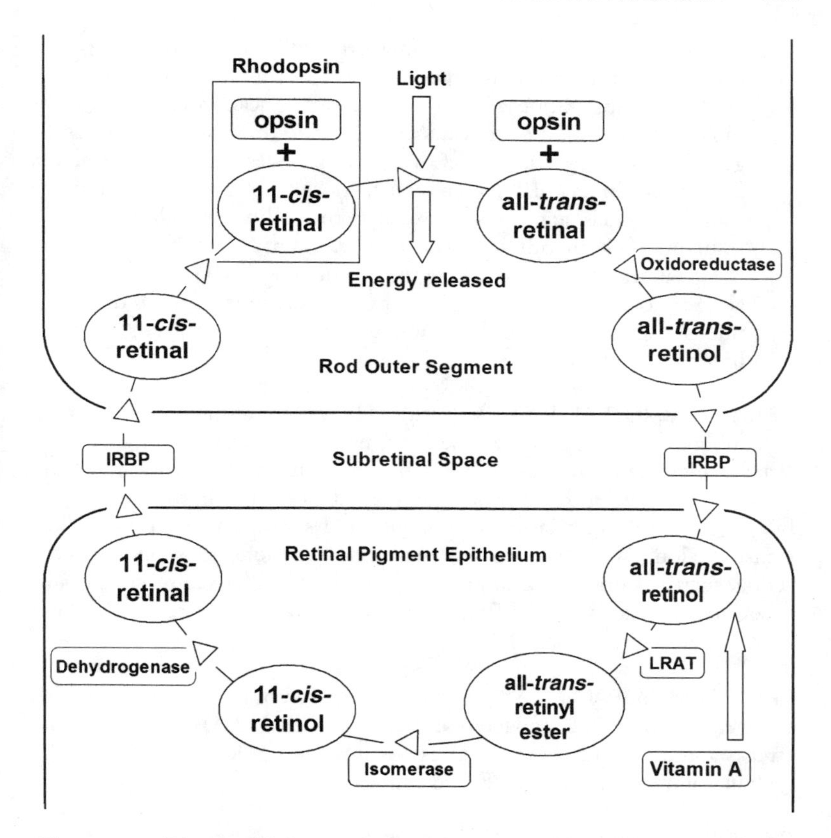

Figure 7–2 Diagram of the visual retinoid cycle in the rod photoreceptor outer segment and retinal pigment epithelium. In cones, the chromophore, 11-*cis*-retinal, is bound to one of three color-sensitive visual pigments instead of opsin. IRBP, intraretinal binding protein; LRAT, lecithin-retinol acyltransferase.

consists of heavily glycogenated inner myoid element next to the cell nucleus and the outer ellipsoid segment containing many mitochondria.

- ○ The outer segment is a "9 + 0" cilium containing multiple, stacked, and separated laminated disks.
- ○ The RPE phagocytizes rod outer segment tips that are shed daily 1.5 hours after light onset (diurnal rhythm) and renewed every 10 days (dark deprivation will quickly cease normal rod disk shedding).

- Phototransduction cascade: protein photopigment opsin is linked to 11-*cis*-retinal, which is the chromophore for all photoreceptors. It is a derivative of vitamin A, and is aligned parallel to the outer segment disk. The chromophore is isomerized by absorption of a photon to the all-*trans* configuration and triggers the amplification cascade, beginning with activation of transducin to activate the outer segment cyclic guanosine monophosphate (cGMP) phosphodiesterase. This results in a decrease in cGMP levels, which close cGMP-gated membrane cation channels and thus decrease permeability to sodium, with a resultant fall in intracellular free calcium. This causes hyperpolarization of the photoreceptor membrane (ERG A-wave). The all-*trans* configuration is oxidized by nicotinamide-adenine dinucleotide phosphate (NADPH) to all-*trans*-retinol that crosses the membrane to the RPE.

RETINAL PIGMENT EPITHELIUM (RPE) Has an apical-apical arrangement with photoreceptors, and the basement membrane is the internal layer of Bruch's membrane. Its desmosomes and tight junctions provide the outer blood–retinal barrier. It is the only pigmented monolayer in the eye (CB is a bilayer, but only one layer is pigmented). Its primary function is heat transfer, along with many other metabolic functions in support of the retina, such as storage of vitamin A. With injury, it is a very reactive tissue. Chorioretinal scar is formed from RPE metaplasia and may recruit Müller's cells to help with repairs.

BRUCH'S MEMBRANE 2–4 μm thick, composed of five layers: RPE BM, collagen, elastic tissue, collagen, and choriocapillaris BM. Site of angioid streaks and drusen (metabolic wastes possibly from phlebosclerosis, causing malnutrition of overlying RPE and retina).

CHOROID Uveal tissue that is the most richly vascularized tissue per gram in the body and is contiguous with the pia of the ON. The innermost layer is choriocapillaris that arises from the short posterior ciliary arteries; it is expansile and radiator-like, with endothelial fenestrations that allow large molecules (e.g., fluorescein) to leak. Outer lamina fusca pigmented cells adhere to the sclera but detach in choroidal effusions. It does not scar with inflammation; thus, following choroiditis, bare sclera are usually seen as punched-out white lesions. Peripheral choroidal lobule arteriole infarction is seen as paving-stone degeneration. Choroid has an increased number of melanocytes with racial pigmentation (unlike skin and conjunctiva, which only have an increased number of melanosomes within the melanocytes). No lymphatics (thus, ocular Kaposi's sarcoma is only in the conjunctiva or eyelid).

ANATOMIC DIVISIONS OF THE RETINA

- Foveola: central 1.2 degrees, rod-free zone. Umbo has only cones and ILM.

- Fovea centralis: central 5 degrees, about 1.5 mm wide (same as optic disk), with 36,000 cells, no ganglion cells, and area of maximal cone density (contributes about 0.5 mV of the ERG), although 90% of the actual number of cones are outside the fovea (100 mV of the ERG). The four layers (ILM, outer plexiform, outer nuclear, and cones) are oriented obliquely away from the foveola. RPE cells are more columnar and have increased melanin and lipofuscin, as well as xanthophyll; this, plus the absence of capillaries, accounts for the perifoveal dark appearance on FA.
- Macula: central 18.4 degrees, comparable number of rods and cones, more than two ganglion cells in thickness.
- Midperiphery: maximal rod density 20–40 degrees eccentric to foveola.
- Periphery: largest anatomic area.

Signs and Symptoms

AMELANOTIC LESIONS OF THE FUNDUS (Mnemonic: learned pathologists should never misdiagnose amelanotic melanomas of the choroid): **l**ymphoid lesions, **p**osterior scleritis, **s**arcoid granuloma (and other inflammatory or granulomatous diseases such as tuberculosis and syphilis), **n**eurolemmoma, **m**etastatic cancer (usually from breast or lung cancer), **a**melanotic **m**elanoma or AMD with a hemorrhagic disciform scar, and **c**horoidal hemangioma or osteoma.

ANGIOID STREAKS Dark reddish brown irregular streaks that radiate from the disk, representing breaks in a thickened and calcified Bruch's membrane. High risk of choroidal rupture or hemorrhage from mild trauma (prescribe safety spectacles), high risk of CNVM (look for subretinal hemorrhage around the disk). FA shows hyperfluorescent streaks early from overlying atrophic RPE. Etiology includes (mnemonic: PEPSI):

- **P**seudoxanthoma elasticum: most common known cause (85% incidence of angioid streaks); associated with ON drusen, peau d'orange retinal appearance, "plucked chicken" skin, widespread vascular malformations that can cause bleeds, and cardiovascular complications. From ATP transporter gene defect.
- **E**hlers-Danlos syndrome: collagen synthesis defect associated with hyperextensible joints, lax skin, ectopia lentis, RD, and blue sclera; risk for corneal or colon rupture.
- **P**aget's disease of the bone: 10 to 15% of cases have angioid streaks and osteoclastic hyperactivity, especially at the base of the skull (patients may have increased hat size from frontal bossing), and long bones (pathologic fractures). Treat with calcitonin.
- **S**ickle cell anemia: 1 to 2% of angioid streaks.
- **I**diopathic: 50% of angioid streaks.

BULL'S-EYE MACULOPATHY Associated with chloroquine (or, less likely, hydroxychloroquine), cone dystrophy, Spielmeyer-Vogt-Batten-Mayou disease, rarely RP, Stargardt's disease, AMD, crystalline retinopathy, and central areolar choroidal sclerosis.

CHERRY RED SPOT Indicative of CRAO, Tay-Sachs disease, Niemann-Pick disease, gangliosides GM1, Farber's disease, sialidosis, and metachromatic leukodystrophy.

CHORIORETINAL FOLDS Etiology: idiopathic (incidental, hyperopia), retrobulbar mass (orbital tumor or implant), scleral inflammation (TRIO, orbital pseudotumor, posterior scleritis), scleral buckle, hypotony, choroidal tumors, CNVM, and ON head diseases (crowded disk, pseudopapilledema). Parallel deep (unlike epiretinal membrane striae; on FA, see hyperfluorescence at apex (thin RPE) and hypofluorescence at trough (RPE bunched and blocks).

CHOROIDAL EFFUSION OR HEMORRHAGE Associated with uveal effusion syndrome, intra- or postoperative from rapid IOP changes, with shearing of choroidal perforating arteries (hypertension and atherosclerosis are primary risk factors), and hypotony.

CHOROIDAL NEOVASCULAR MEMBRANE (CNVM) (Mnemonic: MHATP): **m**acular degeneration, **h**istoplasmosis, **a**ngioid streaks, **t**rauma (choroidal rupture) or toxoplasmosis, **p**athologic myopia. Also ON drusen, choroidal tumors, inflammatory lesions, photocoagulation (if too small [<50 μm] or too hot), hereditary degenerative CNVM, juxtafoveal telangiectasis, multifocal choroiditis, serpiginous choroidopathy, MEWDS, and idiopathic.

CHOROIDAL THICKENING (BY ULTRASOUND) Associated with Sturge-Weber hemangioma, diffuse uveal melanoma, carotid–cavernous sinus fistula, uveitis, VKH, and sympathetic ophthalmia.

COTTON WOOL SPOTS (CWS) Seen with HIV, AIDS, or AIDS-related complex, diabetes, hypertension, cardiovascular disease, anemia, leukemia, vasculitis (SLE, scleroderma), and radiation. From interrupted axoplasmic flow in the NFL, usually ischemic. The nerve fibers whiten from lipid breakdown and some exudation; seen on pathology as necrosis or may see cytoid bodies.

CYSTOID MACULAR EDEMA Fluid collection in cystic spaces in the outer plexiform layer (radiating fibers of Henle), causing decreased VA, loss of foveal light reflection, intraretinal edema, and possible secondary photoreceptor degeneration or lamellar or full-thickness retinal hole.

- Etiology (mnemonic: DEPRIVE NOT): **d**iabetes, **e**piretinal membrane (any vitreous traction) or endophthalmitis (or any severe retinitis, including toxoplasmosis, ARN, CMV, and candidiasis), **p**ars planitis, **r**etinal telangiectasias or radiation retinopathy or RP, **I**rvine-Gass syndrome (pseudophakic or other postsurgical) or idiopathic or iridocyclitis (severe, such as Behçet's syndrome, birdshot choroiditis, and sarcoidosis), **v**enous obstruction (BRVO, CRVO), **e**pinephrine, **n**icotinic acid maculopathy, **o**thers (Goldmann-Favre, juvenile X-linked retinoschisis), and **t**umors. If no leakage is seen on FA, may be from Goldmann-Favre, RP, nicotinic acid, or juvenile X-linked retinoschisis (JXLR).
- Pseudophakic, aphakic, Irvine-Gass syndrome: 10% incidence after ICCE, 5% after ECCE, <1% after uncomplicated phacoemulsification. Associated with ruptured hyaloid face, vitreous to wound, AC IOL, pupillary capture, and inflammation.
- If chronic, becomes macrocystic (usually irreversible) as cysts form between Müller's cells.
- Treat with steroids, NSAIDs, Diamox 500 mg qid (especially in RP and other RPE disturbances but not effective in vasculopathies); relieve vitreous traction or IOL capture, or consider posterior vitrectomy.

DALEN-FUCHS NODULES Associated with sarcoidosis (involves choriocapillaris), sympathetic ophthalmia (spares choriocapillaris), and VKH. Represent T-cell granulomas between Bruch's membrane and retina that look like drusen.

DEAFNESS AND RETINAL LESIONS Seen with Alport's syndrome, choroideremia, Harada syndrome, Hunter's syndrome (MPS II), Sanfilippo's syndrome (MPS III), Laurence-Moon-Bardet-Biedl syndrome, Norrie's disease, Refsum's disease (phytanic acid), rubella, syphilis, Usher's syndrome (Hallgren syndrome), and Waardenburg's syndrome.

DECREASED VISION WITH NORMAL EXAM AND FUNDUS Seen with Stargardt's disease, X-linked retinoschisis, cone–rod dystrophy, amblyopia, and CNS disease.

DIET-ASSOCIATED RP SYNDROMES Associated with Refsum's disease, gyrate atrophy, and Bassen-Kornzweig syndrome.

DRAGGED MACULA Seen with toxocariasis, FEVR, ROP, PHPV, and PDR.

DRUSEN Seen with AMD, juxtafoveal telangiectasia, adult vitelliform, and pattern dystrophy (better prognosis than AMD, not heaped up like vitelliform; autosomal dominant transmission). "Hard" drusen are discrete and small (63 μm, about half retinal vein thickness); "soft" drusen are usually larger and have ill-defined edges. A single lesion is called a druse.

ENDOPHTHALMITIS May be bacterial, fungal, phacogenic, traumatic, or IOL-related. May be exogenous (postsurgery, trauma, etc.) or endogenous (systemic infection, usually in an immunocompromised host or IV drug abuser).

EXUDATIVE, TRANSUDATIVE, OR SEROUS RD Associated with VKH (Harada syndrome), pars planitis, sympathetic ophthalmia, acute hypertension (such as preeclampsia or eclampsia/toxemia), uveal effusion syndrome (usually short eyes with thick sclera), steroid use, ICSR, posterior scleritis, Goodpasture's syndrome, choroidal tumors (75% of uveal melanomas have RD), exudative ARMD, ARN, rheumatic fever, sarcoidosis (Schaumann's syndrome), Stickler's syndrome, toxocariasis, toxoplasmosis, birdshot choroiditis, Crohn's disease, HZV, Coats' disease, and PAN. Characterized by shifting fluid that follows gravity.

FLECKED RETINA (Mnemonic: the "4F's"): **F**undus flavimaculatus (type of Stargardt's disease), **f**amilial dominant drusen, **f**undus albipunctatus (subtype of CSNB), **f**undus punctatus albescens (subtype of RP); also AMD, Doyne's honeycomb dystrophy, Bietti's crystalline dystrophy, toxic reaction (e.g., to tamoxifen), and Alport's syndrome.

GRANULOMA OF THE RETINA Seen with tuberculosis, toxocariasis, sarcoidosis, and toxoplasmosis.

HEMORRHAGE AT ALL LEVELS OF THE RETINA Seen with sickle cell anemia, shaken-baby syndrome, CNVM, trauma, and macroaneurysm.

HEMORRHAGE, INTRARETINAL Many causes, usually vasculopathies (e.g., diabetes, aneurysms, and sickle cell anemia) or trauma.

HEMORRHAGE, SUBRETINAL Many causes, most commonly CNVM. Subretinal hemorrhage is toxic to photoreceptors and may lead to scarring. If large (>1 mm thick), consider vitrectomy with tissue plasminogen activator (tPA) and intravitreal gas injection; if moderate, tPA with or without vitrectomy; if small, observe. May use iron chelation with deferoxamine.

HEMORRHAGE WITH RETINAL NECROSIS Associated with CMV, herpes, toxoplasmosis, and Behçet's syndrome.

INNER RETINAL ATROPHY Caused by retinal ischemia, especially CRAO (inner two thirds of the retina down to the inner nuclear layer depends on the retinal circulation), glaucoma (if advanced, can lead to wipeout of the inner nuclear layer), and toxic-nutritional degeneration.

MUCOPOLYSACCHARIDOSES CAUSING RPE DEGENERATION Hunter's syndrome (type II), Hurler's syndrome (type I-H), Sanfilippo's syndrome (type III), and Scheie's syndrome (type I-S), but not Maroteaux-Lamy syndrome (mucopolysaccharidosis VI).

NEURORETINITIS, LEBER'S IDIOPATHIC STELLATE NEURORETINITIS Macular star and disk swelling caused by cat-scratch disease (*Bartonella*), leptospirosis, mumps, influenza, varicella, or unknown etiology. Usually have spontaneous resolution over several months; 80% of patients regain 20/40 vision or better.

PARAFOVEAL TELANGIECTASIAS Associated with old macular BRVO, DR, radiation, ocular ischemic syndrome, Coat's disease, and acquired parafoveal telangiectasias.

PROLIFERATIVE RETINOPATHY OR NEOVASCULARIZATION PDR, hypertension, sickle cell disease (peripheral seafan NV), CRVO, BRVO, or, less likely, CRAO (you see nothing and patient sees nothing). Also caused by BRAO, carotid disease, blood dyscrasias (Waldenström's macroglobulinemia, polycythemia rubra vera), collagen vascular disorder, inflammmatory disease (syphilis, SLE, Behçet's syndrome, Eales' disease, sarcoidosis, VKH, and pars planitis), radiation, RD with hemorrhage, trauma, FEVR, thrombophilic conditions (microhyperhomocysteinemia, anticardiolipin antibodies, factor V Leiden), and pars planitis (peripheral).

PROLIFERATIVE VITREORETINOPATHY (PVR) Usually seen following RRD, trauma, or any long-standing proliferative retinopathy (see above) caused by fibroglial proliferation into the vitreous framework; if a retinal tear, liberated RPE cells may undergo metaplasia into myofibroblasts that then contract.

PUNCHED OUT LESIONS WITH VITRITIS Seen with panuveitis with subretinal fibrosis, multifocal choroiditis, and sarcoidosis.

RAISED RETINAL LESIONS (Mnemonic: RPE monoliths): **RPE** hypertrophy or hyperplasia (pseudoadenomatous RPE hyperplasia, glandlike RPE scar), **m**elanoma, **o**rganizing hemorrhage, **n**evi or neoplasm, **o**steoma, **l**ate inflammatory changes, **i**diopathic, **t**rauma, **h**emangioma, **s**car (disciform).

RETINAL CRYSTALS Caused by tamoxifen, canthaxanthine, methoxyflurate, talc, and Bietti's crystalline dystrophy.

RETINAL MICROANEURYSMS Caused by diabetes, venous occlusive disease, sickle cell disease, and radiation.

RETINAL VASCULAR TORTUOSITY Caused by fetal alcohol syndrome (FAS) and Fabry's disease.

RETINITIS, RETINOCHOROIDITIS Caused by infections (toxoplasmosis, CMV, toxocariasis, HSV, syphilis, tuberculosis, ARN, progressive outer retinal necrosis (PORN), fungal or candidiasis, septic retinitis or subacute bacterial endophthalmitis, *Bartonella*), and immune diseases (sarcoidosis, birdshot choroiditis, MEWDS, ARPE, SFU, RP).

TRACTION RETINAL DETACHMENT Any fibroproliferative disorder (see above), especially diabetes and ROP, usually with a concave appearance.

ROTH'S SPOTS White-centered hemorrhages that can be seen with any chronic hemorrhage but classically associated with septic emboli (endocarditis, *Candida* bacteremia), as well as leukemia and collagen-vascular diseases.

SALT AND PEPPER FUNDUS Seen with congenital infections (rubella, syphilis, HSV, varicella, mumps), Leber's congential amaurosis, cancer-associated retinopathy (CAR), thioridazine use, and carriers of choroideremia, albinism, or RP.

SCALLOPED RETINAL ATROPHY Associated with gyrate atrophy, high myopia, and choroideremia.

SCLERAL THICKENING (BY ULTRASOUND) Seen with scleritis, hypotony, pthisical eye, and nanophthalmos.

SEROUS RD Associate with idiopathic central serous, ON pits, CNVM, hemangioma, nevi or melanoma, metastatic cancer, and Harada syndrome or other inflammatory disease. See also exudative RD above.

SILENT CHOROID ON FA Associated with Stargardt's disease (lipofuscin in RPE blocks FA) and systemic argyrosis.

STELLATE MACULOPATHY Yellow lipid in outer plexiform layer (OPL) with starlike pattern usually from hypertension, optic neuritis, Coats' disease, hemangioma, or inflammatory disease (especially from *Bartonella*).

UNILATERAL RP Associated with siderosis (retained intraocular foreign body), DUSN, and AZOOR.

VENOUS ENGORGEMENT Seen with cryoglobulinemia, Waldenström's macroglobulinemia, and Takayasu's arteritis.

VESSEL ATTENUATION Caused by Behçet's syndrome, RP, ARN, and CRAO.

VITREOUS HEMORRHAGE PDR (causes 39–54% of VH), retinal break (12–17%), PVD (7–12%), RD (7–10%), and NV (3–10%); also may be seen with X-linked retinoschisis, pars planitis, tumor (RB, melanoma, leukemia), CNVM, trauma, Coats' disease, vein occlusion, sickle cell retinopathy, FEVR, VKH, OHS, Eales' disease, and hypertension. Can lead to hemosiderosis and ghost cell glaucoma.

VITRITIS Associated with Irvine-Gass syndrome, sarcoidosis, amyloidosis, Eales' disease, VKH, pars planitis, any active retinitis (toxoplasmosis), active retinal vasculitis, multiple sclerosis, MEWDS, MCP, birdshot choroiditis, AMPPE, serpiginous choroidopathy, psoriatic, Fuchs' heterochromic iridocyclitis (Fuchs' HIC), Whipple's disease, masquerade syndromes (intraocular lymphoma), spillover from anterior uveitis, recent trauma, retinal detachment, retinal tear, and giardiasis.

Exam and Imaging

ELECTRO-OCULOGRAPHY (EOG) Measures the standing electrical potential of the RPE and the light response of the RPE from depolarization of the basal membrane of the RPE (is thus an indicator of retinal disease). Compares the negative charge of the RPE to the positive charge of the cornea.

- Expressed as a ratio of the maximal light-adapted peak (Lp) to the minimal dark-adapted trough (Dt). The RPE has increased voltage in the light and requires about 8 minutes. Normal Lp:Dt ratio is >2.0; if <1.75, it is abnormal, as in CRAO, ocular ischemic syndrome, ophthalmic artery occlusion, gyrate atropy, and Best's disease.
- EOG usually parallels the ERG, except in Best's vitelliform dystrophy and its carriers, who have normal ERG but abnormal EOG.

ELECTRORETINOGRAM (ERG) Mass response of retina to light (full-field Ganzfeld system). The cornea is in electrical continuity with the front of the retina and the eyelid with the back of the retina.

- ERG waveforms and measurements: no waveform for the ganglion cell.
  - A wave: represents photoreceptor hyperpolarization; a negative deflection from photoreceptor cell inner segment sodium flux.
  - B wave: measures the inner retina (Müller and bipolar cells); positive deflection from increased extracellular $K+$ concentration.

  - C wave: RPE positive deflection.
  - Early receptor potential: small negative deflection at the very beginning of the A wave from rhodopsin cascade initiation in the photoreceptor outer segments.
  - Implicit time: measurement of the trough of the A wave to the peak of the B wave. B-wave implicit times are slowed as the rods dark adapt because rods are a reservoir of vitamin A for cones; thus, widespread diseases with rod loss, such as early RP, may have delayed B-wave implicit time even with normal amplitudes.
- Testing parameters:
  - Scotopic (rod-isolated): single flashes of dim blue light tests rods (100–200 μV, below cone threshold), as the patient is dark adapted.
  - White light: mixed cone and rod response (350–700 μV).
  - Photopic (cone-isolated): white flicker stimulus (30 flashes/sec) tests cones (50–100 μV), as the patient is light adapted to bleach the rods. Rods are unable to cycle quickly enough and fuse at 20 cycles/second. White flicker is mainly extramacular test because 90% of the cones are outside the macula (and are thus not affected by macular scar).
  - Pattern-evoked ERG: small focal ERG using checkerboard pattern, allowing ganglion cell influence (macula tested, not full-field), and thus is abnormal in POAG.
- Selective abnormalities:
  - Selective B-wave reduction: seen in CSNB (defect in rod synapse to bipolar cells), Oguchi's disease, X-linked juvenile retinoschisis (NFL pathology affects Müller end plates and ILM and probably bipolar synapse), quinine toxicity, CRVO and CRAO (flat B wave, but cones are preserved via choroidal circulation).
    - For CRVO that is nonischemic, the B:A ratio is >1.0; for ischemic CRVO, the B:A ratio is <1.0.
    - Flat ERG: seen in ocular ischemic syndrome and ophthalmic artery occlusion.
  - ERG is decreased in myopia and African-American patients (decreased reflection of light). ERG is increased in albino patients.
  - ERG is not affected by glaucoma, ON transection, or cortical disease.

FLUORESCEIN ANGIOGRAPHY (FA) Sodium fluorescein is an orange-red, crystalline, low molecular weight hydrocarbon that is 80% bound to plasma protein. It diffuses through the choriocapillaris but does not leak from intact retinal vessels. It is excited by blue light at 490 nm and emits green light at 530 nm. The camera filters block the blue light and film the light emitted from the fluorescein. Fluorescein, which is excreted by the kidney and liver within 24 hours, may cause yellow skin and urine. Adverse reaction with nausea and vomiting seen in 5% of patients; rarely vasovagal episode or allergic reaction; death reported in 1/250,000. Affects digoxin serum test for 12 hours and cortisol, thyroxine, and quinidine tests for up to 3 hours.

- Normal FA: the choroidal phase begins within 10 to 12 seconds and is very rapid. Arterial phase (from central retinal artery) occurs 1 to 3 seconds later. The arteriovenous phase proceeds 1 to 2 seconds later, and the choriocapillaris is filled. The laminar venous phase occurs 5 to 10 seconds later. The perifoveal capillary network is best seen at 20 to 25 seconds. Recirculation occurs >30 seconds. Late fluorescence is normally seen of choroid, sclera, and edge of disk.
- Hypofluorescence:
  - Blockage: density between camera and choriocapillaris (e.g., blood, exudate), deposited in the retina or choroid.
  - Vascular filling defect: arterial, venous, or capillary defect in retina, disk, or choroid. For example, loss of choriocapillaris seen with staphyloma and choroideremia.
  - Fovea is naturally dark because tall macular RPE cells have increased melanin and lipofuscin, the foveal avascular zone (FAZ) has no retinal capillaries, and fovea has xanthophyll in the OPL.
- Hyperfluorescence:
  - Autofluorescence: ON drusen, astrocytic hamartoma
  - Window defect: focal hyperfluorescence without late leakage from RPE loss, which normally blocks the easily seen lake of choroidal fluorescein (e.g., drusen, laser scar, geographic atrophy).
  - Abnormal vessels: either from the retina (NV, aneurysms, tortuous vessels) or choroid (CNVM, tumor vessels)
  - Leakage: hyperfluorescence that increases with time. May be subretinal from RPE tight junction breakdown (e.g., ICSR, OHS, CNVM), intraretinal from capillary tight junction breakdown (e.g., CME), or vitreal from neovascularization.

VISUAL EVOKED POTENTIAL (VEP) Records the electroencephalogram (EEG) over the visual cortex. Used to gauge visual function (e.g. cortical blindness, malingering) and is abnormal in optic neuritis (prolonged latency but normal amplitude unless there is active disease).

ULTRASONOGRAPHY High-frequency (8–10 MHz) radio signals with short wavelengths used to create images and measure distances in the globe from echos that are generated by acoustic interfaces. Indications include opaque ocular media; can be used to evaluate posterior segment pathology (see also Chapter 2).

- Posterior segment tumors: obtain measurements, determine if solid versus cystic.

- Choroidal detachment: dome-shaped elevation of the retina and choroid; little mobility with eye movement. Detachment may extend to the CB, and is segmental in appearance because the choroid attaches at the vortex veins but not to the ON, as seen with a retinal detachment. If serous, is acoustically clear, in contrast to hemorrhagic choroidal detachment, which has subchoroidal echoes. A-scan shows rapidly rising, usually 100% high, thick or double-spiked echo.
- RD: retina remains attached to the ON and extends to the ora; typically bullous appearance with shifting fluid. Spike amplitude stays same all along the retinal interface and is 100% high and narrow.
- PVD: thin echo spike lessens as it moves toward the ora.
- Also used to evaluate ON cupping, elevation or drusen, IOFB, trauma, endophthalmitis (rule out RD before antibiotic injection or to follow vitritis course). Silicone oil has lower sound velocity, and echos appear much larger.

Fig. 7–3 shows the patterns of some common electrodiagnostic tests.

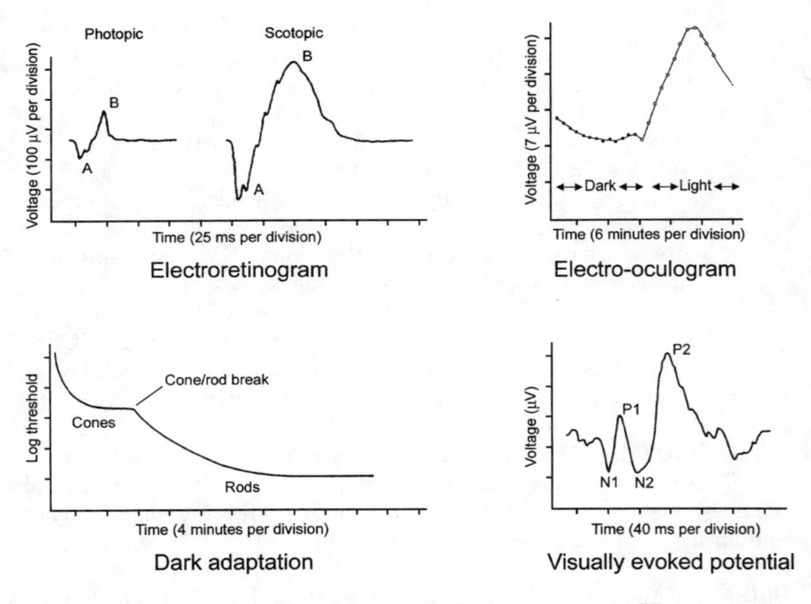

Figure 7–3 Normal patterns of selected electrodiagnostic tests. The electroretinogram (ERG) records the electrical response from the retina and the electro-oculogram (EOG) from the retinal pigment epithelium. Dark adaptation, as tested with the Goldmann-Weekers dark adaptometer, records the time latency for the eye to adjust to scotopic conditions. The visual evoked potential (VEP) is the recorded brainwave activity over the occipital cortex following visual stimulation.

Congenital and Genetic Disease

COATS' DISEASE, CONGENITAL RETINAL TELANGIECTASIAS Nonfamilial developmental vascular anomaly with intra- and subretinal lipid leakage from telangiectatic vessels. Usually presents with leukocoria or strabismus. Ninety percent of cases are unilateral, and 80% are male patients who are usually otherwise healthy. Bimodal distribution: children (18 months to 10 years) and adult (after age 16, associated with hyperlipidemia). Exam shows dilated retinal arteries and veins with aneurysms that may cause circinate lipid exudation; exudative RD in two thirds of patients, with possible CME. FA shows capillary nonperfusion and "light bulb" microaneurysms. Limited form, called Leber's miliary aneurysms, is frequently progressive. Treat early with cryotherapy or laser to obliterate leaking vessels in order to stabilize vision and prevent progression. RD usually needs buckle or vitrectomy.

CONGENITAL HYPERTROPHY OF THE RETINAL PIGMENT EPITHELIUM (CHRPE) Flat, black, well-delineated focal RPE hypertrophy present at birth with no malignant potential. Overlying depigmented lacunae may be present. Multifocal variant shows grouped lesions ("bear tracks"). Pathologically, cells have macromelanosomes (normally, RPE has moderate-size apical melanosomes).

- Gardner's syndrome: multiple, bilateral, variably shaped CHRPE-like pigmented ocular fundus lesions (POFLs) in patients with familial adenomatous polyposis (100% incidence of colon carcinoma by age 50). Patients also have associated benign soft tissue and bony tumors, jaw lesions, and increased risk of thyroid, adrenal, and liver CA. Defect of the adenomatous polyposis coli (APC) gene on chromosome 5q21–22 with a POFL-negative and positive phenotype. Four or more POFLs indicates >90% specific and 70 to 80% sensitive for familial adenomatous polyposis.

CYSTINOSIS Inability of lysosomes to excrete cystine; ranges from benign to nephrotic (renal failure and rickets) severity, with salt and pepper fundus and corneal crystals causing glare and photophobia.

INCONTINENTIA PIGMENTI, BLOCH-SULZBERGER SYNDROME X-linked syndrome at Xp28 in females that has unilateral peripheral retinal degeneration with RD (often presents with leukocoria that may mimic RB), with peripheral capillary nonperfusion, arteriovenous shunts, NV, and isolated cataract. Characteristic "splashed paint" hyperpigmented skin macules with eosinophilic skin infiltration on the trunk and skin erythema, bullae (filled with eosinophils), and verrucae. Patients often have seizure disorder, mental retardation, microcephaly, hydrocephalus, dwarfism, and skull, dental, and palate deformities.

MUCOPOLYSACCARIDOSES Retinal pigmentary degeneration seen in Hurler's, Scheie's, Hunter's, and Sanfilippo's syndromes.

NANOPHTHALMOS, UVEAL EFFUSION SYNDROME Characterized by ciliochoroidal detachment, recurrent choroidal effusions, short axial length, hypermetropia, and glaucoma from thickened sclera (disorder of collagen lamellae) that impedes vortex venous outflow. Treat with partial thickness scleral windows near vortex vein exits in at least three or four quadrants. May also develop uveal effusions with scleritis, hypotony, or postsurgically.

PERSISTENT HYPERPLASTIC PRIMARY VITREOUS (PHPV), PERSISTENT FETAL VASCULATURE (PFV) Caused by arrest in development, which causes a unilateral (75%) small eye. Patients often have leukocoria, cataracts (rare with RB), foveal hypoplasia, retinal folds, RD, and ACG. Observe; consider lensectomy for cataract, but may have hemorrhage from patent hyaloid vessel.

- Anterior: most common presentation; 90% unilateral, with retrolental plaque of tissue (may be fibrous, adipose, muscle, or cartilage) that pulls ciliary processes centrally. Lens may be resorbed or have intralenticular lipid. Associated with leukocoria, secondary ACG, peripheral RD, microphthalmia, cataract, and microcornea. Nearly half of patients have VA 20/200 or worse.
- Posterior: may have features of anterior PHPV plus retinal traction and a nasal retinal fold extending to the periphery, with primary vitreous fibers attached to the retina and potential for RD. Differential diagnosis includes toxocariasis.

PHAKOMATOSES See Chapter 9.

- von Hippel-Lindau disease (VHL): retinal capillary hemangiomas, cerebellar hemangioblastoma; 25% of patients have renal cell carcinoma, pheochromocytomas, and pancreatic and renal cysts.
- Neurofibromatosis (NF) II: choroidal hamartomas (51%)
- Tuberous sclerosis (Bourneville's syndrome): retinal and brain astrocytic hamartomas (50%)
- Sturge-Weber syndrome: choroidal cavernous hemangioma ("tomato catsup" fundus)
- Wyburn-Mason's syndrome (racemose hemangioma): direct AV communication

RETINOPATHY OF PREMATURITY (ROP) Ischemic immature retina in premature infants that leads to proliferative vitreoretinopathy. In normal development, the retina does not have blood vessels until 4 months gestation, when they grow in from the ON toward the ora, reaching the nasal retina edge by 8 months and the temporal retina after birth. Delayed vascularization of especially the temporal retina makes it susceptible to NV, and coincidental O_2 treatment results in vasoconstriction and may compound the ischemia. Differential diagnosis includes FEVR that looks like ROP in an adult.

- Risk factors: primary risk is prematurity (especially birth <32 weeks); also <1500 g (25–35% incidence if <1250 g), poor growth, hypoxia, and sepsis.
- Examine at 4 to 6 weeks of age if birth weight is <1300 g or <30 weeks' gestation (recommendation from the American Academy of Pediatrics). If no ROP, examine every 2 weeks; if avascular zone, examine every week; ROP usually appears at a median conceptive age of 37 weeks. Describe stage, zone, clock hours, and the presence of Plus disease or not.
- Stages of ROP: 85% of Stage 1 and 2 ROP cases regress spontaneously, and only 6% overall reach threshold. Plus disease is dilated tortuous vessels in the posterior pole from AV shunting, poor iris dilation from vessel engorgement and rigidity, and vitreous haze ("Rush" disease).
    - Stage 1: thin white line, demarcating mature and immature retina.
    - Stage 2: wide white line, which is ridge of dilated elevated vessels that do not leak.
    - Stage 3: ridge with neovascular vessels and crossing of this "ragged ridge" shunt area by retinal vessels.
    - Stage 4: tractional detachment. Stage 4a if extrafoveal or stage 4b if macula is involved.
    - Stage 5: funnel RD (10% will recover fix-and-follow visual acuity [F/F]).
- Zones of ROP: anatomic zones are centered on the disk.
    - Zone I: posterior pole, radius 2× disk to fovea (6 mm); more posterior ROP has worse prognosis.
    - Zone II: peripherally from zone I, with radius from disk to nasal ora (cryo-ROP study: a multicenter, randomized prospective trial that studied cryotherapy retinal ablation for ROP; found that cryo-ROP study was a zone II study).
    - Zone III: remaining temporal crescent; most common zone for ROP.
- Treatment: observe prethreshold disease (only 8% progress).
    - Threshold disease: 5 continuous or 8 cumulative clock hours of stage 3 disease (mnemonic: $3 + 5 = 8$) in zone I or II with Plus disease. Treat as soon as detected: obliterate the immature retina with cryotherapy or laser. Apply laser with hot, white, confluent burns anterior to the ridge (use a 28 D lens to get 400 μm spot size).
        - Reexamine 10 days after laser to look for decreased Plus and vessels growing into the avascular retina. Zone I follow-up 1 week, zone II follow-up 2 weeks. Follow patient until maturation is complete to the ora.

        - Usually treat stage 4a with lens-sparing vitrectomy, and stage 4b and possibly stage 5 with vitrectomy with or without a buckle.
    - Cryo-ROP study: cryotherapy to all areas of nonperfused retina in eyes with threshold disease caused 50% decrease in progression and unfavorable outcomes (22% treated vs. 42% untreated). Treatment was cryotherapy for all retina anterior to ridge with contiguous freezes in two or three rows for 360 degrees at −55°C. However, both groups had about the same VA at 5 years (mainly from amblyopia).
    - Goal of treatment is anatomic success, but for visual success, patients will need lifelong care.
- Complications: strabismus, pseudoexotropia (macular dragging, positive angle kappa), retinal fold in macula, progressive myopia in 80% (axial myopia and from forward movement of the lens–iris diaphragm), anisometropia, amblyopia, nystagmus, angle-closure glaucoma (usually at age 10 to 20), RD (may be late-onset), and cataract from laser treatment.

SPHINGOLIPIDOSES Most cause cherry red spot. See Chapter 9.

Hereditary Macular Disorders

BEST'S VITELLIFORM MACULAR DYSTROPHY Autosomal dominant juvenile macular dystrophy that develops about age 4 to 10 years. Defect found on bestrophin gene on chromosome 11q13 that codes for a protein expressed solely in the RPE. Early on, the fundus is normal (previtelliform stage) but the EOG is abnormal. EOG diagnostically shows a diminished light peak (Lp) to dark trough (Dt) ratio <1.5 in affected patients, asymptomatic patients with normal fundi, and asymptomatic carriers. The ERG is normal. Ultimately, the VA is usually 20/100 or worse with no good treatment available.

- Stage 1: subretinal, lipofuscin-like pigment collects in RPE cells and clinically looks like "egg yolk" yellow material in the macula; usually 1–5 DD in size, with good VA.
- Stage 2: "yolk" breaks up and may have macular "pseudohypopyon."
- Stage 3: slowly progresses to atrophy and looks like "scrambled egg."
- Stage 4: AMD-like scarring and severe central loss of vision from subretinal hemorrhage or NV; serous detachment may occur.

CENTRAL AREOLAR CHOROIDAL DYSTROPHY (CACD) Autosomal dominant circular RPE and choriocapillaris atrophy in third decade with mild central vision loss, slow progression, and poor visual prognosis. FA may show zonal choriocapillaris defect. Chromosome 6q defect.

CENTRAL AREOLAR PIGMENT EPITHELIAL DYSTROPHY (CAPE) Autosomal dominant, fine, modeled depigmentation of the fovea in the first decade with good prognosis.

CONE DYSTROPHY Spectrum with rod dystrophies (RP) with early onset cone dysfunction and slowly progressive decreased central VA, photophobia, and defective color vision. Early on, the fundus is normal but later shows a bull's-eye maculopathy, diffuse pigment stippling, and temporal optic nerve atrophy. Often patients later develop rod disease but rarely lose peripheral vision and are not night blind. Usually presents in the first or second decade. Characterized by abnormal photopic ERG with decreased single-flash and flicker and reduced flicker fusion frequency. Ultimately VA is about 20/60–400 and symmetric OU. Most cases are sporadic but when familial are autosomal dominant or X-linked.

DOMINANT DRUSEN, DOYNE'S HONEYCOMB RETINAL DYSTROPHY, MALATTIA LEVENTINESE, FAMILIAL DRUSEN Autosomal dominant chromosome 2p16–21 defect with early (age <55 years) numerous cuticular drusen nasal to disk, atrophy, and linear drusen (especially in ML, where the linear drusen are more peripheral). CNVM is common, and most patients are legally blind by age 70. Has a normal ERG but abnormal EOG. Defect in epidermal growth factor (EGF)–containing fibrillin-like extracellular matrix protein-1.

JUVENILE X-LINKED RETINOSCHISIS (JXLR) Vitreoretinal dystrophy from defective X-linked gene XLRS1 with high penetrance. Presents early in life with parafoveal spokewheel-like radiating retinal folds that progress to macular intraretinal cysts and foveal bullous schisis cavities in the NFL. (In contrast, senile retinoschisis is cleavage of the outer plexiform layer.) Macular degeneration is present in 95% of cases; VH may result from an exposed retinal vessel as the NFL is obliterated. Outer layer holes may lead to RRD; also may have liquefied vitreous, traction bands, and PVD. Fifty percent of patients have peripheral schisis and 100% have foveal schisis. CME shows no leakage on FA. ERG has reduced photopic and scotopic B wave (Müller cell pathology, which causes the NFL schisis) in proportion to the area of schisis with an intact A wave because the photoreceptors are unaffected. Some cases have Mizuo-Nakamura phenomenon (golden yellow sheen when light adapted but disappears when dark adapted), as in Oguchi's disease. Typically, VA is reduced to 20/50–100 or worse.

PATTERN DYSTROPHY RPE dystrophy with yellow-orange deposits under the RPE in a variety of "patterns"; patients are usually asymptomatic or have mildly decreased VA or metamorphopsia. Pathology shows hyperplastic

RPE cells with collagenous periodic acid–Schiff positive deposits between the RPE and Bruch's membrane with no drusen.

- Adult-onset foveomacular dystrophy: solitary, round, yellow spots in the fovea seen in middle-aged patients; may have central pigment with atrophy later, rarely CNVM. Usually unilateral with good prognosis; also called adult Best's disease. Autosomal dominant defect of the retinal degeneration slow (RDS)/peripherin gene that codes for a photoreceptor structural protein.
- Butterfly dystrophy: most common pattern dystrophy that shows bilaterally symmetric "winged" pigmented foveal lesions. Autosomal dominant of the RDS/peripherin gene.
- Reticular dystrophy: coarse, knotted "fishnet" or "chicken wire" pattern in fovea extending to the periphery and later fades. Autosomal recessive.
- Fundus pulverulentus: prominent, coarse, punctate RPE mottling. Autosomal dominant.

SORSBY'S FUNDUS DYSTROPHY Drusen along the arcades; may lead to CNVM. Defect is problem remodeling Bruch's membrane from TIMP-3 gene, chromosome 22q.

STARGARDT'S DISEASE Bilateral progressive macular dystrophy with yellow flecks in the posterior pole. Macula has a "beaten metal" or bronze appearance with pigmentary granularity or bull's-eye appearance that is progressive to atrophy. Patients may be asymptomatic or have central vision loss, but no night blindness or photophobia. All races and both sexes are affected. Same disease but different manifestation as fundus flavimaculatus, which is more peripheral.

- FA shows a silent choroid (lipofuscin in enlarged RPE cells blocks transmittance), and multiple window defects are seen as a mottled hyperfluorescence.
- Fundus flavimaculatus: soft, yellow-white, subretinal, pisciform ("fish-like") flecks surrounding the macula.
- Multiple gene defects identified, including, most commonly, an autosomal recessive form from the ABCR (now ABC4A) gene on chromosome 1p whose product is expressed in rods and cones. Autosomal dominant form has no silent choroid, and mitochondrial DNA inheritence is also reported.
- No treatment has been proven beneficial, including vitamin A supplementation.

Progressive Tapetoretinal Disorders

BIETTI'S CRYSTALLINE DYSTROPHY White crystals in the retina and cornea (crystalline corneal dystrophy); most patients are blind by age 30; most prevalent in China.

CHOROIDEREMIA Pale, peripheral fundus from loss of RPE with islands of pigment. Patients are night blind but usually have 20/20 VA with RP symptoms. Onset: age 6 to 15; M > F, with poor visual prognosis. X-linked recessive disorder of choroidal vasculature with absence of RPE and choriocapillaris except in the macula. CHM gene causes abnormal enzyme-generating protein that cannot anchor fatty acids in the RPE cell membrane. Carriers are asymptomatic, with mottled midperipheral retinal and choroidal atrophy and normal ERG. No treatment effective.

COCKAYNE'S SYNDROME Autosomal recessive defect in DNA repair, with congenital cataract, neurodevelopmental delay, failure to thrive, club feet, poor bony development, dwarfism, progeria, deafness, mental retardation, skin photosensitivity, ocular and orbital degeneration, and usually death before teenage years. Ophthalmic findings include enophthalmos, poor dilation, and pigmentary retinopathy.

GYRATE ATROPHY OF THE CHOROID RPE degeneration beginning in the periphery, with scalloped areas of wiped-out RPE and eventually choriocapillaris with abrupt transition to normal areas. Patients have RP-like symptoms (night blindness, ring scotoma) and progressive myopia in the first decade. From an autosomal recessive chromosome 10q defect in the urea cycle enzyme ornithine aminotransferase (OAT) with elevated serum ornithine. Highest prevalence in Scandinavian Laplanders, with onset at age 10 to 40 and abnormal EOG. Carriers have decreased OAT in skin fibroblasts. Treat with low protein/arginine diet (vegetarian) with creatine supplementation; there is a vitamin B_6 responsive subgroup.

RETINITIS PIGMENTOSA (RP), PIGMENTARY RETINAL DYSTROPHY Diseases characterized by abnormal dark adaptation and night blindness from midperipheral RPE degeneration (bone spicules in the zone of maximum rod concentration) leading to photoreceptor degeneration → decreased NFL and arteriolar diameter → waxy pallor of the disk. May also have ERM and pigment cells in vitreous (differential diagnosis includes uveitis), ON drusen, myopia, glaucoma, and keratoconus. Patients have decreased VF with early inferotemporal scotoma leading to ring scotoma (do not confuse with arcuate defects seen with glaucoma or uncorrected hyperope). The central VA is preserved until late in the disease (usually from atrophic macular degeneration, CME in 50%, or PSC cataract). 1:3500 incidence in the United States. Histopathology shows all retinal layers lost except the ILM.

- ERG: abnormalities precede signs and symptoms, with increased rod threshold with normal cone response and decreased scotopic amplitude and delayed cone B-wave implicit time. Conventional ERG typically "flat," as it cannot detect <10 μV. However, computer averaged ERG can detect down to 0.05 μV. RP averages 1.3 μV at age 32, and although the conventional ERG looks flat, even that low voltage can often carry patients into their 60s.

- Genetics: autosomal dominant in 43% of cases (least severe, varying penetrance), autosomal recessive (20%), X-linked (8%), and isolated (2%). (Older literature still quotes 50% sporadic, 16% autosomal recessive, 22% autosomal dominant, and 9% X-linked recessive.) X-linked is the most rapidly progressive and disabling type, whereas autosomal dominant is least disabling. X-linked carriers have salt and pepper fundus and bronze macular sheen.
  - Rhodopsin gene: first identified RP defect and most common RP mutation, on chromosome 3q, but over 100 other gene defects have been identified. Protein is folded in rod outer segment membrane to create a pocket to hold vitamin A. Pro23his rhodopsin mutation seen in 12% of cases, with average age of RP onset at 37 and average voltage 14.4 μV (thus, patients usually are not blind until age 70).
  - RPGR: X-linked
  - RPE65: autosomal recessive, RPE protein; gene defect also involved in Leber's congenital amaurosis, chromosome 1p.
  - ABCA4 (previously called ABCR): cone and rod degeneration and Stargardt's disease, chromosome 1p defect; unable to pump vitamin A out of RPE (do not give vitamin A).
  - Arrestin: autosomal recessive, chromosome 2q; also in involved in Oguchi's disease.
- Types of RP: most are rod degenerations.
  - Type 1 (rod–cone): primarily rod degeneration, "classic RP;" 20% sine pigmento (no pigmentary changes). Abnormal scotopic ERG.
  - Type 2 (cone–rod): less pigment than type 1 (50% sine pigmento), abnormal photopic ERG.
  - Pigmented paravenous variant: RP along vessels.
    - Differential diagnosis: pigmented paravenous retinochoroidal atrophy (PPRCA) in young males; may be degenerative disorder that is asymptomatic, not progressive, but with ON pallor, attenuated vessels late, and normal ERG.
  - Sector RP: autosomal dominant or recessive, inferior retina, stationary and with a good prognosis. Decreased ERG amplitudes and normal implicit time. Pro-23-his rhodopsin mutation; also with X-linked variant with lyonization.
  - Usher's syndrome: RP associated with sensorineural hearing loss and vestibular dysfunction.
    - Type I: RP, deafness, but no vestibular function.
    - Type II: RP, partial deafness, and normal vestibular function.
    - Type III: RP, progressive hearing loss, and vestibular dysfunction. Several genes are implicated, most commonly myosin VII expressed in photoreceptors and cochlea.

- Treatment of RP: vitamin A palmitate 15,000 IU/day; check fasting serum vitamin A and liver function tests. Avoid vitamin A if serum retinol >100 μg/dL, patient is pregnant or <fifth percentile of body weight. Encourage a well-balanced diet; avoid high-dose vitamin E (>400 IU/day). CME often responds to Diamox. Recommend annual exam and ERG every 2 years. Low vision aids: night-vision pocket-scope provides best monocular daylight vision at night.

SECONDARY RETINITIS PIGMENTOSA Diseases that present with RP-like signs and symptoms but not true dystrophy like RP. Pigmentary retinal degenerations often seen after trauma or inflammation, especially syphilis.

- Abetalipoproteinemia, Bassen-Kornzweig syndrome: rare autosomal recessive disorder, usually presenting in teenage Ashkenazi Jews, with malabsorption and steatorrhea leading to vitamin A deficiency (decreased chylomicrons), acanthocytosis (RBC "burr cells"), ataxic neuropathy, growth retardation, and tiny specks in peripheral retina but usually no bone spicules. Treat with low-fat diet, and replenish vitamins A, E, and K (ERG may reverse).
- Bardet-Biedl syndrome: autosomal recessive, developmental abnormality, characterized by polydactyly, obesity, mental retardation, hypogenitalism (delayed puberty, undescended testes), short stature, and RP, with progressive cone dysfunction early and rods later. Flat ERG. Several genes have been identified; legal blindness by age 20 to 30.
- Friedreich-like ataxia and RP: rare, from decreased serum vitamin E.
- Kearnes-Sayre syndrome, progressive external ophthalmoplegia: mitochondrial inheritance disorder with RP-like disease if severe; associated with facial weakness, ophthalmoplegia, dysphagia, and cardiac conduction defects; usually before age 20.
- Laurence-Moon syndrome: mental retardation, hypogenitalism, short stature, spastic paraplegia, and RP with rod and cone dysfunction. Legally blind usually by age 20 to 30; probably a subset of Bardet-Biedl syndrome.
- Refsum's disease: autosomal recessive disorder of lipid metabolism with decreased phytanic acid alphahydroxylase (chromosome 10p) and accumulation of phytanic acid in the RPE and serum. Patients have atypical RP (granular RPE appearance), cerebellar ataxia, peripheral neuropathy, nerve deafness, anosmia, and EKG conduction defects. Treat with a low phytol diet (no dark green vegetables), and maintain ideal body weight.
- Spielmeyer-Vogt-Batten-Mayou disease (SVBM), neuronal ceroid-lipofuscinosis (NCL): fatal autosomal recessive disorder of abnormal lipopigment deposition in neural tissue. Progressive blindness from RP with a bull's-eye maculopathy; associated with seizures, progressive dementia, and ataxia; seen in very sick children with poor life prognosis. Pathology shows vacuolation of peripheral lymphocytes.

Six clinical subtypes of NCL, of which SVBM is the juvenile form (defect on chromosome 16p).

- Vitamin A and zinc deficiency: vitamin A deficiency may be caused by chronic pancreatitis, cirrhosis, or bowel resection. Insufficient zinc may cause abnormal dark adaptation because it is needed for synthesis of retinal binding protein (RBP).

Stationary Tapetoretinal Disorders

ACHROMATOPSIA, ROD MONOCHROMATISM Autosomal recessive disorder characterized by a total lack of cones. Patients have a complete red-green-blue defect, severe photophobia, and nystagmus from birth with decreased VA 20/200; usually have a normal fundus with paradoxical pupils. Flat photopic ERG (no cone response); EOG is normal.

- Two genetic mutations identified: CNGA3 (cyclic ganglioside alpha-3) chromosome 3 and CNGB3 chromosome 8 (Pingelap Island in the Marshall Islands has a 5% prevalence of CNGB3 achromats). CNG alpha- and beta-1 is in rods, -2 in olfactory nerves, and -3 is in cones. It is an outer plasma membrane cGMP-binding channel to exchange Ca^{++}/K^{+} that regulates voltage of photoreceptor, and a mutated CNG keeps the channel open.

CONGENITAL COLOR BLINDNESS 8% of males are affected. Red and green disorders are X-linked. Blue defects are autosomal dominant on chromosome 7. Disease spectrum from achromatopsia, monochromat (rare, autosomal recessive, consanguinity), dichromat (protanope, deutanope, and tritanope are missing red, green, and blue pigment, respectively), trichromat (normal or protanomalous, deutanomalous, and tritanomalous have color confusion for red, green, and blue, respectively).

- Deuteranomaly (5%) and protanomaly (1%) have mild red-green confusion. Deuteranopia (1%) and protanopia (1%) have severe red-green confusion. Tritanopia (0.2%) has blue-yellow confusion, and tritanomaly is not yet reported.
- Blue cone monochromatopsia: autosomal dominant disorder that is difficult to distinguish from rod monochromat (both have flat ERG flicker response, but achromatopsia is autosomal recessive). Demonstrates a reverse Purkinje shift (instead of dark adapting at 500 nm, then shifting forward to light adapt at 570 nm; instead, it shifts backward in light to 480 nm).

CONGENITAL STATIONARY NIGHT BLINDNESS (CSNB) Infantile onset of night blindness with nonprogressive nyctalopia, normal fundus, paradoxical pupils, normal VF, but a nearly nonrecordable scotopic ERG. X-linked form is the most common and has high myopia. Also autosomal recessive form with an abnormal fundus and autosomal dominant variants.

- Oguchi's disease: autosomal recessive CSNB from chromosome 2q arrestin and other gene defects. Shows the Mizuo-Nakamura phenomenon, where the fundus has a golden-brown metallic sheen in light that disappears and normalizes 6 to 8 hours after it is dark adapted.
- Fundus albipunctatus: autosomal recessive CSNB from chromosome 12q defect in 11-*cis*-retinol dehydrogenase; characterized by white-yellow, round flecks radially scattered but sparing the macula.

LEBER'S CONGENITAL AMAUROSIS Profound retinal blindness from birth, presenting with nystagmus within the first few months, poor pupillary reflexes, oculodigital reflex (unlike achromats), and normal fundus initially, with late pigmentary changes (one third of cases have a normal retina, one third a salt and pepper appearance, and one third atrophic macular coloboma). Also associated with hyperopia, keratoconus, cataract, strabismus, and enophthalmos. Causes 10 to 25% of all congenital blindness. Do not confuse with Leber's optic atrophy. Shows absent ERG amplitudes. Six known gene defects (AIPL1, GUC24D, RPE5, RPE6, CRX, RETGC-1) account for only 45% of cases (all involved in the visual transduction cycle); will end up with probably 20 or more responsible genes.

NORTH CAROLINA MACULAR DYSTROPHY Autosomal dominant chromosome 6 completely penetrant disorder present at birth with lesions ranging from few macular drusen to severe macular coloboma, well-delineated subretinal scar tissue, and risk for CNVM, although most patients have good VA.

Congenital and Genetic Vitreoretinopathies

AUTOSOMAL DOMINANT VITREORETINOCHOROIDOPATHY (ADVIRC) 360 degrees of coarse peripheral pigmentatary degeneration posterior to the equator with a discrete border. Associated with retinal and vitreous opacities, cataract, NV, and choroidal atrophy.

FAMILIAL EXUDATIVE VITREORETINOPATHY (FEVR) Autosomal dominant 11q13 defect causing the failure of the temporal retina to vascularize, leading to peripheral ischemia and neovascularization that resembles retinopathy of prematurity. Patients also may have cataract or tractional RD; 73% are asymptomatic.

GOLDMANN-FAVRE SYNDROME Rare, autosomal recessive disorder with varied presentation of RP-like peripheral degeneration, liquefied vitreous with traction bands and PVD, central or peripheral retinoschisis with inner holes, beaten copper macula, progressive cataract, myopia, AC cell, late optic atrophy, and CME that does not leak on FA. ERG is nonrecordable late; abnormal EOG (unlike X-linked retinoschisis). M = F.

JANSEN'S SYNDROME Optically empty vitreous, like Stickler's syndrome, but no systemic manifestations.

KNIEST SYNDROME Collagen mutation that presents like Stickler's syndrome. Characterized by RD in 50% of cases, ectopia lentis, bone dysplasia, short stature, stiff joints, cleft palate, and deafness.

KNOBLOCH'S SYNDROME Autosomal recessive chromosome 21q22.3 defect (may be seen with Down syndrome) of collagen 18 gene that causes vitreoretinal degeneration, similar to Stickler's syndrome, with high myopia, RD, nystagmus, cataract, ectopia lentis, occipital scalp defect, or encephalocele.

NORRIE'S DISEASE X-linked (Xp11) disease of abnormal ectoderm and disorganized retina; patients are usually blind from birth and have delayed-onset deafness and mental retardation in 50%. Often presents with leukocoria; differential diagnosis includes RB. Milder phenotype is like X-linked FEVR.

SNOWFLAKE DEGENERATION Autosomal dominant, rare disorder causing fibrillar degeneration of the vitreous with small yellow-white opacities in the peripheral retina, with white without pressure (WWP) and potential RD.

STICKLER'S SYNDROME, HEREDITARY ARTHRO-OPHTHALMOPATHY Autosomal dominant abnormality of type II collagen (COL2A1 gene on chromosome 12), presenting by the second decade with optically empty vitreous, lattice retinal degeneration (often radial), high myopia, retinoschisis, and RD in 35% of cases that is difficult to treat. Also associated with cataract, glaucoma, optic atrophy, orofacial and basilar skull abnormalities (flat facies, cleft palate and uvula, Pierre Robin sequence), hearing loss and frequent otitis media, tall stature, and joint hyperextensibility (marfanoid habitus). ERG is depressed. Poor long-term visual prognosis.

WAGNER'S VITREORETINAL DYSTROPHY No systemic manifestations; chromosome 5q defect with optically empty vitreous, vitreous membranes that drape over retina, moderate myopia, atrophy of choroidal vessels, and typical peripheral cystoid degeneration (TPCD). RD is unusual, but cataract is common.

Infectious Disease

AIDS RETINOPATHY, HIV MICROANGIOPATHY Background microvasculopathy that is noninfectious but is the most common intraocular manifestation of AIDS. Mainly presents with CWS but also may have hard exudate (HE) and vessel sheathing. Correlates with the patient's immune status; is nonprogressive and resolves.

ACUTE RETINAL NECROSIS (ARN) Rapid, painful vision loss from HSV or HZV with signs and symptoms of acute anterior uveitis, severe vitritis (unlike PORN), and retinal arteritis with multiple focal white peripheral lesions (usually spares the posterior pole). Starts slow and becomes confluent in 2 to 3 weeks, resolving in 3 to 4 weeks with hemorrhages, sheathing, capillary dropout (unlike CMV and PORN), and optic neuritis. One third of cases are bilateral (called BARN) and spread via the chiasm; with second eye infected usually within 6 weeks.

- Pathology shows necrosis of the retina with strictly intranuclear inclusions (unlike CMV). M = F; patients are usually 30 to 70 years old and in good health unless the ARN is central, which is usually seen in immunosuppressed patients (compare with CMV and PORN in which most patients have AIDS).
- Seventy-five percent of patients develop RRD, generally within 2 years, which is difficult to repair. Retinal detachment should be anticipated and prevented if possible with extensive retinopexy. Treat with IV acyclovir 1.5 g/kg/day. Poor visual prognosis; only 30% are better than 20/200.

CANDIDIASIS Vitrial or subretinal yellow-white fluffy infiltrates that cause floaters or decreased VA usually in immunosuppressed patients, patients on hyperalimentation, or those with a history of IV drug abuse. Blood cultures are usually positive; ocular infection found in 30% of systemically positive patients. Treat with IV and intraocular amphotericin B or ketoconazole, and consider vitrectomy to debulk vitritis.

COCCIDIOIDES IMMITIS Choroiditis present in 10% of disseminated cases; pulmonary is usually the primary site (95% resolve). Fungus is inhaled as a mold and becomes a spherule, which ruptures, releasing endospores.

CYSTICERCOSIS *Cysticercus cellulosae* is larval form of pork tapeworm *Taenia solium*; 13 to 46% of infected patients have ocular involvement after ingestion of eggs, usually in pork meat. Larvae then invade the intestinal walls and migrate to the CNS, eye, skeletal muscle, and heart and grow into a cystic structure that is usually well tolerated by the body until the parasite dies, causing marked inflammation. Predilection for the macula; may see translucent white cysts with dense white spot formed by invaginated scolex. Serologic tests help if positive (but negative result does not rule out disease); eosinophilia is uncommon, and stool samples may be negative. No effective drug treatment available; may laser the larvae, but death will produce inflammation. Surgical removal of cyst may be possible.

CYTOMEGALOVIRUS (CMV) RETINITIS Most common ocular opportunistic infection in AIDS, although relatively rare now. Usually seen when the CD4 count is <50 (otherwise, think about other causes of retinitis, e.g., toxoplasmosis) or in neonates, malignancy, or other immunocompromised states. May also be congenitally aquired, causing systemic infection with fever, hepatosplenomegaly, anemia, thrombocytopenia, and cataract, peripheral retinal lesions, and optic atrophy. Is a clinical diagnosis, as most individuals are already serologically positive.

- Usually asymptomatic, but may have floaters, photopsias, or decreased VA, without redness or pain. Hemorrhagic necrotizing retintis of all layers with CWS in vascular distribution ("cottage cheese and ketchup," "pizza pie" fundus) with only mild vitritis (unlike toxoplasmosis), and rarely frosted branch angiitis. Significant retinal atrophy may lead to multiple small holes and RD in 25% of cases (difficult to treat; usually needs vitrectomy with silicone oil). May also have brushfire variant with slowly advancing white lesion at border of atrophic retina or granular variant without significant hemorrhage, usually in partially treated cases.
- Pathology: "owl's eye" intranuclear and intracytoplasmic DNA-positive viral inclusion bodies (unlike herpes virus, which has intranuclear inclusions).
- Treatment: 40% of patients lose central VA in both eyes by time of death (blindness was leading cause of suicide in AIDS patients).
    - Gancyclovir used IV, PO, vitreous injection or Vitrasert implant (controls CMV better than other modes but does not protect other eye and requires signficiant surgery with a 6 mm sclerotomy). Can stop gancyclovir when CD4 count rises above 50 and continue highly active antiretroviral therapy (HAART).
    - Can also use foscarnet (good response but needs slow infusion; use limited by nephrotoxicity), cidofavir (monthly intravitreal injection; may cause hypotony, uveitis), and Famvir, all of which are virostatic, not virocidal. Isis is an intravitreal reverse transcriptase CMV drug.
- Highly active antiretroviral therapy (HAART): fewer opportunistic infections (CMV, PORN, etc.), but more atypical presentations, such as immune recovery vitritis (symptomatic vitritis with CME, seen with inactive CMV retinitis and increased CD4 from HAART).

DIFFUSE UNILATERAL SUBACUTE NEURORETINITIS (DUSN) See Chapter 5.

FUNGAL Insidious onset with localized vitreous abcess "snowballs" or choroidal granuloma. See candidiasis above.

HISTOPLASMOSIS, OCULAR HISTOPLASMOSIS SYNDROME (OHS) *Histoplasma capsulatum*, endemic in the Ohio/Mississippi River valleys, causes a systemic fungal infection that is usually asymptomatic. Most patients are 20 to 45 years old and may have pulmonary scars; >90% have positive histoplasmin skin test. May have choroid involvement with a classic triad of peripapillary atrophy, "histo" spots, and juxtapapillary CNVM; may also have linear chorioretinal scars, but no vitreous cell. Treat with Amsler grid monitoring.

- CNVM: usually classic lacy "cartwheel" or "seafan" appearance. Risk of second eye developing CNVM is 1% if normal fundus and 25% over 3 years if there is a macular disciform scar.
- Macular Photocoagulation Study, a multicenter, randomized controlled trial (1990–1995), showed benefit to treat juxtafoveal and extrafoveal CNVM; patients tend to do better than CNVM related to AMD. Ten percent of treated extrafoveal CNVM lost >6 lines at 3 years (compared with 47% AMD) versus 45% of untreated patients (62% of AMD). May also respond to sub-Tenon's Kenalog (STK); submacular surgery gives better results in OHS than AMD.

NOCARDIA ASTEROIDES Acid-fast bacteria that may cause panuveitis, choroiditis, retinitis, or vitritis with abcess formation.

PNEUMOCYSTIS CARINII CHOROIDITIS Rare protozoan infection typically unique to AIDS patients, with multiple creamy-yellow, round, plaquelike, choroidal lesions with sharp borders in the posterior pole, with no vitritis. Treat with Bactrim or equivalent.

PROGRESSIVE OUTER RETINAL NECROSIS (PORN) Rare, necrotizing retinitis, usually from HZV (two thirds of patients have antecedent cutaneous zoster) and in AIDS patients (second most common retinal infection in AIDS), characterized by multifocal, full-thickness, deep (outer) retinal lesions (see retinal vessels overlying the lesion), with minimal intraocular inflammation that is rapidly progressive, with a predilection for the ON and macula. One quarter of cases are bilateral, and 70% of patients have RD. NLP in two thirds of patients by 4 weeks. No established therapy; usually try intravitreal antiviral injections at high concentrations.

RUBELLA, GERMAN MEASLES With active maternal rubella infection, 25 to 50% of exposed infants will have retinitis with a salt and pepper fundus and optic atrophy; also associated with cataract, esotropia, mental retardation, congenital heart disease, and deafness. Often also have signs of uveitis with AC reaction, glaucoma, iris atrophy, poor dilation, posterior synechiae, and vitreous haze. The fundus changes do not usually cause vision loss. Has normal ERG and abnormal EOG.

RUBEOLA, MEASLES Similar to rubella; acquired cases may have decreased VA 6 to 12 days after measles rash appears, with measles maculopathy, retinal edema and macular star, leading to a pigmentary retinopathy with attenuated vessels, or subacute sclerosing panencephalitis (SSPE).

SYPHILITIC RETINITIS Especially seen in AIDS patients with nongranulomatous fibrinoid anterior uveitis, mild to severe vitritis, retinal phlebitis, papillitis, deep necrotizing retinitis, and choroiditis. Diagnose with positive Ab test and positive reagin test (VDRL or RPR), and treat for neurosyphilis with penicillin 2.0 million units IV every 4 hours for 1 week. With effective treatment, VDRL should decline to 1:4 within 6 months. Congenital syphilis shows segmental pigmentation of the peripheral retina with a salt and pepper fundus usually without active chorioretinitis. See Chapter 5.

TOXOCARIASIS *Toxocara canis* or *Toxocara cati* nematode larvae ingested by children, allowing second-stage larvae to migrate to the eye. May present with endophthalmitis or a localized, peripheral, eosinophilic granuloma that forms around the dead worm. A peripheral lesion may have retinal traction with temporal macular dragging, causing an apparent XT. Usually incidental finding or presents with leukocoria (differential diagnosis includes RB). Humans are accidental hosts, usually children (ages 2 to 10) who come in contact with contaminated soil or feces (life cycle in dog); also may be acquired from improperly cleaned vegetables. May also have flulike symptoms, with affected lungs or liver. Check ELISA titers (any positive titer is significant). On pathology may see chitin exoskeleton with birefringence. No calcium on CT (unlike RB). Usually no treatment is necessary.

TOXOPLASMOSIS See Chapter 5.

WHIPPLE'S RETINITIS See Chapter 5.

Infectious Endophthalmitis

SIGNS AND SYMPTOMS Pain (from long posterior ciliary nerve, CN V thus radicular-like pain) and decreased VA (25% are light perception [LP]), red eye, hypopyon (if small, may be seen only as the patient looks down), and vitritis (decreased red reflex).

POSTOPERATIVE 75% of cases. If acute but mild, most likely *Staphylococcus epidermidis*. If acute and severe, most likely *S. aureus*, streptococcus, or gram-negative. If chronic, most likely *S. epidermidis*, *Propionibacterium acnes*, or fungal.

- Endophthalmitis Vitrectomy Study (EVS): a multicenter, randomized controlled trial (1990–1995), which looked at endophthalmitis within 6 weeks of cataract extraction. Showed that IV antibiotics in addition to intravitreal antibiotics added no benefit. Also, immediate vitrectomy versus just vitreous tap or biopsy was not beneficial unless the patient was LP. For LP vision at presentation, 33% of the vitrectomy patients vs. 11% of the biopsy patients achieved 20/40 or better VA. Overall, patients had a good prognosis: 53% were 20/40 or better, and 75% were better than 20/100; only 5% NLP at 1 year. Five percent of patients had RD, 1% had increased IOP, and 3% developed pthisis. Fifty percent of cases were *S. epidermidis*, and only 4% were gram-negative organisms.
- Localized, chronic, low-grade, late postoperative inflammation: consider *Propionibacterium acnes* or *Candida parapsilosis. P. acnes* is a facultative anaerobe that may be sequestered in the lens bag; seen as a white capsular plaque and on pathology with Gram and periodic acid–Schiff stains. YAG laser may increase dispersion of organism.
- Blebitis may lead to endophthalmitis, especially after trabulectomy with MMC, thin walled bleb, or inferior location. Likely from streptococcus, *S. epidermidis*, or *Haemophilus influenzae*.

POST-TRAUMATIC 15 to 20% of cases. Usually seen in a rural setting, delayed repair, or with a foreign body or organic material contamination. Likely from *Staphylococcus* species, but also consider *Bacillus cereus*.

ENDOGENOUS, METASTATIC Accounts for 5 to 10% of endophthalmitis, usually seen in premorbid medical conditions or in transplant patients (especially liver). OD is affected 2× more often and is bilateral in 25%. May present with discrete white nodules on the iris, retina, or choroid or with fulminant diffuse panuveitis. Ultrasound the posterior pole if poor view is present in order to evaluate the density of vitritis, and rule out RD, IOFB, or abcess. Obtain CBC, blood cultures, and consider aqueous or vitreous tap.

- Fungal organisms are most common: *Candida* (three quarters of fungal cases) and *Aspergillus* (second most common, usually from pneumonia).
- Bacterial: Group B streptococcus (newborns with meningitis), Group G streptococcus (elderly patients with wound infection or malignancy), Group A streptococcus (skin infection, diabetic, or renal failure patients), *Streptococcus pneumoniae*, *Bacillus cereus* (IV drug abuse), *Clostridia* (malignancy), gram-negative bacteria (urinary tract infection or diabetes), and *Nocardia* (immunocompromised patients with pneumonia).

TREATMENT Perform intravitreal tap, and inject ceftazidime 2.25 mg/0.1 ml or cefazolin 2.25 mg or vancomycin 1.0 mg/0.1 ml plus amikacin 400 μg or gentamicin 100 μg, and consider dexamethasone 200–400 μg. If fungal infection is suspected, inject amphotericin B 5–10 μg.

Neoplastic Disease

ASTROCYTIC HAMARTOMA Benign, stable, glial tumor from the retina or ON, often juxtapapillary, which is white or glistening yellow appearance (contains calcium), at the level of the NFL. No dilated, tortuous vessels like a hemangioma; vessels "ignore" an astrocytic hamartoma. FA shows early hypofluorescence with corkscrew vessel at its base. Usually presents in the first decade; may be acquired or associated with tuberous sclerosis.

BILATERAL DIFFUSE UVEAL MELANOCYTIC PROLIFERATION (BDUMP) Systemic infection or visceral neoplasm that stimulates melanocytic proliferation, mimicking a diffuse uveal melanoma, but it is not a malignancy.

CAPILLARY HEMANGIOMA Distinct red-orange tumor, 2–3 mm high, with dilated afferent arteriole and efferent venule that is a benign vascular hamartoma from proliferation of retinal capillaries. May leak exudates and have exudative RD. Rapid flow on FA. Often inherited as autosomal dominant, presenting age 15 to 40, or may be isolated or part of VHL if associated with renal cell carcinoma, pheochromocytoma, and cerebellar hemangioblastoma. May observe, or if <2.5 DD, may cryotherapy or laser.

- Primary vasoproliferative tumor: presumed acquired capillary hemangioma in an elderly patient; usually inferotemporal with no feeder vessel, little exudate, stationary, no family history, and safely observed.

CAVERNOUS HEMANGIOMA OF THE RETINA Rare, benign, unifocal, vascular hamartoma of the inner retina with reddish blue grapelike vascular clusters, usually flat and localized along the course of a vein. May have VH or gliosis. FA shows blood layering in the sacs, with slow circulation (independent of retinal circulation). Usually presents about age 30, M = F; stable, excellent prognosis. May be part of phakomatosis with cutaneous or CNS lesions, or may be autosomal dominant.

CHOROIDAL HEMANGIOMA Congenital isolated red-orange benign vascular hamartoma in the posterior pole, usually peripapillary, 2–3 mm thick and 5–10 mm diameter, with overlying RPE disturbance; may have exudative fluid with RD. FA shows early filling of large choroidal vessels and late staining. Echography shows high internal and initial reflectivity. Most are well circumscribed and have no associated systemic abnormalities, although some are diffuse and associated with Sturge-Weber syndrome. May photocoagulate over hemangioma to decrease exudation.

CHOROIDAL MELANOMA Primary intraocular malignancy in the United States (RB in Africa), and the only intraocular tumor that is routinely fatal. Most present asymptomatically on routine exam, or with blurred VA, floaters, photopsias, VF alteration, or ocular pain (2% of patients presenting with decreased vision and obscured fundus view have MM; thus, get B-scan). Unilateral (if bilateral, consider metastasis or BDUMP), well circumscribed (rarely is diffuse, which is more aggressive), pigmented nodule (base diameter is 2× thickness; pigmentation does not correlate with prognosis, and 25% are amelanotic). May break through Bruch's membrane, causing a mushroom shape, and may have rapid enlargement from venous obstruction. May cause CNVM (better tumor prognosis, as it indicates chronicity), CME, serous RD, sectoral cataract, lens subluxation or lenticular astigmatism, rubeosis, and scleral sentinel vessel, especially with ciliary body melanoma. Typically presents at age 50 to 60.

- Risk factors: Caucasian, ocular and oculodermal melanocytosis, NF, nevi, possibly pregnancy.
- Work-up: get echography (false-negative [FN] and false-positive [FP] rates 0.3%) to confirm diagnosis, characterized by high surface spike with low internal reflectivity (homogeneous), high posterior spike (acoustic hollowing), and sometimes reverberation vascular pattern, and quantify thickness. A scan is most accurate if tumor height is >2.5 mm. May see size and location of tumor with transillumination. FA is not necessary but may show "double circulation" sign (also in hemangioma, ectopic disciform scar), or a "hot spot," which is not predictive of growth. CT and MRI imaging are not as good as echography. Phosphorus P32 (malignant cells incorporate P32) testing is not beneficial. Check liver function tests (gamma-glutamyltransferase [GGT] is the most sensitive), and if >5 mm high, check CXR and abdomen CT.
- Differential diagnosis:
  - AMD with hemorrhage: blocks on FA; echo shows high internal reflectivity; may see drusen in the fellow eye.
  - BDUMP: see above.
  - Choroidal detachment, effusions, or suprachoroidal hemorrhage: transilluminates; usually blanches with pressure, typically from hypotony, postoperative or trauma.
  - Choroidal hemangioma: peripapillary location with orange color; high reflectivity with echo because it is a solid tumor.
  - Choroidal metastatic cancer: creamy color, corrugated surface, and often multifocal; echo shows medium to high reflectivity with heterogeneity.
  - Choroidal nevi: may have associated SRF.

- Choroidal osteoma: 75% are in young females; usually bilateral, juxtapapillary, and yellow-orange color with calcification.
- CHRPE: flat, jet-black tumor, sharp borders; lacunae.
- ON melanocytoma: jet-black tumor arising from the optic nerve, with fibrillated margins; large polyhedral cells on pathology; equal incidence in African-American and Caucasian patients.
- Posterior scleritis: may have elevated choroidal lesion.
- *Toxocara* granuloma: usually peripheral.

- Pathology: tumor cells arise from dendritic melanocytes in the choroid or rarely (1 in 10,000) choroidal nevi transformation into MM. May also arise from iris (less likely, <1%, to metastasize) or ciliary body. Modified Callender classification identifies three cell types:
  - Spindle A: more benign, looks like a coffee bean or hot dog and with a chromatin stripe; found in nevi.
  - Spindle B: cells are plumper, round, with prominent nucleoli.
  - Epithelioid cells: large irregular cells with large nucleoli; are more malignant.
- Worst prognosis: larger tumor size, location anterior to the equator (discovered later), pure epithelioid, <2 mm from the ON. Risks for growth: larger tumor, presence of orange pigment, absence of drusen, absence of adjacent RPE changes, mushroom shape, associated SRF, and lymphocytic reaction.
- Treatment: more aggressive course is typical for younger patients. If no metastatic disease, then historically patients have been enucleated (Zimmerman's hypothesis: intraocular manipulation may shower tumor cells and cause metastatic cancer). However, today, tumors are often treated with radiation therapy.
  - Observation if small until documented growth.
  - Photocoagulate if <3.5 mm and posterior.
    - Transpupillary thermotherapy (TTT): heat treatment, best for low diffuse melanoma; several treatment sessions needed to "cook" the tumor down to sclera.
    - Xenon (is a bright light and not really a laser, penetrates deeper) has a 15% 2-year recurrence rate, which is better than the argon laser; 60% 2-year recurrence.
  - Radiation is standard treatment.
    - Brachytherapy: most commonly used because melanomas are relatively radioresistant and plaque delivers ionizing radiation close to the tumor (3000 rads to tumor base, 800–1000 at the apex). Cobalt 60 in use the longest; 90% of tumors are responsive, and 60% have radiation complications (retinopathy, cataract, optic neuropathy, NVG, scleral necrosis, dermatitis, etc.).
    - Charged particle radiation: proton beam (90% responsive, 32% complications) or helium ion.

  - External beam radiation: may slow growth, but frequent side effects.
- Resection: if anterior tumor, lamellar sclerouvectomy (partial thickness sclera, 78% 5 year survival), or full-thickness wall resection. If posterior, some have attempted internal tumor resection.
- If extrascleral extension (8–14%), usually seen with advanced patient age and larger tumors; treat with enucleation and orbital radiation if nodular. If orbital invasion, usually all patients die within 2.5 years regardless of treatment. If systemic metastatic cancer, the 1 year mortality rate is 71%, but may add 3 to 9 months with palliative radiation to the eye and site of metastatic cancer with or without chemotherapy.

- Collaborative Ocular Melanoma Study (COMS): a multicenter, randomized clinical trial that began in 1986, and is ongoing, to evaluate brachytherapy (iodine 125) versus enucleation. For medium-size tumors (2.5–10 mm), plaques increase time to enucleation, but no mortality difference in surgery versus observation groups.
- Overall, one third to one half of patients die from their melanoma. Table 7–1 presents size characteristics and mortality of melanoma. The 15 year mortality is 75% for epithelioid histological type, 25% for pure spindle cell, and 50% for mixed cell types. Following enucleation, the average time to demise is 2 years. Tumor prefers direct invasion via emissary channels. Rarely metastatic, only 1 to 3% at diagnosis, and metastasizes almost always to the liver.

CHOROIDAL OSTEOMA Yellow-white to orange-red, well-defined, juxtapapillary lesions that arise from osteoblastic activity (bony trabeculae, not tissue calcification) of unknown cause, usually in white females. Most are 0.5–2.5 mm thick, and degeneration of the overlying RPE and retina may cause gradual visual loss. Eighty percent are better than 20/30 initially, and 24% deteriorate to 20/200 in 2 to 5 years. FA shows early patchy hyperfluorescence with diffuse late staining. Ultrasound demonstrates

TABLE 7–1

Characteristics of Uveal Nevus and Melanoma

Size	Height	Base	5-Year Survival
Nevus	<2 mm	1:2 height to base ratio	100%
Small melanoma	2–3 mm	4–6 mm	95%
Medium melanoma	3–5 mm	6–0 mm	75%
Large melanoma	5–8 mm	10–16 mm	50%
Extra large melanoma	>8 mm	>16 mm	<50%

high spike from inner surface with acoustic shadowing. Tumors are bilateral in 30% of cases. No treatment necessary unless laser needed for the 33% that have CNVM.

COMBINED HAMARTOMA OF THE RPE Rare, benign, unilateral, nonfamilial tumor of disorganized RPE, retina and vitreous elements, usually juxtapapillary. Looks like a disorganized gray and pigmented sessile mass with secondary traction. Average age of presentation is 15 years old. Associated with vision loss in 60% of cases, strabismus (18%), retinal vascular tortuosity (93%), hyperpigmentation (87%), and ERM. Heavy leakage on FA. Treat amblyopia if presenting at an early age, and consider vitrectomy with MP. Forty-five percent are 20/40 or better, and 40% are 20/200 or worse.

INTRAOCULAR LEUKEMIA Usually B-cell acute myelogenous leukemia (most common leukemia in adults and highest eye involvement); 33 to 62% of patients with systemic disease have intraocular involvement. Most commonly presents with choroidal infiltrates, and may have serous RD and RPE changes ("leopard skin" appearance). May also have retinal or ON infiltrates, anemic and thrombocytopenic retinal hemorrhages or CWS with vascular tortuosity, hyperviscosity with mild CRVO, or opportunistic infections (CMV, HSV, toxoplasmosis, fungi, etc.). Treat with chemotherapy, and consider ocular radiation therapy.

LARGE CELL LYMPHOMA, PRIMARY INTRAOCULAR OR HISTIOCYTIC LYMPHOMA, RETICULUM CELL SARCOMA B-cell lymphoma (non–Hodgkin's lymphoma) caused by chromosome 14–18 translocation, presenting with deep, multifocal, yellow-white, sub-RPE infiltrates with vitritis, intermediate uveitis, decreased VA, floaters, CME, exudative RD, pseudohypopyon, iris mass, NVI, or NVG. The CNS is the primary site, and the eye is the "septic tank" where the brain dumps some of the cancer; this is in contrast to systemic lymphoma, which has visceral signs and symptoms and may metastasize to the choroid. Bilateral in 75%; usually seen in older patients (average age 65 but reported as young as 15). May initially respond to steroids and thus masquerades as uveitis; delayed diagnosis for 18 to 24 months is common. Schedule work-up with CNS MRI, lumbar puncture, vitreous biopsy, and cytologic analysis by experienced eye pathologist with flow cytometry (70% positive). Is a tissue diagnosis that is treated with bilateral ocular and probable CNS radiation (4000 cGy fractionated), intrathecal methotrexate, and may consider IV ARA-C. Median survival time is 3 years.

MEDULLOEPITHELIOMA Unilateral, nonfamilial, yellow-pink tumor that arises from the nonpigmented epithelium of the ciliary body or pathologically from the retina or ON. Found in children usually age 4 to 5. May contain cartilage (highly reflective on echography) or cause lens coloboma (lack of zonular support), surface or vitreous cysts, cyclitic membrane cataract, or NVG. Tumor may make vitreous. Classified as either teratoma or nonteratoma (also called diktyoma).

MELANOCYTOMA Benign, jet-black, magnocellular nevus with fibrillated margins. Unilateral; 50% have contiguous choroidal nevus. APD in 30%, and may have enlarged blind spot. Up to 50% occur in African-American patients; rare malignant degeneration.

METASTATIC CHOROIDAL TUMORS Most common intraocular malignancy, found in 10% of all cancer deaths. May be asymptomatic or the presenting feature of systemic malignancy with blurred VA, ocular pain, VF defect, or photopsias. Usually yellow-white lesion deep to the retina, which is relatively flat, and may be associated with serous RD. Most are in the posterior pole; 20% are bilateral and 20% multifocal.

- In females, usually from breast (80%), lung, or unknown primary. In males, most commonly from lung (54%), unknown, or skin melanoma primary tumor.
- FA not particularly helpful, and generally shows hypofluorescence early with progressive hyperfluorescence. B-scan shows a solid, ill-defined, convoluted tumor with overlying RD. A-scan has moderate-high internal reflectivity.
- Treatment: if tumor threatens disk or macula or is causing disturbing visual symptoms, consider radiation therapy with 3000–4000 cGy, fractionated. Breast cancer may respond to chemotherapy or hormonal therapy. Average survival overall is 8 to 23 months. Lung cancer average survival is 3 months.

PARS PLANA CYSTS 18% prevalence at autopsy (usually represent a degeneration), but may also see with multiple myeloma (cysts filled with lambda light chains). May cause forward rotation of ciliary body and angle-closure glaucoma.

RACEMOSE HEMANGIOMA Direct arteriovenous communication seen as extremely tortuous and dilated posterior pole vessels. No treatment.

- Group 1: interposed arteriolar or capillary plexus between the major artery and vein; asymptomatic, not associated with CNS lesions.
- Group 2: no interposed capillary elements, stationary; not associated with CNS lesions.
- Group 3: many anastomosing channels, poor VA, perivascular sheathing, exudation, pigmentary degeneration. Fifteen to 25% are part of Wyburn-Mason's syndrome, with midbrain vascular abnormalities or facial lesions.

RETINOBLASTOMA (RB) Most common intraocular tumor in children (1/15,000 births) from loss of cancer suppressor gene. Ninety-four percent are sporadic, 6% familial. No gender predilection. Presents most commonly by age 2 with leukocoria (90%), followed by strabismus (35%), NVI (up to 50%), unilateral dilated pupil (1%), hyphema, NVG with heterochromia irides, pseudoinflammatory (pseudohypopyon or orbital cellulitis-like in 2%), or orbital mass (common in developing countries). Lens and cornea remain clear. Bilateral RB present in 33%.

- May be endophytic from the inner retina that seeds the vitreous or exophytic if it arises from the outer retina that presents as solid mass (or rarely diffuse and infiltrative, usually 7 to 8 years old); most cases are a mix of the two.
- Work-up: CT to look for calcification and rule out orbital extension; any intraocular calcification in a child is RB until proven otherwise (is elemental, intracellular calcium, not chunks, and is thus uniformly white). MRI the pineal gland in bilateral cases to rule out "trilateral" tumors. Examination under anesthesia (EUA) and ultrasound (echography shows high internal echoes with rapid attenuation of orbital pattern with or without shadowing). Consider bone marrow biopsy, lumbar puncture cytology, and gene studies if enucleated. Can screen serum by testing for leukocyte esterase D activity, as it is tightly linked with RB gene.
- Genetics: chromosome 13q14 defect (intact gene protects against malignancy). Autosomal recessive gene, but because of 100 million neurons in the retina, it behaves like autosomal dominant with incomplete penetrance. E2F transcription factor needs RB gene protein to control cell reproduction ($G_0 \rightarrow G_1$), and RB gene suppresses this division. Mutation in the RB gene causes unchecked cell growth. Knudsen's two-hit hypothesis showed that mutations in both RB genes is necessary for RB; although the spontaneous mutation rate is $< 10^{-7}$, the retina develops with 10^8 divisions, thus making two hits plausible. Bilateral tumors = heritability (if bilateral, then the patient is heterozygous, but the opposite is not necessarily true). RB is associated with advanced paternal age.
  - Sporatic somatic mutation: 66% of cases (75% of sporadic cases). Patients inherit RB/RB (two healthy genes), then need two hits; thus, almost always unilateral, presenting at 18 to 24 months, and not transmitted.
  - Sporadic germinal mutation: 21% of cases (25% of sporadic cases). Patients inherit RB/RB, but early in embryogenesis one hit changes to RB/rb (may be in all cells or a mosaic), then later needs only one more somatic hit. Tumors may be bilateral; mutation is the beginning of a familial transmission.
  - Familial: accounts for 5 to 10% of cases. Patients inherit RB/rb in all cells; thus, need one somatic hit. Seventy percent are bilateral;

presents at 10 to 12 months (have a genetic headstart) but is not congenital.
  - 13q-chromosome deletion syndrome: RB (<5% of RB cases) associated with holoprosencephaly, mental retardation, low ears, thin upper lip, broad nasal bridge, gastrointestinal or genitourinary abnormalities, and sarcomas.
- Pathology: tumor staining shows red (necrosis), white (calcium, which actually stains purple), and blue (tumor). Other features include dystrophic calcification in the tumor necrosis and pseudorosettes (multicellular structures seen at low power, with central vessel and surrounding tumor until the tumor outgrows its nutrient supply). Rosettes are well-differentiated, monocellular features of RB. Three types:
  - Flexner-Wintersteiner rosettes: have a lumen with 9 + 0 cilia configuration, like nerve tissue; represent early photoreceptor differentiation. Also seen in medulloepithelioma, pineal tumors, and glioma.
  - Homer-Wright rosettes: central tangle instead of lumen; seen also in neuroblastoma and medulloblastoma.
  - Fleurettes: bouquet-like cellular structures that are more benign representations of advanced photoreceptor differentiation; seen with retinocytoma, which is thought to be benign, involuted RB.
- Abramson staging for retinoblastoma:
  - Stage I: Intraocular disease—a. Retinal tumor(s); b. Extension into choroid; c. Extension up to lamina cribrosa; d. Extension into sclera.
  - Stage II: Orbital disease—a. Orbital tumor that may be 1. Suspicious (pathology of scattered episcleral cells) or 2. Proven (biopsy proven orbital tumor); b. Local nodal involvement.
  - Stage III: ON disease—a. Tumor beyond lamina but not up to cut section; b. Tumor at cut section of ON.
  - Stage IV: Intracranial metastasis—a. Positive CSF only; b. CNS mass lesion.
  - Stage V: Hematogenous metastasis—a. Positive marrow/bone lesions; b. Other organ involvement.
- Treatment: most important prognostic factor is whether there is extension into the ON. In general, treat small tumors with radiation therapy, photocoagulation, or cryotherapy, plus chemotherapy, and enucleate larger tumors. If recurrent, usually presents within 2 years.
  - Photocoagulate: if <2.0 mm thick and no vitreous seeding; laser applied around the base, not over the surface, with 69% cure rate. Cryotherapy if anterior to equator and <2.5 mm thick and no vitreous seeding. May also use cobalt plaque.
  - Chemotherapy: often vincristine, etoposide (1–2% risk of blood malignancy), and Cytoxan are used in combination. Also cyclophosphamide (hyperthermia increases chemotherapy uptake),

VP-16, carboplatin, and VM-26. Chemotherapy shrinks tumor and allows for more effective use of radiation, photocoagulation, or cryotherapy.
  - If large tumors, enucleate with 5–10 mm of ON removed. If bilateral, enucleate the worse eye with vison-sparing treatment to the better eye.
  - Radiation: RB is very radiosensitive; radiation usually used for the fellow eye after enucleation with 3500–4000 cGy, fractionated.
  - Radiation or chemotherapy regression pattern: Type I—"cottage cheese" appearance; II—"fish flesh" appearance; III—combination of the first two; IV—total tumor wipeout.
- Reese-Ellsworth classification for RB: predicted eye survivability and visual prognosis after radiation (1950s).
  - Group I: a. Solitary tumor, less than 4 disk diameters in size, at or behind the equator; b. Multiple tumors, none over 4 disk diameters in size, all at or behind the equator. Very favorable visual prognosis; 95% of eyes survive.
  - Group II: a. Solitary tumor, 4 to 10 disk diameters in size, at or behind the equator; b. Multiple tumors, 4 to 10 disk diameters in size, behind the equator. Favorable visual prognosis.
  - Group III: a. Any lesion anterior to the equator; b. Solitary tumors larger than 10 disk diameters behind the equator. Doubtful visual prognosis for tumors anterior to the equator.
  - Group IV: a. Multiple tumors, some larger than 10 disk diameters; b. Any lesion extending anterior to the ora serrata. Unfavorable visual prognosis.
  - Group V: a. Massive tumors involving over half the retina; b. Vitreous seeding. Very unfavorable visual prognosis; 32% eye survival.
- Prognosis: overall, 90% child survival. Reese-Ellsworth classification predicts the survival of the eye (see below). Tumors may involute spontaneously. If advanced, the tumor prefers to infiltrate the ON to the brain, rarely hematogenous spread to lungs, bone, brain, or orbit or subarachnoid extension or spread via conjunctival lymphatics. Metastatic disease usually occurs within 2 years. Mortality odds ratio if choroid, sclera, orbital invasion is 21.6; if invades ON, is 8.7.
  - Thirty percent risk of secondary tumors by 30 years (1% per year) especially if patient received radiation (occurs 5 years earlier than nonradiation patients, and most tumors occur in the field of radiation). Main secondary tumor is osteogenic sarcoma usually of the orbit or femur. Also, radiation increases risk of poor performance of orbital grafts and implants and causes hypoplastic orbits.
  - Follow patients with exam every 3 months for 18 months or until 3 years old, then annual B-scan or CT.
  - Ensure family receives genetic counseling (Table 7–2).

TABLE 7–2

Genetic Counseling for Retinoblastoma (RB)

Genetics	Parent Affected?	Offspring Affected?	Laterality	Focality	Chances of Next Sibling Affected
Sporadic	Unaffected	<1% affected	40% bilateral	100% multifocal	5%
(90% of cases)			60% unilateral	15% multifocal	<1%
				85% unifocal	
		99% unaffected	NA	NA	
Familial	Bilateral RB tumors	45% affected	85% bilateral	100% multifocal	45%
(10% of cases)			15% unilateral	96% multifocal	
				4% unifocal	
		55% unaffected	NA	NA	
	Unilateral RB tumor	7–15% affected	85% bilateral	100% multifocal	45%
			15% unilateral	96% multifocal	
				4% unifocal	
		85–93% unaffected	NA	NA	7–15%

NA, not applicable.

Metabolic and Degenerative Disease

AGE-RELATED MACULAR DEGENERATION (AMD) The major cause of irreversible, severe, central vision loss in developed countries. Affects 18% of persons >60 years old (2.2% of whom are blind), or about 10 million Americans. Disease is characterized by drusen deposits in Bruch's membrane, RPE disturbance, and potential violation of Bruch's with resultant CNVM.

- AMD risk factors: age, Caucasian, light-colored irides, cardiovascular disease, family history of AMD (especially Malattia Leventinese or Doyne's honeycomb retinal dystrophy; also, ATP-binding cassette rim (ABCR) gene mutation as in Stargardt's disease is found in 8–16% of AMD), extensive light exposure, smoking, and poor nutrition.
    - Risk factors for vision loss: age, hyperopia, positive family history, soft confluent drusen (especially in the second eye), pigment clumping, focal hyperpigmentation, and retinal pigment epithelial detachment (PED).
    - Favorable prognosis: normal blood pressure, nonsmoker, and with exudative disease, blood or blocked fluorescein on foveal side (e.g., no extension of CNVM into the FAZ).
- Differential diagnosis: ICSR, pattern or adult vitelliform dystrophy (yellow spot in macula), any bull's-eye maculopathy, basal laminar drusen (good prognosis), melanoma (may look like extrafoveal disciform scar), and macroaneurysm.

"DRY," NONEXUDATIVE, OR ATROPHIC AMD Comprises 90% of AMD and only 10% of severe vision loss; characterized by usually mild loss of central VA that is slowly progressing from macular drusen, RPE changes, or geographic atrophy of the RPE (GARPE).

- Drusen: excrescences of lipoproteins in and thickening of Bruch's membrane: "hard" drusen are small <63 μm, distinct, and flat; "soft" drusen are larger, more diffuse or basal laminar (nodular, cuticular), and are usually found in younger patients.
- RPE pigmentary changes: may be hyperfluorescent (window defect) or hypofluorescent (blocking defect) on FA; pigment clumping is a risk factor for exudative disease.
- Geographic atrophy of the RPE (GARPE or areolar atrophy): central, large (>175 μm), demarcated atrophic RPE with loss of choriocapillaris and overlying photoreceptors; see large choroidal vessels underneath the GARPE lesion.
- Treatment: no proven therapy for dry ARMD. Antioxidant vitamins and nutritional supplements may play preventive role. Amsler grid monitoring for development of CNVM; however, only 10% progress to exudative disease. Encourage sunglass wear, and consider low-vision aids.

"WET," EXUDATIVE, OR NEOVASCULAR AMD Characterized by severely decreased central VA from CNVM, PED, disciform scars (fibrovascular wound-healing scar associated with CNVM), or rarely VH. Makes up only 10% of AMD but is responsible for 90% of severe vision loss.

- RPE detachment (PED): orange-yellow dome-shaped elevation; FA shows sharp borders, with slow pooling of fluorescein (like a dimmer switch turning on), and may have a "notch" blocking defect. May lead to RPE tears; the free edge may roll over on itself, blocking on FA, leaving a "half moon" shape of early hyperfluorescence in the area devoid of RPE. One third of patients with PED develop CNVM within 5 years.
- Choroidal neovascular membrane (CNVM): patient reports blurred or distorted vision (metamorphopsia) or scotoma. Exam usually shows subretinal hemorrhage and exudate with a gray-green crescent or membrane, and possible localized serous RD. May be difficult to detect clinically (17% of AMD patients with CNVM will have a "normal" exam by retina specialist); obtain FA to diagnose.
  - Classic CNVM: 13% of exudative cases, showing a well-defined CNVM on FA, with early hyperfluorescence that increases in size and intensity (unlike RPE window defects), as well as progressive leakage and late staining.
    - Extrafoveal: >200 μm from the center of the FAZ. Sixty-three percent of patients lose six lines of vision by 3 years.
    - Juxtafoveal: 1–199 μm from the center of the FAZ. Seventy-one percent of patients suffer severe vision loss in 21 months.
    - Subfoveal: 64% of patients with initially good VA lose six lines of VA at 2 years.
  - Occult CNVM: also called fibrovascular PED or diffuse leakage of undetermined origin; poorly defined on FA, with speckled late hyperfluorescence. Consider indocyanine green angiography (ON looks black), which may show a "treatable" lesion in 40% of cases. A "hot spot" (well-defined small bright area within 3 to 5 minutes; lasts 20 minutes but loses definition with time) on ICG is very helpful in guiding laser treatment.
  - CNVM risk factors: bilateral drusen (14% risk over 4.3 years), larger more confluent drusen (30% risk to fellow eye over 5 years), extensive drusen (five or more within the central macula), RPE hyperpigmentation (alone carries a 30% risk of CNVM in the fellow eye over 5 years; if with large drusen, then 60% risk), exudative disease in fellow eye (about 10% risk per year), hypertension, low serum levels of antioxidants and micronutrients, smoking, and hyperlipidemia.
    - Risk of CNVM in fellow eye: 10 to 12% per year, especially if multiple, soft, confluent drusen or RPE clumping is present.

        - Decreased CNVM risks: high carotenoids, estrogen replacement therapy
    - Gass classification: type 1 CNVM grows within the sub-RPE space, as in exudative AMD in older patients with a "sick" RPE; type 2 grows through a focal defect of Bruch's membrane and RPE into the subretinal space and may induce reactive RPE response, as in OHS (Submacular Surgery Trial: ongoing multicenter, randomized controlled trial).
- Treatment: standard treatment is laser photocoagulation of the CNVM (see Macular Photocoagulation Study recommendations below). Technique: have a current FA; consider a retrobulbar block if necessary; adjust power to apply confluent white laser burns usually with 200 μm spot and 0.5 second; repeat angiography in 2 to 3 weeks.
    - Macular Photocoagulation Study: laser treatment was beneficial for classic CNVM (52% of lesions in the study were purely classic, 35% mixed, 13% occult).
        - Extrafoveal CNVM: laser treatment, in general, considered beneficial. Twenty-five percent of treated eyes had severe vision loss at 18 months versus 69% of untreated eyes; at 5 years, 46% of treated versus 64% of untreated eyes had severe vision loss. Recurrent CNVM found in 54% of treated eyes at 5 years.
        - Juxtafoveal CNVM: in general, laser treatment considered beneficial if no systemic hypertension is present. Fifty-two percent of treated eyes had lost six lines of vision loss at 5 years (average 20/200) versus 61% of untreated eyes (average 20/250). CNVM was persistent within 6 weeks after treatment in 32% (vs. 10% extrafoveal). Recurrent CNVM seen in 69% of treated patients at 3 years, 79% at 5 years. Average VA in treated eyes at 4 years was 20/80, 20/200 if persistent CNVM, and 20/250 if recurrent.
        - Subfoveal CNVM: only well-defined subfoveal CNVM <3.5 DD was treated in the study, and occult lesions were excluded. At 3 months, 20% of treated versus 11% of untreated eyes lost six lines of vision, but at 24 months, 20% of treated versus 37% of untreated eyes lost six lines. Fifty-one percent of treated eyes had persistent or recurrent CNVM at 24 months. Occult lesions may be stationary.
    - Photodynamic therapy (PDT): The Treatment of Age-related Macular Degeneration with Photodynamic Therapy (TAP) study (a multicenter, randomized ongoing controlled trial) showed that Visudyne safely reduces visual loss in AMD with subfoveal CNVM that is at least >50% classic for patients with VA

20/20–400. Sixty-one percent of treated versus 46% of untreated eyes lost <15 letters on the ETDRS chart. Sixteen percent of treated versus 7% of untreated eyes had > one line increase in VA.

- Age-Related Eye Disease Study (AREDS): high levels of antioxidants and zinc reduce the risk of vision loss from advanced AMD by 19%. No benefit found for minimal AMD, and does not prevent the initial development of AMD or improve vision (also showed no benefit to prevent or slow progression of cataracts). Doses used:
  - Vitamin C 500 mg
  - Vitamin E 400 IU
  - Beta-carotene 15 mg (avoid in smokers, as it is linked to lung cancer)
  - Zinc oxide 80 mg plus copper 2 mg (cupric oxide): high-dose zinc is associated with copper deficiency.

AMYLOIDOSIS Eight percent of patients with primary familial disease have ocular involvement, often with retinal hemorrhage, exudates, CWS, peripheral NV, and extracellular vitreous opacities adjacent to retinal vessels with wispy edges. Associated with polyneuropathy, skin and heart involvement.

ASTEROID HYALOSIS Unilateral vitreous opacities representing calcium soaps (calcium hydroxyapatite). Asymptomatic; may be associated with diabetes.

CHOLESTEROLOSIS BULBI, SYNCHYSIS SCINTILLANS Cholesterol crystals in liquefied vitreous that settle inferior after a large VH; seen as yellow, glistening bodies attached to the vitreous framework.

EPIRETINAL MEMBRANE (ERM), MACULAR PUCKER, CELLOPHANE MACULOPATHY, SURFACE WRINKLING Disruption of the ILM with glial proliferation and differentiation into myofibroblasts that may contract, causing retinal surface wrinkling.

- Most cases are asymptomatic but may have metamorphopsia, decreased VA, diplopia, or central photopsias (especially with vitreomacular traction). Exam may show cellophane wrinkling, vessel tethering or straightening, retinal hemorrhage, CWS, macular pucker or pseudohole, and CME (if seen on preoperative FA, portends a lower prognosis for visual recovery after surgery). Eighty-five percent of patients have VA better than 20/70.
- Prevalence 5% (20% by age 75). Idiopathic is leading cause (associated with PVD, 30% bilateral) but also seen with RD (examine peripheral retina for holes), vascular occlusion, inflammation, trauma, postoperative.

- Treat with vitrectomy plus membrane peel if VA 20/40 or worse; 80% regain two lines of vision. Fifty to 60% of phakic patients develop cataract after surgery. Five to 7% of cases are recurrent.

HIGH MYOPIA, MYOPIC DEGENERATION Progressive thinning of the choroid and RPE in the macula that may cause loss of central VA, usually at about age 50. May be associated with posterior staphyloma, RPE atrophy, tilted disk, extensive PPA, increased IOP, RD, and the following:

- Fuchs' spot (also known as Förster-Fuchs' spot): a raised circular pigmented lesion that represents a small, aborted CNVM.
- Lacquer cracks: linear breaks in Bruch's membrane that may present acutely as photopsias follwed by decreased VA. May have hemorrhage; CNVM in 72% of cases.
- CNVM: usually close to fovea, small size, and less likely to respond to laser than in AMD. Sixty percent of patients have VA <20/200 but higher spontaneous resolution; does not behave as poorly as AMD.

IDIOPATHIC CENTRAL SEROUS RETINOPATHY (ICSR) Acquired macular disease with serous elevation of the neurosensory retina; 80% are male, usually age 20 to 60, presenting with metamorphopsia, micropsia, or mildly decreased VA that improves with pinhole. Exam shows absent foveal reflection, occasional PED or RPE clumping from prior episodes, possible subtle elevation of the retina, and document that there is no ON pit. FA shows a hyperfluorescent expanding dot in 80% of cases or the classic smokestack in 10 to 20% of cases and window defects from prior lesions. Fifty percent recover within 6 weeks but may need a temporary hyperopic correction. Sixty-six percent of patients eventually recover 20/20 VA, but up to 50% of cases recur. Laser treatment may accelerate resolution but does not improve VA or recurrence rate and carries the risk of CNVM. Corticosteroid treatment may greatly worsen the condition.

IDIOPATHIC MACULAR HOLE Tangential traction on the fovea by posterior cortical vitreous that creates a retinal dehiscence. Women 60 to 80 years old are most commonly affected. Ask about prior trauma; 25% are bilateral. Stage 3 and 4 holes are often treated with vitrectomy plus membrane peeling to relieve tangential traction; may use tissue adhesives such as autologous serum, transforming growth factor β (TGF-β), plasmin, or fibrinogen.

- Stage 1: impending hole that is a foveal detachment by cortical vitreous contraction but no actual retinal break. May see a yellow spot or ring, mildly decreased VA; 50% resolve.
  - Differential diagnosis: vitreomacular traction, ICSR, pattern dystrophy, phototoxic maculopathy, post-traumatic, drusen, CME, and parafoveal telangiectasis.
- Stage 2: hole that is <400 μm, and the posterior hyaloid is attached.

- Stage 3: hole >400 μm with an operculum; see yellow spots at the level of the RPE (macrophages with lipofuscin), and the posterior hyaloid is attached.
- Stage 4: large full-thickness hole with complete separation of the posterior cortical vitreous. May have a cuff of SRF, yellow deposits within the defect, and RPE atrophy with window defects. Differential diagnosis includes ERM with pseudohole (negative Watzke-Allen test), impending macular hole, lamellar hole from aborted macular hole (hyperfluorescence on FA), and chronic CME.

PERIPAPILLARY STAPHYLOMA Unilateral deep excavation with well-defined normal disk from scleral weakness, usually in high myopes.

PERIPHERAL RETINAL DEGENERATIONS

- Cystoid degeneration: small intraretinal cysts near the ora that increase with age; not associated with retinal tears.
  - Typical peripheral cystoid degeneration (TPCD): cystic spaces in the outer plexiform layer that may coalesce into a retinoschisis cavity (may see a gray band posterior to the ora serrata, usually temporal; may have Blessig-Iwanoff's cysts).
  - Reticular: cystic spaces in the NFL, usually more posterior than TPCD.
- Lattice degeneration: equatorial band of retinal thinning ("stretch marks") seen as a white "snail track" or reddish crater with overlying sclerosed retinal vessels; has an 8 to 10% prevalence, mostly in myopes. Found in association with 25% of RDs (is the cause of 30–45% of RDs in young myopes). Retinal tears usually occur at the end of or posterior to the lattice lesion. Twenty-five percent of cases have small atrophic holes within the lattice (usually does not cause RD). Lattice is usually not treated unless patient has a history of RD.
- Pars plana cysts: usually normal finding, although may be associated with multiple myeloma.
- Paving stone or cobblestone degeneration: round chorioretinal atrophy with pigmented borders that represent an infarction of a peripheral choroidal lobule, usually inferiorly; overall 22% prevalence, and incidence increases with age. May protect against RD because there is an adhesion between the retina and the choroid.
- Retinoschisis (degenerative, acquired, or senile): splitting of the retina in the outer plexiform layer (thus predisposed by TPCD) from a partial vitreous detachment with oblique traction on the retina. Seventy percent are inferotemporal, and 66% are bilateral. The elevated inner retina may have tiny white dots (Müller foot processes) and is very translucent (can see choroidal details, unlike RRD). If a hole is present in the inner retinal layer only (often pinpoint), there is no RD risk. However, a hole in the outer layer of the schisis (usually has rolled

TABLE 7–3
Characteristics of Retinal Detachment versus Degenerative Retinoschisis

Characteristic	Retinal Detachment	Retinoschisis
Surface	Bullous, corrugated	Convex, smooth
Transparency	No choroidal details seen	Transparent
Pigmentation	Demarcation line	None
Fluid	Shifting	None
Progression	Progressive	Stable
Usual location	Near retinal break	Inferotemporal
Scotoma	Relative, sloping	Absolute, sharp
Response to laser	No uptake (retina is off the RPE)	Uptake

edges) may cause RD (causes up to 3% of RD), and RD usually remains localized unless there is an inner and outer hole. Usually stable or very slowly progressive. May treat with laser photocoagulation or vitrectomy if threatening the fovea. (See Table 7–3 for a comparison of retinal detachment and degenerative retinoschisis.)

- o Differential diagnosis: reticular retinoschisis with involutional splitting of the NFL or secondary schisis seen with Coats' disease, trauma, intermediate uveitis, tumors, and vitreomacular traction.

POSTERIOR VITREOUS DETACHMENT (PVD) Separation of the posterior cortical vitreous from the retina, as evidenced by a Weiss ring. Common, age-related degeneration of the vitreous as hyaluronidase is replaced by water (syneresis, also accelerated after intraocular surgery and with high myopia); 63% incidence in patients >70 years old and only 27% of patients 60 to 69 years old. Patients may complain of new-onset floaters or photopsias (from retinal traction). PVD may cause splinter hemorrhage, VH, or retinal tear. The more recent the symptoms, the more urgent the need for examination. Risk of retinal break is 10 to 15% if patient is symptomatic with photopsias, 2 to 4% if no VH, and 70% if VH is present. Seventy percent of PVD-associated tears are between 10 and 2 o'clock, usually at the vitreous base, where the vitreous attaches firmly to the retina and the pars plana epithelium. If there is a VH but no tear is seen, then reexamine within 2 weeks to look for tear.

- Vitreomacular traction (VMT) syndrome: partial PVD but still attached to macula, causing edema, striae, thickening, or RD; if traction is on the disk, may cause "fleshy donut" sign. May need vitrectomy.

RETINAL HOLES AND TEARS Often present with floaters and photopsias, may have Schaeffer's sign (pigmented cells in anterior vitreous).

- Atrophic retinal holes: round, often in areas of typical peripheral cystoid degeneration; seen in 5% of the population. Rarely progress to RD; thus, no laser treatment is necessary.
- Dialyses: circumferential tear at the ora; accounts for 75% of traumatic tears, usually seen in young patients. Typically do well with scleral buckle.
- Giant retinal tear: a tear that extends 90 degrees or more around the circumference of the fundus (usually at the posterior border of the vitreous base, compared with dialyses, which occur at the ora serrata). Usually nontraumatic (77%) and seen in young males; also carries a very high risk of RD in the fellow eye. Difficult to treat, usually with vitrectomy and unfolding the often inverted posterior retinal flap.
- Horseshoe tear (HST): partially torn retinal flap; almost always points toward the posterior pole, with vitreous traction on the flap that is attached at its anterior edge. Thiry-three to 55% of HST will progress to RD if left untreated; thus, treat all HST with laser. Apply hot laser at least two rows around the tear; if SRF is present, consider cryotherapy. Have patient avoid exertional activity until scar forms.
- Operculated round tear: retinal hole with the operculum of the retina seen in the vitreous. If patient is asymptomatic and there is no current vitreous traction, <5% progress to RD. No treatment is usually needed unless the patient is a high myope, has a personal or family history of RD, or is aphakic or pseudophakic. Treat all symptomatic holes, as 5 to 17% will progress to RD if untreated.
- Evidence-based treatment recommendations: type I strong evidence, type II substantial, type III consensus. Always treat symptomatic HST (I). Almost always treat all dialysis (III). Sometimes treat symptomatic operculated tear (II), lattice in fellow eye of tear (II), and all asymptomatic HST (III). Rarely treat asymptomatic hole (II), symptomatic hole or lattice (II), asymptomatic holes or operculated tear in myope/fellow eye of tear/aphakic patient (III). No treatment needed for asymptomatic operculated tear or asymptomatic lattice in phakic or myopic eye (II).

RHEGMATOGENOUS RETINAL DETACHMENT (RRD) Most common type of RD, occurring from a break in the retina and often causing photopsias or loss of vision, like a curtain, veil, or shade coming across the vision. Retina often maintains its viability if it is repaired in a timely fashion. If chronic, the retina becomes macrocystic and often inoperable, as fixed cysts form between Müller's cells.

- Evaluation: perform history, and ask about symptom duration, trauma, family history, and previous surgery. Do full eye exam and obtain the BCVA; check IOP (usually low), APD, EOM (prior to buckle), and note lens status, then do careful DFE (find the tear; always presume that there are other tears).

- RRD etiology: myopia (40–55%), aphakia (30–40%), trauma (10–15%), genetic predisposition (family history and certain races, e.g., Egyptian ancestry), PVD, pseudophakia/other intraocular surgery, scleral perforation, intraocular inflammation (ARN 75% have RD, CMV 25%, etc.), and inherited disease (Wagner syndrome, Jansen's disease, Stickler's syndrome, Goldmann-Favre syndrome). One third of RD is believed to be from myopia, one third from trauma, and one third from other causes.
    - RRD prevalence: 1 in 15,000 overall; high myopes (5%, mainly from lattice degeneration), aphakic patients (2%), vitreous loss after ECCE (10%; 50% are within the first year).
    - RRD personal risk factors (in order): RD in fellow eye (15%), myopia (7–8%), family history, lattice degeneration
- Anatomical risks: meridional complex or tufts (fold in the retina up to a dentate process or oral tooth), lattice degeneration (tears begin at edge of lattice; tears within lattice are usually atrophic), degenerative retinoschisis and cystoid degeneration, retinal break (full thickness, 5–18% prevalence), retinal tear (traction present), retinal hole (operculated with no traction and low risk of RD), giant retinal tear (>90% have RD)
- Pathology: early in the course, inner retinal edema is seen, followed by photoreceptor disruption and outer layer degeneration by 4 weeks; cysts are present by 10 weeks, then fixed retinal, folds. May also see proliferative vitreoretinopathy, pathologic drusen, and hyperplasia of RPE, often seen as a diffuse pigment proliferation or demarcation line (pigment line at the ora serrata is called *ringschweile*).
- Treatment: surgical options should be considered in light of whether the patient is symptomatic or asymptomatic, presence of a tear or a hole, whether the patient is high myope, pseudophakic or phakic, or needs cataract extraction or not; also, whether there is a history of RD in the other eye, RD location (superior location has risk of macular detachment, vs. inferior location, which is usually harder to treat), and, patient reliability and access to care. Final vision is determined by duration of RD and whether the macula is "on" or "off." Treatment options include observation, retinopexy alone (with cryotherapy or laser), scleral buckle procedure (SBP), pneumatic retinopexy, temporary buckle (Lincoff balloon, gelatin, etc.), and vitrectomy with or without lensectomy, membrane peel (MP), perfluorocarbon (PFC), retinotomy, fluid–gas exchange (FGX), and SiO.

SEROUS, EXUDATIVE RD Characterized by bullous, shifting, subretinal fluid. Usually from breakdown of the blood–retinal barrier, RPE disturbance or disturbance of the subretinal pump. Determine and treat etiology.

- Congenital ON pit: usually inferotemporal disk; may use laser to demarcate between fovea and ON.
- Choroidal tumors: such as hemangioma, metastatic cancer, leukemia, melanoma, and osteoma
- Retinal hole in high myopes: macular holes usually just have a cuff of SRF, but in high myopes, fluid does not resolve and may need vitrectomy with gas placement.
- Vasculopathy: malignant hypertension (often with bilateral ON swelling), toxemia of pregnancy, collagen vascular disease, disseminated intravascular coagulation (DIC), etc.
- Choroidal inflammatory disease: Harada's disease (often have pinpoint hyperfluorescent spots that leak), sympathetic ophthalmia, and other posterior uveidites
- Others: idiopathic uveal effusion, ocular contusion, AMD, chronic steroid use (thick and cloudy SRF, with many RPE defects), and syndrome of RRD, choroidal effusions, hypotony, and panuveitis (treat with steroids first, then fix RD).

TRACTIONAL RETINAL DETACHMENT (TRD) Second most common type of RD; from vitreoretinal fibroproliferative membranes that mechanically pull the retina away from the RPE. Typically presents with a smooth retina that is concave toward the anterior segment; usually confined, and rarely extends to the ora serrata. Retinal tears may result in combined TRD and RRD.

VITAMIN A DEFICIENCY Results in night blindness; patients are prone to measles and smallpox, which may lead to severe corneal scarring.

Systemic and Vascular Disease

ACQUIRED PARAFOVEAL OR IDIOPATHIC JUXTAFOVEAL TELANGIECTASIAS Mild vasculopathy with retinal thickening usually temporal to the macula, characterized by right-angle venules (horizontal vessels that dive deep into the retina). Patients typically are age 40 to 65, F > M, and have mildly decreased VA from CME or rarely from CNVM. Types Ia, Ib, II (most common). May be thought of as "localized Coats' disease"; FA shows dilated capillaries with late leakage. Disease is slowly progressive and associated with diabetes. Does not respond well to treatment, but may try focal or grid laser.

ARTERIOSCLEROSIS Begins as arteriolar-venous nicking that becomes more marked, then "copper wiring" (hypercellularity), and finally "silver wiring" (collagen deposition).

BRANCH RETINAL ARTERY OCCLUSION (BRAO) Superficial retinal whitening along a blocked arteriole; 90% occur in the temporal arcades. Good prognosis; 80% improve to 20/40 VA or better. May occur from thrombosis or emboli. Emboli may be Hollenhorst plaques, yellow cholesterol emboli from the carotid (check carotid duplex) or less commonly calcific plaques from a cardiac valve (check echocardiogram).

- Susac syndrome: multiple recurrent BRAOs from microangiopathy of unknown etiology affecting brain, retina (usually bilateral), and cochlea. Onset usually at age 30; self-limited disease over 4 years. May treat with steroids, antiplatelets, and calcium channel blockers.

BRANCH RETINAL VEIN OCCLUSION (BRVO) Blocked retinal vein (usually temporal arcades) most commonly from compression at an arteriovenous crossing (because they share a common adventitial sheath). Typically presents with painless decreased VA in 75% (40% are better than 20/50, 66% better than 20/200) or VF loss with pie-shaped distribution of retinal hemorrhages (usually flame), microaneurysms, CWS, edema, distended and tortuous veins, and slightly decreased IOP. Occurs in M = F, average age 65; from hypertension (70%), arteriosclerosis, and POAG (12%). May be ischemic (>50%).

- Fifteen to 20% have occlusion in the fellow eye within 5 years. Usual course is gradual resorption of the hemorrhage and edema over months; however, may have occlusion of macular capillaries with chronic CME, retinal NV in 20%, NVD 10% (only 1% have NVI), or RD. If >4 DD of nonperfusion, then 62% have NV. Overall, 1% of nonischemic versus 54% of ischemic BRVOs have retinal NV, usually within 2 years.
- Macular branch retinal vein occlusion: superior vein in 85%; CME treatment with laser.
- Treat underlying conditions. Photocoagulation for CME or NV. Complications may include a rapid progression to "90-day glaucoma" (retinal ischemia, leading to NV, then NVI and glaucoma).
- BVO Study (multicenter, randomized controlled trial, 1977–1985): use grid laser after 4 months for CME if VA is 20/40 or less and there is good macular perfusion. Sixty-three percent of treated versus 36% of untreated eyes gained two or more lines of VA; follow-up at 3 years showed average VA 20/40 for treated versus 20/70 for untreated eyes (neither group returned to 20/20). Segmental PRP is recommended only for NV (only 12% of ischemic BRVO developed significant VH).

CANCER-ASSOCIATED RETINOPATHY (CAR) Paraneoplastic process of decreased retinal function that may have normal-appearing fundus, associated with systemic cancer. Typically presents with scintillations, acquired nyctalopia, or decreased vision or visual field.

- Bone marrow transplant (BMT) retinopathy: combination of radiation and chemotherapy toxicity.

CENTRAL RETINAL ARTERY OCCLUSION (CRAO) Painless, profound vision loss over seconds (may have history of amaurosis fugax or transient visual obscuration) with immediate APD, macular cherry red spot, and opaque inner retina; may have thinned arteries or "box carring." Emboli in arterial system seen in 20% of cases (poor prognostic sign; 59% mortality within 9 years); 25% have sparing of cilioretinal artery with preserved VA. Irreversible damage occurs within 90 minutes. FA shows delayed arterial filling, delayed AV transit time, normal choroidal pattern (unless there is an ophthalmic artery occlusion), and late disk staining. Loss of inner retina is noted by a decreased ERG B wave. VF may show a remaining temporal island. Rubeosis occurs in 15% of cases, NVG in 11%.

- Etiology: atherosclerosis (leading cause in older patients), often accompanied by hypertension (67%), carotid atherosclerosis (45%), and diabetes (25%). Cardiac valvular disease causes 25% of cases; rule out GCA. Mean survival status post-CRAO is 5.5 years, compared with 15.4 years for age-matched controls. In younger patients, migraine causes one third of CRAO. Other causes include trauma (especially male patients), hypercoagulable state (oral contraceptives, pregnancy, etc.), embolic source (carotid, cardiac, intravenous drug abuse), cocaine use, collagen vascular disease, hyperhomocystinemia, and sickle cell disease.
- Treatment: no proven best therapy, but emergently may try to decrease IOP (ocular massage, AC paracentesis, beta-blockers, Diamox, mannitol), increase retinal oxygenation (carbogen, hyperbaric chamber), or improve vascular flow with fibrinolytic agents (intra-arterial tissue plasminogen activator).

CENTRAL RETINAL VEIN OCCLUSION (CRVO) Second most common retinal vascular disorder after diabetes. Retinal hemorrhage is seen in all four quadrants from venous thrombosis at the cribriform plate. May also have hemicentral or hemispheric retinal vein occlusion if the superior or inferior retinal vein is occluded.

- Signs and symptoms: decreased VA (usually from CME) or loss of VF with CWS, NFL hemorrhages, and dilated and tortuous vessels, often described as "blood and thunder"; may have slightly lower IOP in affected eye and delayed venous filling on FA.
    - Signs of prior CRVO (once resolved, fundus may look nearly normal): collateral vessels on the disk (not NV vessels that leak) and vessels that cross the midline raphae.
    - If the thrombosis is behind the cribriform plate, patients usually have more disk swelling but less retinal ischemia as they develop more collateral vessels and have a better visual prognosis. If

thrombosis is anterior to the cribriform plate, there is less disc swelling, but more retinal hemorrhage and ischemia and more decreased VA.

- Etiology: hypertension (60%), atherosclerosis (25–50%), diabetes (15–30%), POAG (6–20%), hyperopia, tight cup, and hypercoagulable state; rule out GCA. Most patients are usually >50 years old (if age <50, most are a result of head trauma or hypercoagulable state from estrogen).
- Order work-up if etiology is not obvious, especially in young patients: RPR/MHA-TP, CBC, electrolytes, lipids, ESR, coagulation panel, protein S and C deficiency, ANA, glycohemoglobin, antithrombin III factor, factor V Leiden, anti-phospholipid antibody; rule out hyperhomocystinemia.
- Nonischemic: accounts for up to 66% of CRVO. Seen in younger patients; characterized by milder signs with venous tortuosity, mainly affecting the posterior pole with retinal hemorrhages, rare CWS, and mild CME, and only 10 to 20% progress to ischemic. ERG B:A >1.0 (normal). Follow every 2 months for 1 year; majority of patients are 20/50 or better. No treatment is usually indicated.
    - Papillophlebitis is type of CRVO from inflammatory venous vasculitis with nonischemic occlusion and residual vessel sheathing and optociliary shunt vessels.
- Ischemic: accounts for up to 33% of CRVO. Seen in older patients; characterized by severe loss of VA and VF, with confluent intraretinal hemorrhages in the posterior pole (flame hemorrhages predominant), engorged venous tree, and numerous CWSs (a marker for ischemia; if >10, then 75% develop NVG). Severe capillary dropout is seen on FA; ERG B:A <1.0.
    - Outcome: hemorrhage, CWS, and venous tortuosity gradually resolve; may have residual optociliary shunt vessels, arteriolar narrowing, optic atrophy, or APD. Twenty-five percent of patients will have a contralateral occlusion within 5 years. Retinal NV is rare, but NVI is more common, and 50% develop NVI, NVA, then NVG (especially if >50% capillary nonperfusion), which may occur as early as 2 weeks, but 92% occur within 6 months (thus, follow patients closely early).
- Treat underlying systemic conditions (does not affect CRVO outcome except possibly hyperviscosity etiology). Not beneficial: anticoagulants, fibrinolytics, carbogen, steroids, hyperosmotics, vitamins, and prostacyclin. May consider ON sheathotomy.
    - Scatter photocoagulation should be offered if >50% nonperfusion on FA with 1000 to 1200 spots; prevents and regresses NV, but no effect on final visual outcome (unlike BRVO).
    - Central Vein Occlusion Study (CVOS) (multicenter, randomized controlled trial, 1988–1994): do not offer prophylatic PRP; wait

until NVI or NVA develops. Risk factors to develop 2 o'clock hours of NVI or NVA: 36% if 30 to 74 nonperfused disk areas on FA, 52% if >75 disk areas, retinal hemorrhage > standard photo 2a, <1 month duration, and female gender. FMG not recommended for CME.
- ○ Complications: acute angle-closure glaucoma from increased posterior pressure and "90 day glaucoma"; neovascular glaucoma can occur as late as 24 months.

CILIORETINAL ARTERY OCCLUSION Artery is present in 32% of normals and fills in the choroidal phase of the FA, as it is a branch of the posterior ciliary artery. Blockage causes decreased VA from macular ischemia and possible CME. Forty percent are isolated cases; do work-up like CRAO, and rule out GCA. Ninety percent improve to 20/40 or better. Forty percent are combined with CRVO probably from ON edema compressing the cilioretinal artery, and 70% return to 20/40 or better. Fifty percent are associated with ischemic optic neuropathy with poor vision (20/400 to NLP), as both are from posterior ciliary artery insufficiency.

DIABETIC RETINOPATHY (DR) Diabetes causes a diffuse vasculopathy and is the leading cause of preventable blindness in the United States. Vasculopathy is symmetric (only 5% of PDR have high-risk characteristics in one eye and less than moderate NPDR in the fellow eye) and classified as nonproliferative or proliferative. Nonproliferative disease is characterized by dot-blot hemorrhages (deep retina), microaneurysms, hard exudates (distinct yellowish lipoprotein deposits deep in retina), NFL infarcts (called CWSs, but they are not soft exudates), intraretinal microvascular abnormality (IRMA; localized NV confined to the retina that does not leak on FA). Proliferative DR adds the characteristic of retinal NV and fibrous glial proliferation with possible tractional RD. Vision loss may be due to retinal hemorrhages, macular ischemia, diabetic macular edema, tractional RD, or lens edema with myopic shift (lenticular retention of sorbitol from elevated blood sugar). Vascular endothelial cell growth factor (VEGF) injected into mice causes NV. PRP destroys tissue to decrease VEGF.

- Pathology: loss of pericytes (supporting cells for capillary endothelial cells), leading to capillary leakage and dropout, and basement membrane thickening. A classic ophthalmic finding is lacey vacuolization of the iris pigment epithelium.
- Two types of diabetes:
  - ○ Insulin-dependent diabetes, type 1, adolescent-onset: typically from premature failure of pancreatic islet cells to produce insulin. Twenty-five percent of patients have DR after 5 years with the disease, 60% at 10 years, and 80% at 15 years, and 25%

of these have proliferative diabetic retinopathy (PDR). Examine these patients within 5 years of diagnosis. Growth hormone released during adolescence may be associated with progression of retinopathy.
    - Non–insulin-dependent diabetes, type II, adult-onset: usually from acquired insulin resistance. Initial ophthalmic exam should follow the diagnosis.
- Risk factors for DR progression: elevated serum glucose or glycosylated hemoglobin, hypertension, years with disease, nephropathy, and hyperlipidemia. Factors that retard DR progression: ipsilateral glaucoma, ipsilateral chorioretinal scarring, but not ipsilateral carotid stenosis.
    - Diabetes Control and Complication Trial (DCCT): showed delayed onset of DR, nephropathy, and neuropathy in type 1 diabetic patients with tight glucose control.
    - Wisconsin Epidemiological Studies of DR (WESDR): showed that patients with intensive glucose control (glucose <180), as well as hypertension and hyperlipidemia control, had 80% less progression of DR in patients with no retinopathy, 65% less progression in patients with mild to moderate DR; patients with more severe DR had the same risk reduction as patients with milder DR but showed a temporary "early worsening" effect.
    - Sorbinil Retinopathy Trial (SRT): showed that aldose reductase was not effective.
    - Early Treatment of Diabetic Retinopathy Study (ETDRS): looked at aspirin use and VH risk, and defined treatment parameters for clinically significant macular edema (CSME) and PRP for NPDR.

DIABETIC RETINOPATHY: CLINICALLY SIGNIFICANT MACULAR EDEMA (CSME) Diabetic macular edema (DME) may be focal, diffuse, or cystoid (outer plexiform or inner nuclear layers) and is the most common cause of diabetic vision loss.

- CSME is a clinical criterion that the ETDRS showed benefited from focal laser, with a 50% decreased moderate vision loss (doubling of visual angle). CSME diagnosis requires one of the following:
    - Elevated or thickened retina within 500 μm of the FAZ
    - HE within 500 μm of the FAZ associated with thickening
    - Thickened retina >1 DD and within 1 DD of the FAZ
- Although CSME is a clinical diagnosis, obtain FA to further define the leakage prior to laser treatment and to rule out macular ischemia. Poor visual prognosis includes central capillary occlusion, HE in the fovea, VA <20/200, and fixed chronic cysts; if excessive exudate, is present, rule out hyperlipidemia.

DIABETIC RETINOPATHY: NONPROLIFERATIVE (NPDR) Diabetic vasculopathy that is usually confined to the posterior pole and has not progressed to neovascularization. Usually asymptomatic or has vision loss from CSME or macular ischemia.

- Minimal: 1 microaneurysm (Ma)
- Mild: 1 Ma plus a retinal hemorrhage, CWS, or HE
- Moderate: HE or Ma that is > ETDRS standard photo 2a in one quadrant and IRMA or CWS or venous beading
- Severe NPDR: any one of the following "4-2-1 rule" (very severe NPDR is two of these):
  - Four quadrants of Ma or HE > photo 2a
  - Two quadrants of venous beading > standard photo 8b
  - One quadrant of IRMA > standard photo 8a
- ETDRS showed that PRP is effective for severe and very severe NPDR, as 15% of severe and 45% of very severe NPDR cases progress to PDR each year. Severe and very severe NPDR and early PDR cases have a 2 to 7% risk of severe vision loss within 2 years and thus warrant at least partial PRP.

DIABETIC RETINOPATHY: PROLIFERATIVE (PDR) Progression of vasculopathy from NPDR to neovascularization. The Diabetic Retinopathy Study (DRS) showed benefit of PRP for PDR.

- Early: any NV not meeting criteria for high risk
- High risk: 25 to 40% risk of severe vision loss (VA <5/200 on two exams 4 months apart) within 2 years usually from VH. PRP decreases the 5-year loss of vision risk by 50%. High-risk PDR has at least three of these criteria:
  - Any NV
  - NV on or within 1 DD of the disk
  - Moderate or severe NV (either of the following findings):
    - Neovascularization of the disk (NVD) $>\frac{1}{3}$ DD, as in photo 10a
    - Neovascularization elsewhere (NVE) $>\frac{1}{2}$ DD
  - Preretinal hemorrhage or VH
- Advanced: tractional RD involving the fovea or VH obscuring ability to grade NV
- Vitreous hemorrhage: Diabetic Retinopathy Vitrectomy Study (DRVS) showed that early vitrectomy is beneficial for insulin-dependent diabetic patients with VH; 25% regain 20/40 VA or better. ETDRS showed that oral aspirin use does not increase a patient's VH risk.

DISSEMINATED INTRAVASCULAR COAGULATION (DIC) Systemic platelet and fibrin thrombi in small vessels, causing choriocapillaris occlusions and serous RD, with late multiple RPE changes. Over 100 different causes reported (septicemia, amniotic fluid embolism, snake bite, etc.).

EMBOLIC VASCULOPATHY Temporary blockage of artery may cause amaurosis fugax, typically from cholesterol embolus (Hollenhorst plaque) that lodges at an arteriole bifurcation.

GIANT CELL ARTERITIS (GCA), TEMPORAL ARTERITIS May cause choroidal nonperfusion via short posterior ciliary arteries with nasal or temporal choroidal ischemia, in addition to temporal arteritis, CRAO, AION, or posterior ischemic optic neuropathy (PION). Treat with IV steroids, then temporal artery biopsy. See Chapter 8.

HYPERLIPIDEMIA A risk factor for atherosclerosis and vascular occlusions; if severe, may cause intraretinal lipid exudation. Lipoproteins have a lipid core surrounded by a plasma membrane containing cholesterol and apolipoproteins (high-density lipoprotein, beta-low-density lipoprotein). Secondary lipoproteinemia is more common than primary and is less severe; usually seen with diabetes, hypothyroidism, nephrotic or hepatic dysfunction, or pancreatitis. Five types of primary hyperlipidemias:

- Type 1: increased cholymicrons with very elevated triglycerides; higher incidence of lipemia retinalis.
- Type 2: increased cholesterol, beta-lipoprotein; higher incidence of coronary artery disease and arcus senilis but no lipemia
- Type 3: increased cholesterol, increased triglycerides
- Type 4: increased triglycerides, increased pre-beta-lipoprotein
- Type 5: very elevated triglycerides, increased cholymicrons and pre-beta-lipoprotein

HYPERTENSIVE RETINOPATHY Elevated blood pressure may cause acute or chronic retinopathy or choroidopathy.

- Acute, acclerated, or malignant hypertension: retinopathy is not as prominent as choroidopathy because of protective retinal vasoconstriction. Mostly see choroidopathy, as the choroid cannot autoregulate; thus, expect infarction of choroidal lobule and overlying RPE changes (Elschnig's spots), serous RD, and hyperplastic RPE over sclerotic choroidal vessel (Siegrist's streaks). May have fibrinoid necrosis of the choriocapillaris endothelium with hemorrhage, edema, and exudates. May have optic neuropathy and disk swelling from ischemic axonal swelling.
- Four stages of hypertensive retinopathy:
  - Narrowing of arteries
  - Focal arteriolar constriction
  - Hemorrhage and exudates
  - Papilledema
- Chronic hypertensive retinopathy: hyalinization of vessel media with arteriolar narrowing, increased light reflection seen as "silver wiring" (sclerotic phase from collagen deposition), and arteriovenous

compression or "nicking" (Gunn's sign), as the arteriole and venule share a common adventitia. Increased incidence of BRVO, BRAO, CRVO, and macroaneurysm.

IDIOPATHIC POLYPOIDAL CHOROIDAL VASCULOPATHY (IPCV) Usually seen in African-American female patients with CNVM from choroidal vascular anomaly; often found peripapillary, and may see the abnormal vessels better with ICG angiography.

MACROANEURYSMS Acquired arteriolar dilatations in the posterior pole within first three orders of retinal bifurcations, most commonly superotemporal. Usually seen in elderly female patients with hypertension and atherosclerosis. Linear breaks in the vessel wall may lead to hemorrhage at any retinal level, especially subhyaloid "boat-shaped" hemorrhages; may also have CME, exudate, or vitreous hemorrhage if a subhyaloid hemorrhage ruptures.

- Group I hemorrhagic form (vs. exudative group II) tends to be larger and occur closer to the disk. FA shows a "light bulb" appearance that fills completely in the arterial phase with progressive late leakage.
- Usually resolves spontaneously. If macular exudation is present, may photocoagulate directly over the lesion with low energy, long duration, large spot laser. Krypton yellow is probably best, as the laser energy is absorbed by RBCs, but laser may cause hemorrhage, BRAO, ERM, or macular hypoperfusion.

OCULAR ISCHEMIC SYNDROME (OIS) Globally poor ocular perfusion, usually from high-grade carotid stenosis (usually >90% on duplex ultrasound) or chronic ophthalmic artery occlusion. The disease is usually related to atherosclerosis, but it also may be from Eisenmenger's syndrome, carotid dissection, GCA, or other inflammatory vasculitide. Age is usually >55, and is bilateral in 20%.

- Signs and symptoms: gradual decreased VA or amaurosis, ocular angina, or prolonged recovery after bright light. May present with limbal flush, AC cell (20%), NVI (two thirds of patients), or NVA or NVG (although usually has decreased IOP early secondary to decreased ciliary body perfusion), retinal artery narrowing, dilated but not tortuous veins, dot-blot midperipheral hemorrhages or microaneurysms, NVD, or CME (hypoxic capillary endothelial cells leak).
- FA demonstrates delayed filling characterized by decreased arteriovenous transit time (in 95% of patients), delayed mid or laminar phase, last vein to fill >15 seconds, delayed choroidal filling (60% of patients), prominent vascular staining (95%), or CME. Ophthalmodynamometry shows decreased central retinal artery perfusion; ERG may show decreased A and B waves.

- Complications: marker for vascular disease: 50% of patients have ischemic cardiovascular disease, 25% history of stroke, 20% peripheral vascular disease, increased stroke rate; overall, a 5-year mortality of 40%. If NVI is present, 90% are blind within 1 year.
- Treatment: PRP for NVI is effective in 35% of patients, as well as carotid endarterectomy (CEA), unless the vessel is 100% occluded. Note: CEA may suddenly increase the ciliary body perfusion and cause an increased IOP.
  - North American Symptomatic CEA Trial (NASCET) showed that patients with a history of amaurosis fugax, TIA, or stroke and who had a 70 to 90% carotid stenosis have a 2-year stroke rate of 9% after CEA versus 26% in control patients who were treated only with antiplatelet therapy.

OPHTHALMIC ARTERY OBSTRUCTION Abrupt, severe vision loss (may be NLP), with a lower IOP, and intense inner and outer retinal whitening with no cherry red spot resolving over several weeks with RPE disturbance and severe optic atrophy. No A or B wave on the ERG. Grim visual prognosis.

- Saturday night retinopathy: prolonged prone position with pressure on the globe that causes decreased ophthalmic artery perfusion. So named because patients may awake blind from a drunken stupor.

SICKLE CELL RETINOPATHY Abnormal red blood cell hemoglobin causes vascular sludging and occlusions. Hemoglobin in RBCs is normally in solution; however, with hypoxia or acidosis, the abnormal hemoglobin molecules become inflexible and precipate as rods within the red blood cells. The sickled, deformed RBCs then block arterioles. The most severe eye disease is seen with SC (homozygote for Hgb-C) and sickle cell thalassemia (Sthal) because the anemia is milder, thus causing more viscous blood and more vaso-occlusions. However, more severe systemic disease with homozygous sickle cell (Hgb SS) disease characterized by sickle cell "crises" with severe pain from microvascular occlusions, bone infarcts, leg ulcers, and autoinfarction of the spleen (susceptible to bacterial infections). Disease usually presents at age 30 to 40 years, especially in African-American patients; diagnose with hemoglobin electrophoresis.

- Ten percent of African-Americans have abnormal hemoglobin: 8.5% have sickle cell trait (AS), 2.5% Hgb-C trait (AC), 0.4% homozygous sickle cell disease (SC), 0.2% sickle cell Hgb-C (SC), and 0.03% sickle cell thalassemia (Sthal).
  - Hemoglobin is comprised of two alpha and two beta chains. In sickle cell anemia, or S disease, a single amino acid substitution (valine for glutamic acid) in the sixth position of the hemoglobin beta chain causes an abnormal hemoglobin molecule (Hgb-S). Homozygotes have 85 to 95% Hgb-S and severe anemia (SS

disease), whereas heterozygotes (sickle cell trait, AS disease) have 40 to 45% Hgb-S and the rest is normal hemoglobin.
  - Another mutation, substituting lysine for glutamic acid in the sixth position, causes sickle cell C disease (Hgb-C). Homozygotes have SC disease, and heterozygotes are considered to have sickle cell C trait (AC disease).
  - The thalassemias are a group of inherited disorders of hemoglobin metabolism in which there is a decrease in the net synthesis of a particular globin chain without a change in its structure.
- Nonproliferative retinopathy: characterized by arteriovenous tortuosity from peripheral vascular shunting, retinal hemorrhages in any layer. Subretinal hemorrhage may have a "salmon patch" appearance that is >1 DD and may resolve with black chorioretinal scars from RPE hypertrophy ("sunbursts") or intraretinal hemosiderin seen as iridescent spots. May also see "wedge sign" from arteriolar occlusions (usually SS disease) or "depression sign" from focal retinal thinning. Also associated with CRAO (especially in hyphema patients), choroidal occlusion, "sickle disk" sign (red spot on retinal surface), and angioid streaks (risk of CNVM). On the rest of the eye exam, patients may have conjunctiva sickle sign (comma-shaped capillaries) and iris atrophy, and are prone to hyphema.
- Proliferative retinopathy: neovascularization is usually peripheral and in a classic "seafan" pattern. NV may lead to vitreous hemorrhage and tractional RD. Staged like retinopathy of prematurity: I (peripheral occlusions), II (AV anastamosis), III ("seafans"), IV (VH), and V (RD).
- Treat with segmental PRP in the anterior periphery of the areas with capillary nonperfusion. "Seafans" often autoinfarct; thus, follow closely. RD usually requires vitrectomy; avoid buckles, as they increase anterior ischemia.

SUPRACHOROIDAL ARTERIAL HEMORRHAGE Rupture of arteriole (usually atherosclerotic and hardened) as it passes from the sclera into the choroid, usually from sudden hypotony (e.g., surgery or penetrating injury). Hemorrhage fills the suprachoroidal space, creating a hemorrhagic choroidal detachment, and may be expulsive, with the loss of intraocular contents and pain from globe expansion. Risk factors include age, atherosclerosis, hypotony, hypertension, chronic glaucoma, axial length >26 mm, and tachycardia.

VITREOUS HEMORRHAGE (VH) From many causes; may resolve with complications such as ocher membrane that may mimic RD, organization with fibroblast recruitment and contraction leading to tractional RD, cyclitic membrane on the anterior hyaloid face with traction on the ciliary body and hypotony, or ERM from glial cell proliferation. See Signs and Symptoms section for list of etiologies.

Physical Disease

POSTERIOR SEGMENT TRAUMA There are approximately 2.4 million eye injuries each year in the United States; 40,000 patients are left with significant vision impairment. Before the 1970s, only 6% of patients suffering penetrating injuries recovered 5/200 VA or better; today, that figure is about 75%. Globe injuries may be classified as closed or open (laceration, IOFB, etc.).

- Emergency evaluation: AMPLE history and physical (patient **a**llergies and **m**edications, **p**ast medical and history, **l**ast meal, then **e**xamination). Check the VA before touching the patient (legal concerns); if VA is 5/200 or better, then there is a 28×-increased chance of salvaging acuity versus NLP, which has a very poor visual prognosis.
- Early treatment is directed toward ocular stabilization as dictated by the injury. Late surgical goals include clear the ocular media, remove vitreous scaffold from any laceration, remove posterior hyaloid, and identify and treat retinal tears and breaks.
- Late complications of globe injuries (and reasons for surgical failure): proliferative vitreoretinopathy, tractional RD, ciliary body shut down and phithis, cyclitic membrane, overwhelming injury, or infection (e.g., *Bacillus*).

CLOSED GLOBE INJURY Injuries may be classified as direct, such as commotio, RPE contusion, choroidal rupture, macular hole, chorioretinitis sclopetaria, ON evulsion, traumatic tears, or dialysis. Injuries may also be indirect, such as Purtscher's disease, Terson's syndrome, shaken baby syndrome, Valsalva's maneuver, fat embolism, and whiplash injury. Associated conditions include contusion, lamellar laceration, superficial foreign body, hyphema, subluxated lens, vitreous hemorrhage (rule out RD; not an independent adverse prognostic factor).

- Commotio retinae, Berlin's or contusion edema: diffuse retinal whitening, not in a vascular pattern, from disruption of photoreceptor outer segments, with edema of all retinal layers; may have hemorrhage. Typically reversible, but may have late atrophy and variably decreased VA; may progress to macular hole or RPE disturbance.
- Contusion of the RPE: like commotio, but no white discoloration, and RPE edema may have overlying serous RD. No early hypofluorescence on FA, but may have patchy RPE staining. Usually resolves.
- Choroidal rupture: seen as a white scleral curvilinear streak concentric to the disk, generally temporal and single, with overlying retinal damage. May be from direct or indirect (anterior injury causing posterior contusion) injury with a tear in Bruch's membrane, as it is not very elastic. May have associated hemorrhage or commotio. Fibrovascular ingrowth seals the rupture within 4 to 6 weeks. Give

an Amsler's grid with close follow-up, as CNVM risk is 10% within 5 years.

- Traumatic macular hole: common after trauma, predisposed by the avascularity of the macula. Occurs days to years postinjury, with variably decreased VA, usually 20/70–400 (patient fixates at the edge of the hole). Unlike idiopathic macular holes, traumatic holes are usually larger (¼–⅓ DD), sharply delimited, with a cuff of SRF; represents actual loss of retinal tissue, not just dehiscence. Classic treatment is observation, but patient may benefit from vitrectomy (85% closure, 20% improved VA); rarely leads to RRD.
- Chorioretinitis sclopetaria: simultaneous rupture of retina and choroid without scleral rupture from passage of a high-velocity missile near the globe, causing coup-contrecoup injury. Characterized by poor VA with extensive hemorrhage and necrosis, and a "clawlike" break in Bruch's membrane with late pigmentary changes and glial proliferation. Rarely RRD.

FAT EMBOLISM SYNDROME Present in 5% of patients with long bone fracture; fatal in 20% of severe cases, retinal lesions in 50%, mostly CWS and small blot hemorrhage (looks like Purtscher's disease). Majority are asymptomatic.

NONACCIDENTAL TRAUMA (NAT), SHAKEN BABY SYNDROME Multiple circumpapillary retinal hemorrhages in any layer, often with Roth's spots (indicates chronicity), CWS, perimacular folds, VH, retinoschisis, and subdural hemorrhage. Retinal injuries occur from rapid accelerating-decelerating injury. Occurs in 30 to 40% of child abuse cases. Differential diagnosis: Purtscher's disease, Terson's syndrome, but is not caused by CPR.

- Commonly has associated neurologic damage, intracranial hemorrhage, and seizures; seen in lethargic and irritable patients who are not septic. Also have high suspicion if you see hyphema, periorbital contusions, incompatible injuries, delay in presentation, multiple admissions to different hospitals, wounds in different stages of healing, mouth wounds, or skin burns. Also may occur in association with cultural therapies, such as hot spoon or coin burns, cupping, salting, moxibustion, and maqua (therapeutic burn).
- Risks for NAT: lower socioeconomic status, irritable and sick babies (who are abused more often)
- NAT masquerades: osteogenesis imperfecta, copper or vitamin A or C deficiency, congenital syphilis, and congenital sensory neuropathy. Differential diagnosis of bruises: mongolian spot, coagulopathies, malignancy (neuroblastoma), Hermansky-Pudlak syndrome, Ehlers-Danlos syndrome, vasculitis, and aspirin use.

- No specific treatment. Document injuries with photos, and observe chain of custody. Be very specific in write-up: stay in your area of expertise, and do not comment on the rest of body.

OPEN GLOBE INJURY May be penetrating (into the globe), perforating (through the globe), or blunt rupture (sclera is weakest at limbus, under rectus muscles, and at the SO insertion and lamina cribrosa). Also can categorize as laceration (penetrating, IOFB, perforation) or rupture.

- Signs of globe rupture: severe hemorrhage (chemosis, hyphema, VH), VA LP or worse, APD, shallow or deep AC, peaked pupil, IOP <5, or unable to visualize globe
- Poor prognostic signs: APD, wound >10 mm, vitreous hemorrhage, wounds extending posterior to the muscle insertions. Zone 1 (cornea): better prognosis. Zone 2 (5 mm ring around cornea) and Zone 3 (posterior to Zone 2): worse prognosis.
- Treatment (mnemonic: TICS) **t**etanus, **I**V antibiotics, **C**T **s**can; and shield the eye. Avoid ointment, and use only sterile drops prior to surgery. Even in overwhelming trauma try to suture what you can, and if necessary, do enucleation later to allow for psychological adjustment. For globe laceration, there is no outcome difference in waiting up to 36 hours. Once initial repair is completed, if secondary surgery is needed, usually wait at least 7 days for vitrectomy but not later than 14 days.
  - Surgery goals: determine extent of injury, restore structural integrity of globe, avoid iatrogenic damage, and decide to excise or reposit (all retina) prolapsed contents.
  - Surgery principles: close corneal lacerations with 10.0 nylon; fully explore scleral lacerations, excise vitreous and uvea from wound, and close with 7.0 nonabsorbable suture, but do not close small posterior wounds. Explore beneath muscle insertions, but do not insert an instrument blindly into a laceration. Prophylactic cryotherapy or scleral buckle is not recommended.
- Intraocular foreign body (IOFB): 10% risk of infection, 30% if farm injury. Evaluate with x-ray or CT (not MRI).
  - Copper: causes chalcosis with deposits in basement membranes, causing sunflower cataract, Kayser-Fleischer ring, and retinal degeneration; may reversibly suppress the ERG. Mild inflammation from copper amalgams (often contain nickle or other metals or brass, which contains copper); higher concentration of copper causes severe suppurative endophthalmitis.
  - Inert foreign bodies: sand, plastic, glass, stone, and ceramic are well tolerated.
  - Iron: poorly tolerated; causes siderosis with deposits in epithelium, causing RPE and inner retinal degeneration (photoreceptors are spared until late). ERG early shows reduced B wave and altered loss of early receptor potential, becoming flat later.

- Wood: brisk inflammatory reaction; high risk of infection.
- Zinc-aluminum: minimum inflammation; often become encapsulated.

PHOTIC, SOLAR, SUNGAZING, OR PSEUDOPHAKIC MACULOPATHY Usually bilateral if sungazing or unilateral if postoperative. Initially presents as a yellow spot in the foveola, then reddish appearance; may lead to lamellar hole (RPE rematins intact). VA usually 20/40–70 and improves over 3 to 9 months. On FA, damaged RPE may stain acutely (no leakage) and with healing leaves window defects. Reported with surgery as short as 55 minutes, from a natural "hot spot" of microscope light focused by the cornea and lens onto the fovea.

PURTSCHER'S RETINOPATHY From severe compression injury to the trunk, with sudden increased intrathoracic pressure with or without air or fat emboli or complement-mediated granulocyte aggregation (often coincidence with pancreatitis), causing bilateral peripapillary HE, CWS, venous congestion, few NFL hemorrhages, and occasionally ON atrophy or macular pigmentary changes. Most patients recover without visual sequelae.

RADIATION RETINOPATHY Looks like, predisposed by, and treated like diabetic retinopathy.

TERSON'S SYNDROME Twenty percent of patients with spontaneous or traumatic subarachnoid hemorrhage have sub-ILM hemorrhage that may break through into the vitreous. Vitreal or subhyaloid blood is not from direct communication with the arachnoid space but from increased venous pressure secondary to increased intracranial pressure. Usually resolves with normal VA.

TOXIC PHOTORECEPTOR RETINOPATHIES Multiple etiologies are seen:
- Cardiac glycosides (digoxin, Lanoxin): used to treat congestive heart failure and arrhythmia; may cause blurred VA, yellow vision, scintillating scotomas from a direct, reversible photoreceptor toxicity; potentiated by concurrent quinidine treatment.
- Sildenafil (Viagra): impotence drug that is selective inhibitor of phosphodiesterase-5 (PDE5), which modifes transduction cascade, causing a rise in cGMP. Characterized by bluish or hazy vision peaking 1 to 2 hours after ingestion in 3% of patients taking 25–50 mg, up to 50% taking > 50 mg. No long-term visual complications.

TOXIC RPE RETINOPATHIES Drugs bind to melanin in the RPE, leading to pigmentary changes and atrophy.
- Thioridazine (Mellaril): most toxic drug for the RPE, causing initial decreased central VA, with brownish discoloration of vision, and

central or ring scotoma. Characterized by initial salt and pepper fundus, followed by pigment clumping in plaquelike fashion, with later RPE atrophy. Usually safe up to 800 mg/day, and toxic if >1 g/day; maximal daily dose is more critical than accumulative dose. Needs fundoscopic exam every 6 months during administration.

- Chlorpromazine (Thorazine): binds strongly to melanin, infrequent toxicity. Nonspecific fundus granularity with pigment clumping seen when dose is >800 mg/day. Also may cause pigment dusting on the lens with mild stellate cataract and brown bulbar conjunctiva deposits (pathognomic).
- Chloroquine (Aralen): used as an antimalarial drug, as well as for treatment of RA and SLE. Characterized by early asymptomatic perifoveal granularity with loss of foveal reflection (reversible), followed by "bull's-eye" thinning of foveal RPE (nonreversible) and late tapetoretinal degeneration. Patients notice decreased VA with paracentral scotoma and field constriction. Maximum safe dose is 4 mg/kg/day. If total dose >300 g, 70% of patients have some degeneration, but daily dose is more critical than accumulative dose. Follow Amsler's grid, and examine every 6 months (FA not needed routinely); may have supranormal EOG and decreased color. Can progress even after drug is discontinued.
- Hydroxychloroquine (Plaquenil): significantly safer than chloroquine because it does not cross blood-retinal barrier; also used for treatment of RA and SLE. Toxic dose variable, but up to 400 mg/day is generally safe. Causes a cone dystrophy from transynaptic degeneration with classic "bull's-eye" maculopathy and dyschromatopsia. Screen at least every 2 years with exam, central VF monitoring, and color plates or D-15.
- Desferrioxamine: used to treat iron overload; may cause RPE alterations, cataract, and optic atrophy.

TOXIC VASCULAR RETINOPATHIES Drug causes vascular occlusion with secondary ischemic damage.

- Ergot alkaloids (ergotamine, methysergide): adrenergic blockers used in migraine and postpartum hemorrhage can cause CRVO or macular edema.
- Interferon-alpha retinopathy: numerous CWS, intraretinal hemorrhage, vessel occlusion, and ischemic optic neuropathy.
- Oral contraceptives: less systemic thromboembolic disease today, as there is less estrogen concentration than in the past. May see disturbances in color vision, arteriolar occlusion, CRVO, retinal hemorrhage, and CME.
- Quinine sulfate: antimalarial and muscle relaxant; also occasionally used as abortifactant or suicidal agent. Toxic dose is >4 g, causing blurred VA, decreased VF, nyctalopia, and photophobia. Initially

subtle fundus findings, followed by disk pallor and vessel attenuation that resembles an old CRAO. Patients may need hemodialysis or vasodilating agents.

TOXIC EDEMATOUS RETINOPATHIES Drugs that cause CME or retinal edema.

- Nicotinic acid (niacin): used in hyperlipidemia; may cause megavitaminosis and atypical CME without leakage on FA with dosage >3 g/day; reversible.
- Sulfa drugs (especially chlorthalidone, Diamox, hydrochlorothiazide): drug-induced myopia from ciliary body edema, with anterior movement of the lens–iris diaphragm, or transient CME with retinal or choroidal folds.

TOXIC CRYSTALLINE RETINOPATHIES Drugs cause deposition of intraretinal crystals.

- Methoxyflurane (Penthrane): anesthetic may cause secondary hyperoxalosis with calcium oxalate crystals in the RPE and inner retina; resembles flecked retina (pisciform throughout the posterior pole); may also have renal failure.
- Tamoxifen (Nolvadex): antiestrogen used in breast CA; 1 to 6% of cases develop bilateral intraretinal refractile opacities ("doughnut ring" in macula); not reported in cumulative doses <10 g. Patients may be asymptomatic to blurred VA; can continue therapy with close follow-up. May have cataract from blockage of chloride channels.
- Talc: usually from intravenous drug abuse with end arteriole deposition, causing macular ischemia, secondary NV, or choroidal infarction.
- Canthaxanthine (Orobronze, Riviera): carotenoid use in food coloring; also found in mushrooms and sometimes used as suntanning agent. Yellow, birefringent, glistening crystals in "doughnut" ring in the macular RPE.
- Nitrofurantoin (Macrodantin): intraretinal crystals reported.

TRAUMATIC RETINITIS Post-trauma, patients may have RP-like RPE changes.

TRAUMATIC TEARS, RETINAL DETACHMENT OR DIALYSIS Twenty percent of RD is from trauma, usually seen in younger males (average age 28 years old). Most are closed globe injuries to lower lateral eye, with coup (inferior temporal) and contrecoup (superior nasal) pathology.

- Dialysis is the most common lesion, seen as a "bucket handle" appearance behind the lens; 31% are inferotemporal, and 22% are superonasal. Giant retinal tears (>180 degrees) are seen in 16%.
- Posterior flap tears with attached vitreous are seen in 11% of cases. Also, tears seen around lattice or meridianal folds. Most tears are

found later: 12% initially, 30% by 1 month, 50% by 8 months, and 80% by 24 months.

- Penetrating injuries usually have a retinal break opposite the injury, and proliferative vitreoretinopathy may cause a traction band away from the break.
- For litiginous evaluation, may need to determine if trauma is causal: suspect traumatic cause if patient has unilateral pathology with dialysis or giant tear in a nonmyope <40 years old without otherwise prior history of trauma within 2 years.

VALSALVA RETINOPATHY Hemorrhagic detachment of ILM that is circumscribed, and juxtapapillary, from a sudden rise in the intrathoracic or abdominal pressure, with increased venous pressure and rupture of superficial capillaries. Also may have transient increased IOP ("brass players' glaucoma") from increased choroidal engorgement. Can occur with unrecognized Valsalva stress (e.g., intercourse). No treatment needed, and good prognosis can be expected, but if nonclearing, can consider YAG laser disruption of posterior hyaloid to drain hemorrhage into the vitreous.

WHIPLASH RETINOPATHY Immediate mild decreased VA (usually about 20/30) with gray swelling of the fovea. FA may show a tiny area of hyperfluorescence that may look like solar retinopathy. Typically resolves with little long-term changes.

Inflammatory and Immune Disease

See Chapter 5.

Surgery: Laser

FOCAL PHOTOCOAGULATION Used to ablate CNVM, tumors, vascular lesions (capillary or choroidal hemangioma, retinal artery macroaneurysm, etc.), parasites (DUSN, cysticercosis, etc.), destroy sick RPE in ICSR, create chorioretinal adhesions for retinal tears, or "wall off" RD or necrotic CMV or ARN retina.

GRID PHOTOCOAGULATION, FOCAL MACULAR GRID (FMG) Used to treat macular edema for diabetic CSME (ETDRS) or after BRVO (BVOS). Settings usually use argon green, 100 μm, 0.1 second, and 100 mW (often begin lower). Light burns (for blond fundus, may begin at 50 mW), one burn width apart. Full grid for diffuse edema ("doughnut"-shaped ablation 500 μm around fovea) or partial laser over edema. Increased spot size increases cataract risk.

PANRETINAL PHOTOCOAGULATION (PRP) Used to cause regression of NV, destroy ischemic tissue that is producing VEGF, or improve oxygenation from the choroid such as for PDR, sickle cell retinopathy, NV following BRVO, or NVI after CRVO. Settings often about 200 mW, 0.2 seconds, 200 μm spot. Power density, and thus tissue damage, increases as the spot size is decreased, wattage is increased, or time is decreased. Partial PRP usually leaves two laser spots between burns; in contrast, extensive PRP tightens the pattern to one spot separating burns. Usually deliver argon PRP <900 spots per session, in two or three sessions, and complete PRP is around 2000 spots. Treat inferior retina first; focally treat NVE. If FMG is needed, complete it first.

- Complications: 11% of patients lose one line of VA. May also have nyctalopia (especially warn diabetic patients) and field constriction (rare complaint with PDR, as the peripheral retina is already ischemic). With extramacular treatment, the patient will have a negative scotoma that is not noticed as much as a positive scotoma, which occurs with a macular lesion. Also may have CME (treat the temporal "C" last and avoid temporal retina within 2 DD of the fovea), foveal traction, choroidal rupture (apply gentle pressure on globe if any bleeding is seen), and serous choroidal detachment (avoid by delivering in several sessions). May also have posterior synechia if iris is burned when treating the retinal periphery, cornea or lens burns, CNVM or foveal burns, transient retinal edema (improves after 3 weeks), retinal thinning, and holes (especially in high myopes). Persistent mydriasis and paresis of accommodation have been reported from ciliary nerve damage (the 3 and 9 o'clock location in the retina).

PHOTODYNAMIC THERAPY (PDT) Intravenous photosensitizing agent (e.g., verteporfin or Visudyne, peak sensitivity at 690 nm) accumulates in proliferating neoplastic or NV tissue (possibly from LDL receptors on proliferating cells), which is then activated by irradiation at wavelength specific for the molecule's peak absorption. Photochemical reaction (not photocoagulation) produces tissue damage by free radical formation (type 1 injury) and reactive singlet oxygen molecules (type 2 injury) that causes vascular endothelial damage and thrombus formation.

TRANSPUPILLARY THERMOTHERAPY (TTT) Subthreshold laser to "cook" vascular lesions, such as CNVM and melanomas. Laser wavelength is 810 nm (choriocapillaris level), usually with 3.0 mm spot size, 60 seconds, and 820 mW. Several sessions needed.

Surgery: Operative

GASES AND FLUIDS USED INTRAOPERATIVELY Used to maintain vitreous space and pressure (Table 7–4).

TABLE 7–4
Expansile Gas Properties

Gas	Duration	Expansion	Nonexpansile Concentration
Air	1–3 days	0	NA
SF_6 (sulfur hexafluoride)	10 days–2 weeks	2×	20% (can rapidly increase IOP)
C_2F_6 (perfluoroethane)	4 weeks	3×	NA
C_3F_8 (perfluoropropane)	6 weeks–2 months	4×	16%

NA, not applicable.

- Intraocular gases: specific gravity of the gases are much less than water. Also, blood nitrogen diffuses into the gas; thus, do not use N_2 with inhalational anesthetics during surgery.
- Perfluorocarbons (PFCs): used in proliferative vitreoretinopathy, giant retinal tears, retinopathy of prematurity, and to remove posteriorly displaced lens fragments or IOL. Characterizewd by high specific gravity, with transparency, high surface tension, and low viscosity. Potential toxicity seen in subretinal space and anterior segment with retained intraocular PFC. Four PFCs commonly in use, most commonly perfluoro-N-octane (PFO), which has a relatively low viscosity (0.8 Cs at 25°C) and a high vapor pressure (50 mmHg at 37°C). Low viscosity allows for easy injection and aspiration via a 20-gauge needle, and high vapor pressure allows evaporation of small droplets of residual PFO during air–fluid exchange.
- Silicone oil (SiO): surface tension is less than for gases, and SiO is buoyant in fluid-filled eye (inferior peripheral iridectomy is needed). Use for long-term tamponade, especially with recurrent RD, when 180 degree retinotomy is performed, air travel is anticipated, etc.

INTRAVITREAL INJECTION Useful for antibiotic and steroid delivery, for subfoveal hemorrhage >1 mm (may inject TPA), and for pneumatic displacement.

- Endophthalmitis tap and inject: usually place retrobulbar block, then use empty tuberculin syringe or other small syringe with 23 gauge needle placed 3 mm posterior to limbus, observing through the pupil (indirect light works well) as the needle is advanced about 1 cm, and aspirate about 0.5 mL. Then use a new site and 30 gauge needle on TB syringe to inject 0.1 cc of antibiotics in the midvitreous.

RETINAL DETACHMENT SURGERY Goal is to find the retinal holes and close them, then relieve vitreoretinal traction. Three common errors: failure to find the hole, failure to find the other holes, and failure to close them. If macula is on and RD is peripheral, then do surgery within a few days. If RD is near macula, then perform surgery as early as possible, and within hours if macula is threatened or giant retinal tear is present (>1 quadrant). If macula is off, then can wait 1 or 2 days if history suggests that the RD is recent or up to 1 or 2 weeks if it is a chronic RD.

- Pneumatic retinopexy: best for single break or group no larger than 1 clock hour within the superior 8 clock hours. Intraocular gas temporarily closes the break and displaces the retina toward the eye wall; holes are treated with cryotherapy or laser. Successful in 75% of cases.
- Scleral buckle procedure: conjunctival peritomy, pass bridle suture around each rectus muscle, and inspect sclera. Scleral depress and localize all breaks, and mark externally on sclera. Create chorioretinal adhesion with laser or cryotherapy (most commonly used), with cryoreactions touching each other without a gap, "toe in" (avoid indenting eye with shaft), do not cryotherapy in middle of flap tear, surround each tear with 2–3 mm of cryotherapy, and treat the entire lattice lesion if applicable. Apply the buckle to indent the sclera and choroid toward the retina, relieve vitreous traction, and displace SRF. Then place sutures to anchor the exoplant. Drain SRF if needed, where the RD is most elevated usually, anterior to the equator and superior or inferior to the horizontal rectus muscles; expose choroid by radial scleral incision and peforate choroid with a 27 gauge needle diagonally (ensure IOP is not elevated; relieve tension on traction sutures). Tighten the buckle, and irrigate with Marcaine for pain relief. Carefully close conjunctiva and Tenon's capsule.
  - Complications: scleral rupture from cryotherapy, retinal perforation, retinal incarceration (do not try to push back in; put gas or air into eye to flatten out), redetachment, buckle exposure, anterior segment ischemia, strabismus, and induced myopia. Proliferative vitreoretinopathy is most common cause for failure (5–10% for RRD); PVR is usually an "inferior disease" (gravity dependent).
  - Eighty to 90% scleral buckle success for RD, with permanent support of the vitreous base and less proliferative vitreoretinopathy. Ten to 20% require more than one surgery. Eighty-five percent of patients who present with 20/20 VA keep that following surgery, and 15% have decreased VA usually from CME or ERM. If macula is on preoperative, then 80 to 85% of patients are 20/50 or better following surgery. If macula is off preoperative, then there is only a 20 to 40% chance of 20/50 VA or better (one third will be 20/200 or worse).
- Vitrectomy with gas: used for posterior breaks.
- Vitrectomy with scleral buckle: used for complicated RD, such as with proliferative vitreoretinopathy, traction RD, and giant tears.

VITRECTOMY Performed for nonclearing VH with severe PDR in insulin-dependent diabetes, complicated RD, removal of ERM or other posterior segment lesions, and CME (vitreous holds cytokines against macula, blocks medications getting to macula, and is a reservoir for antigens and cells). The microvitreoretinal (MVR) blade passes through the sclera, stroma of pars plana, pigmented then non-pigmented epithelium, sometimes zonules, and into the vitreous base. If a VH occurs after vitrectomy, consider anterior hyaloid vascular proliferation around the sclerotomy site.

CHAPTER 8

Neurologic

Anatomy and Physiology

EMBRYOLOGY Migrating axons from retinal ganglion cells converge to the optic stalk, which later becomes the optic disk, and reach the ON by the seventh week. They continue centrally, guided by CNS pigment, to synapse at the lateral geniculate nucleus (LGN). Myelination starts proximally at the LGN in the seventh month. Neuroglial cells of the optic stalk support the axons and gradually obliterate the optic stalk lumen.

CRANIAL NERVES (Figs. 8–1 and 8–2) CN I and II are found in the diencephalon, III and IV in the midbrain, V, VI, VII, and VIII in the pons, and IX, X, XI, and XII in the medulla.

- I. Olfactory nerve: may be affected by meningioma in association with Foster Kennedy syndrome.
- II. Optic nerve: length is 1 mm intraocular, 25 mm intraorbital, 10 mm intracanalicular, and 17 mm intracranial to the chiasm (mnemonic: telephone number 125–1017).
  - Disk vasculature: laminar and prelaminar portions of the disk are supplied by the posterior ciliary artery (watershed area and site of AION); the intraorbital ON is supplied by the central retinal artery and pial vessels. The ophthalmic artery is nasal to the vein at the disk.
  - Nerve vasculature: peripheral, larger ON axons are metabolically supported by CSF and pial vessels (thus, they are relatively protected from toxins because of the blood–brain barrier). Central, smaller macular axons are supplied by the central retinal artery, which lies central within the ON within 12 mm of the globe.
  - The subdural space of the ON does not communicate with the subdural space of the cranium, as it fuses with the periosteum of the optic canal and is only a potential space. The dura is then contiguous with the sclera.
- III. Oculomotor nerve: nucleus lies in the dorsal midbrain at the level of the superior colliculus. The levator nucleus is central and thus gives bilateral innervation; the SR fibers cross to innervate the contralateral muscle. All other subnuclei give ipsilateral fibers. CN III also supplies parasympathetic fibers from the Edinger-Westphal nucleus (afferent

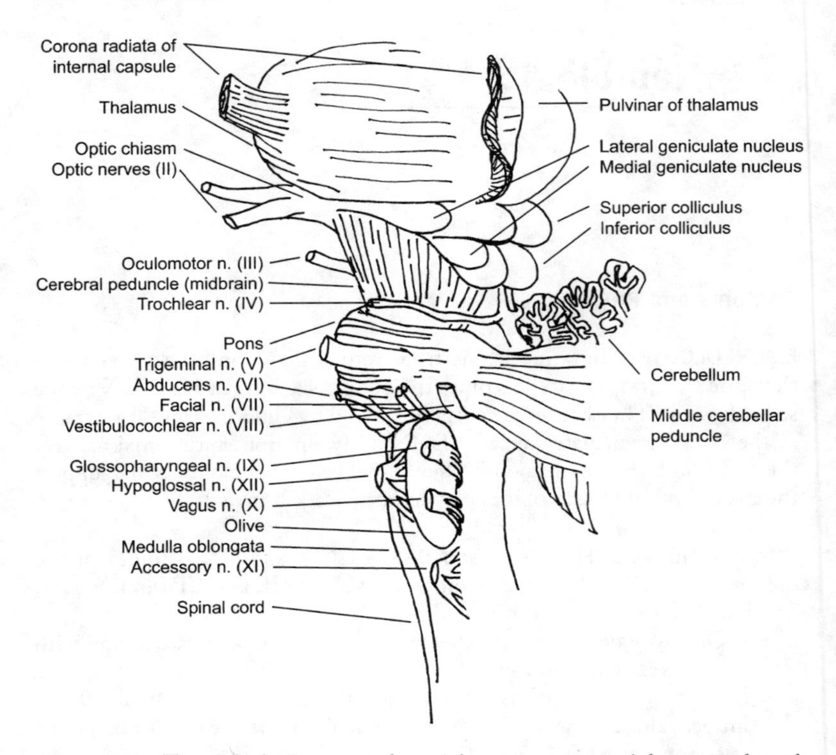

Figure 8–1 The right brainstem and cranial nerve anatomy, right posterolateral view.

input to the Edinger-Westphal nucleus is from the retina). CN III fasciculus exits the brainstem in the subarachnoid space, travels to the cavernous sinus, then through the SOF as a superior division (supplying SR and levator muscles) and inferior division (innervating IR, IO, and MR muscles and carrying parasympathetics to the pupil sphincter and ciliary body).

- IV. Trochlear nerve: longest intracranial course innervating the SO. The nucleus lies in the midbrain tegmentum at the level of the inferior colliculus, near the midline but ventral to the cerebral aqueduct. Axons exit dorsally and cross (thus contralateral innervation), curving around the cerebral peduncle, then passing between the posterior cerebral and superior cerebral arteries along with CN III. They course anterior, piercing the dura at the tentorium cerebelli, then into the cavernous sinus and through the SOF, crossing medially to innervate the SO.

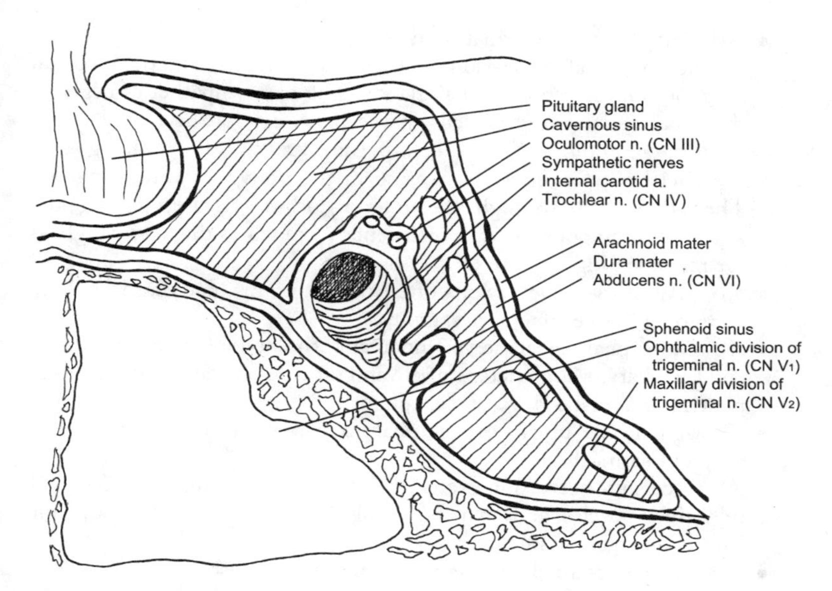

Figure 8–2 Left cavernous sinus and associated structures, coronal section.

- V. Trigeminal nerve: provides facial and ocular sensation and also innervates the muscles of mastication (temporalis, masseter, and pterygoids), the tensor veli palatini, the tensor tympani, the anterior belly of digastric, and the mylohyoid muscle.
  - Three divisions: CN V_1 (ophthalmic), CN V_2 (maxillary), and CN V_3 (mandibular).
  - Lesions of CN V_1 are often neoplasm (especially acoustic neuroma); CN V_2, usually orbital trauma, or maxillary sinus disease (often the first sign of nasopharyngeal CA); and CN V_3, often involved with nasopharyngeal tumor or middle fossa disease. Also trigeminal neuralgia or Raeder's paratrigeminal neuralgia (CN V palsy plus Horner's syndrome).
- VI. Abducens nerve: most commonly injured by increased intracranial pressure or hydrocephalus (also known as the "tumor" nerve). The nucleus lies in the pontine tegmentum, close to the midline, just ventral to the fourth ventricle. Axons exit ventrally, then pass through the subarachnoid space, up the clivus through Dorello's canal, through the petrous space, and into the cavernous sinus. In the cavernous sinus, CN VI floats in the lumen, joined briefly by sympathetics, and enters the orbit through the inferior division SOF, to innervate the LR muscle.

- VII. Facial nerve: originates in the pontine nucleus to supply the muscles of facial expression and provide parasympathetic input to secretory salivary and lacrimal glands. The parasympathetics begin in the superior salivatory nucleus in the pons, exit as the nervus intermedius, and join CN VII before they branch off as the greater superficial petrosal nerve, synapsing in the pterygopalatine ganglion. They then pass through the inferior orbital fissure, joining the zygomaticotemporal nerve, which sends a branch to the lacrimal gland for reflex tearing.
- VIII. Auditory nerve: lesions often cause tinnitus, decreased hearing, vertigo, and a peripheral nystagmus.
- IX. Glossopharyngeal nerve: innervates the stylopharyngeus muscle and the pharynx constrictor muscle and provides sensation to the upper pharynx and distal third of the tongue.
- X. Vagus nerve: innervates the pharynx, larynx, heart, lungs, esophagus, and stomach.
- XI. Accessory nerve: innervates the sternocleidomastoid (SCM) and trapezius muscles and may be involved in myotonic dystrophy or Meigs' blepharospasm.
- XII. Hypoglossal nerve: innervates the tongue muscle.

RETINAL ORGANIZATION Main retinal function is to convert information about brightness (luminance) into information about contrast. Retinal organization is only concerned about relative quantities, except the pupillary control cells, which travel to the pretectum and need direct luminance information.

- Simplified, the retina functions as five main layers:
  - Photoreceptors (rods and cones): respond to light or color by hyperpolarization (in the dark, normally have a graded depolarizing response with the release of neurotransmitter glutamate) and project to the horizontal and bipolar cells.
  - Horizontal cells: located in the outer plexiform layer and respond to glutamate neurotransmitter from the photoreceptors with a graded release of inhibitory gamma-aminobutyric acid (GABA) neurotransmitter; function as a lateral connector of the photoreceptors and bipolar cells to detect center-surround contrast.
  - Bipolar cells: located in the inner nuclear layer and respond to glutamate neurotransmitter from the photoreceptors; project to amacrine and ganglion cells.
  - Amacrine cells: lateral connector of bipolar and ganglion cells with various types of cells, neurotransmitters, and functions, including sensing movement and direction; located in the inner plexiform layer.
  - Ganglion cells: carry the visual information to the brain and generate an action potential (not a graded response) when depolarized by glutamate released from bipolar cells.

- Bipolar receptive field: all parts of the retina that affect activity in a particular bipolar cell depolarize that cell if directly connected (comprise the "center" of receptive field) or hyperpolarize and oppose it if indirectly connected to it by a horizontal cell ("surround" of receptive field). Each bipolar cell may be a depolarizing cell as described above or a hyperpolarizing cell, which responds to objects that are darker than the background, and thus are hyperpolarized by light in the center and depolarized by light falling on the surround.
  - "Off" bipolar cells: depolarized by glutamate released by photoreceptors in the dark
  - "On" bipolar cells: hyperpolarized by glutamate, and thus are depolarized by the decreased photoreceptor release of glutamate in light
- Color: certain horizontal cells are excited by green-absorbing cones and inhibited by red cones (and vice versa); other horizontal cells are excited by blue cones and inhibited by red and green cones, known as red/green and yellow/blue opponent color cells.
- Ganglion cell functional division: ganglion cells have a receptive field concentric center/surround organization like bipolar cells: "on" center ganglion cells are excited by "on" center bipolar cells, and "off" center ganglion cells are excited by "off" center bipolar cells.
  - Magnocellular (M) cell axons: large diameter; carry information about dim illumination and motion to the LGN layers 1 and 2.
  - Parvocellular (P) cells: small axons; are responsible for color and fine detail (because they receive input from a small number of bipolar cells and thus have small receptive fields) and travel to the LGN layers 3, 4, 5, and 6.

OPTIC NERVE Optic disk is a vertical oval (average dimensions 1.78 mm × 1.90 mm) with an optic cup that is normally a horizontal oval. Axons receive glial support from astrocytes in the NFL and laminar and prelaminar layers. Oligodendrocytes in the retrolaminar ON produce myelin. The lamina cribosa is composed of stacked, fenestrated collagen and laminin plates.

- Axons: 1.2 million axons arise from 5 million to 100 million ganglion cells and respect the horizontal raphae (vs. optic tract fiber organization that respects the vertical meridian).
  - Macular axons travel in the papulomacular bundle (PMB); temporal axons curve above and below the PMB (thus, the optic disk is thickest at the superior and inferior poles as more fibers enter from the periphery of the retina), and nasal fibers enter the disk more directly.
  - Peripheral axons travel deep in the NFL and enter the disk peripherally. Macular central axons lie superficial in the retina and pass into the center of the disk and nerve.

  - Macular axons occupy the temporal wedge of the distal ON, then are diffusely oriented in the chiasm. Inferior ON fibers pass into the chiasm and continue in the medial optic tract. Superior ON fibers pass into the lateral optic tract.
- Vascular (Fig. 8–3): the NFL is supplied from the central retinal artery, prelaminar and laminar layers from short posterior ciliary arteries, and the retrolaminar layer from the central retinal artery. No normal disk vessels leak on FA because of the blood–brain barrier (formed by cellular tight junctions, pericytes, and nonfenestrated endothelium).

RETINA PROJECTS TO FOUR SUBNUCLEI The majority of fibers synapse at the LGN; however, a small number of fibers do not synapse at the LGN

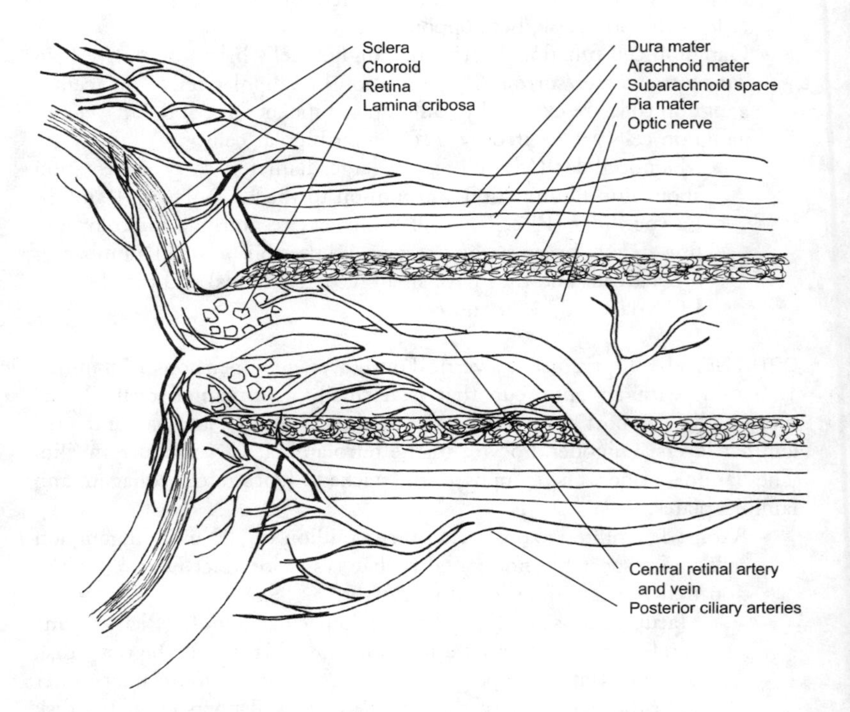

Figure 8–3 Cross section of the anterior optic nerve, showing branches from the central retinal artery supplying the retrolaminar portion of the nerve and the NFL, and the prelaminar and laminar areas of the nerve supplied by the short posterior ciliary arteries.

but instead travel to the superior colliculus, pretectum, and suprachiasmatic nucleus.

- Lateral geniculate nucleus (LGN): responsible for object perception but is mainly a gateway and does little processing. It does have "on" and "off" center cells similar to the retina and and also yellow/blue and red/green coded cells. The LGN projects to the primary visual cortex (also known as the striate pathway because on gross specimen it is seen as a stripe):
  - Primary visual cortex has six layers: tract fibers enter at layer IV and project to layers II and III, which project to layer V, which projects to the superior colliculus and layers II, III, and V, which project to layer VI, which projects to secondary visual cortical centers and feedback loop to the LGN.
  - Secondary visual cortical centers:
    - Temporal cortex: concerned with shape and *what* information
    - Parietal cortex: concerned with color and movement and *where* information
- Superior colliculus: involved with eye movement control. Projects to the pulvinar, then to the cortex (extrastriate pathway).
- Pretectum: concerned with pupil control and near synkinesis. Projects to incalated neurons, which are excitatory to the Edinger-Westphal nucleus (unlike cortical and spinal-reticular input and sleep and coma states that are inhibitory to the Edinger-Westphal nucleus).
- Suprachiasmatic nucleus: involved with diurnal rhythms and hormonal control.

BRODMANN'S AREAS Number 17: primary occipital cortex (the macula is inside on the banks of the calcarine fissure in a watershed zone between the posterior and middle cerebral arteries). Number 18: splenium, which connects the right and left occiputs. Number 19: occipitoparietal area.

Fig. 8–4 shows the superior view of right cerebral blood vessels and the anterior/posterior visual pathways.

EYE MOVEMENT CONTROL Purpose is to stabilize gaze and put the object of interest on the fovea. Retinal slip velocity describes the smooth pursuit eye movement system that uses retinal information about the image-slip-velocity of the target to match the gaze-velocity to the actual target velocity (need a gain of 1 to keep image on the retina).

- Gaze control: horizontal gaze includes pursuits (ipsilateral parietal origin) and saccades (fast movements from the contralateral frontal lobe).

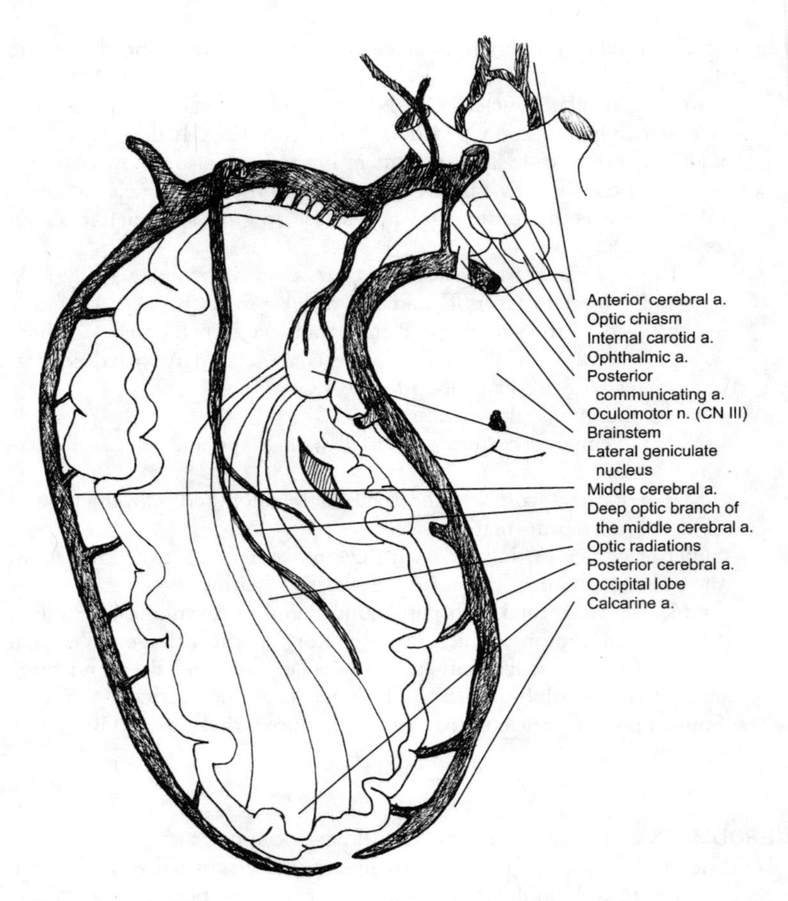

Figure 8–4 Superior view of selected right cerebral blood vessels and their relationship to the anterior and posterior visual pathways.

- Horizontal gaze control: cortical input from the contralateral frontal eye fields, ipsilateral parietal lobe, and vestibular apparatus project to the ipsilateral paramedian pontine reticular formation (PPRF) adjacent to the CN VI nucleus. This input stimulates the ipsilateral LR muscle, which then projects interneurons, crossing into the medial longitudinal fasciculus (MLF) to the CN III nucleus (stimulating the contralateral MR muscle), with the result that the eyes look toward the ipsilateral side (Fig. 8–5).
- Vertical gaze control: originates in the frontal eye fields or superior colliculus that projects to the rostral interstitial nucleus

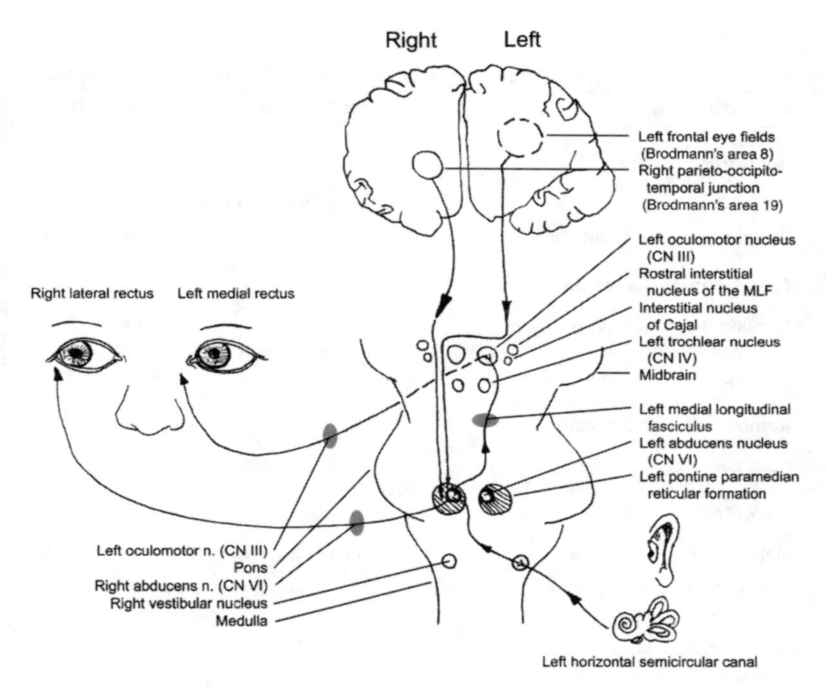

Figure 8–5 Schema of nuclei and neural pathways involved with horizontal eye movement control. The rostral interstitial nucleus of the MLF (riMLF), interstitial nucleus of Cajal (INC), and the trochlear nucleus (CN IV) are involved with vertical eye movment control.

of the MLF (riMLF) and then to CN III and IV nuclei. The interstitial nucleus of Cajal (INC) is involved with vertical pursuits.

- Gaze acquisition mechanisms:
  - Saccades: voluntary eye movements with about 200 msec of latency. Initated from the PPRF, saccades have two components: initial pulse (burst of neuronal firing from burst cells), followed by step (to maintain the smooth movement, the firing neuron must overcome the viscous drag of muscle and the elastic restraining forces of orbit). The neural integrator keeps the burst and step in the same frequency and is located in the nucleus prepositus hypoglossi (NPH) and the medial vestibular nucleus (MVN) for horizontal movement and the interstitial nucleus of Cajal for vertical saccades.
  - Quick phases of nystagmus: fast 500 degrees/second.

TABLE 8–1

Comparison of the Sympathetic and Parasympathetic Autonomic Nervous System

Sympathetic Nervous System	Parasympathetic Nervous System
Neurotransmitter	
Preganglionic: acetylcholine	Preganglionic: acetylcholine
Postganglionic: norepinephrine	Postganglionic: acetylcholine
Production of Neurotransmitter	
Tyrosine (tyrosine hydroxylase) → dopa → dopamine → norepinephrine → epinephrine	Choline + acetylcoenzyme A (choline acetylase)
Removal of Neurotransmitter	
Reuptake, COM-T, MAO	Acetylcholinesterase
Receptors	
$alpha_1$: smooth muscle and glands	Nicotinic: ganglia and skeletal muscle
$alpha_2$: presynaptic receptors	Muscarinic: smooth/cardiac muscle and glands
$beta_1$: increased heart rate, decreased heart contractility, lipolysis	
$beta_2$: vaso- and bronchodilatation	
Pupillary Autonomic Nerve Pathways	
Cervical sympathetic chain	Oculomotor nerve (CN III)
Superior cervical ganglion	Ciliary ganglion
Long ciliary nerves	Short ciliary nerves
Dilator fibers of iris	Ciliary body and iris sphincter
Medication Effects	
Adrenergic (sympathomimetic)	Cholinergic or anticholinesterase
Mydriasis	Miosis via iris sphincter muscle
Decreased IOP (alpha receptors)	Accommodation (ciliary muscle)
Increased IOP (beta receptors)	Increased aqueous outflow
Adrenergic blocking drugs	Cholinergic blocking drugs
Block production of aqueous	Mydriasis, cycloplegia

COM-T, catechol-o-methyltransferase; dopa, dihydroxyphenylalanine; IOP, intraocular pressure; MAO, monoamine oxidase.

- Gaze stability mechanisms: from vestibular apparatus (labyrinthine) with a short latency (<16 msec vs. visually mediated movements that have >70 msec latency). Combined movements of head and eye require cancellation of the vestibulo-ocular reflex (VOR).
  - Angular movement: mediated by the semicircular canals responsible for torsional motion. Vestibular input projects ipsilaterally to the MVN, then to the contralateral PPRF and CN VI nucleus, then back across the midline to the ipsilateral MLF and CN III nucleus. Also controlled by midline cerebellar structures (anterior vermis) and cervical neck receptors.
    - Example: a head turn to the right stimulates the right semicircular canals and thus stimulates the left CN VI nucleus and the left LR and the right CN III nucleus and the right MR, with the result that the eyes turn to the left.
    - Destruction of vestibular apparatus causes the opposite inner ear to stimulate gaze toward the side of the lesion.
  - Linear movement: mediated by the otoliths (utricle and saccule), concerned with translational motion.
- Gaze-shifting mechanisms: primarily from visually mediated mechanisms (pursuit, optokinetic, vergence); supplement the VOR and stabilize the gaze during sustained head movements (e.g., optokinetic nystagmus and full-field movement) and VOR (e.g., brainstem function and doll's eyes).
- Vergence movements: arise from midbrain control and include fusional vergences, resting state, and horizontal and vertical vergences. Other horizontal vergence movements include accommodative for near work, tonic for everyday use, and proximal or instrument (e.g., when looking through a microscope).

Table 8–1 presents a comparison of the sympathetic and parasympathetic autonomic nervous system.

Signs and Symptoms

ABERRANT REGENERATION Seen with axons that become misdirected during the repair phase, such as that following CN III palsy from trauma, tumor, or aneurysm (but not ischemia). May manifest as crocodile tears, Adie's pupil, pseudo-Graeffe's sign (lid elevation with down gaze), and pseudo–Argyll Roberston pupil. Distinguish from dyskinesis.

ABNORMAL DISK WITH ELEVATION Pale disk, papilledema, pseudopapilledema, and swollen disk

ACQUIRED CRANIAL NERVE PALSY Ischemia, tumor, aneurysm, inflammation, and infection

AFFERENT PUPILLARY DEFECT (APD) Usually from unilateral or asymmetric ON disease. Mild APD may also be seen with contralateral optic tract damage (52% of chiasmal fibers cross) or contralateral pupillomotor fiber damage in the midbrain. ON may lose 40 to 50% of fibers before APD develops and does not show a change in pupil size.

ANISOCORIA Asymmetric pupil size (>1 mm of difference between the eyes). Figure 8–6 shows flowchart for amiscoria dignosis.

- Anisocoria greater in light (larger than normal pupil): suggests parasympathetic paresis such as that seen in Adie's tonic pupil, CN III lesion (e.g., uncal herniation), postictal seizures, migraine, siderosis, or pharmacologic reactions. A larger pupil may also be seen with acute glaucoma, iris trauma, or sympathetic hyperactivity.
  - Adie's pupil: parasympathetic denervation in the ciliary ganglion with aberrant regeneration of the fibers that normally travel to the ciliary body to control accommodation now innervating the iris sphincter. Thus, patients have light-near dissociation and vermiform iris movements. The iris is hypersensitive to weak pilocarpine; if acute, may not constrict to pilocarpine and may mimic pharmacologic dilation.

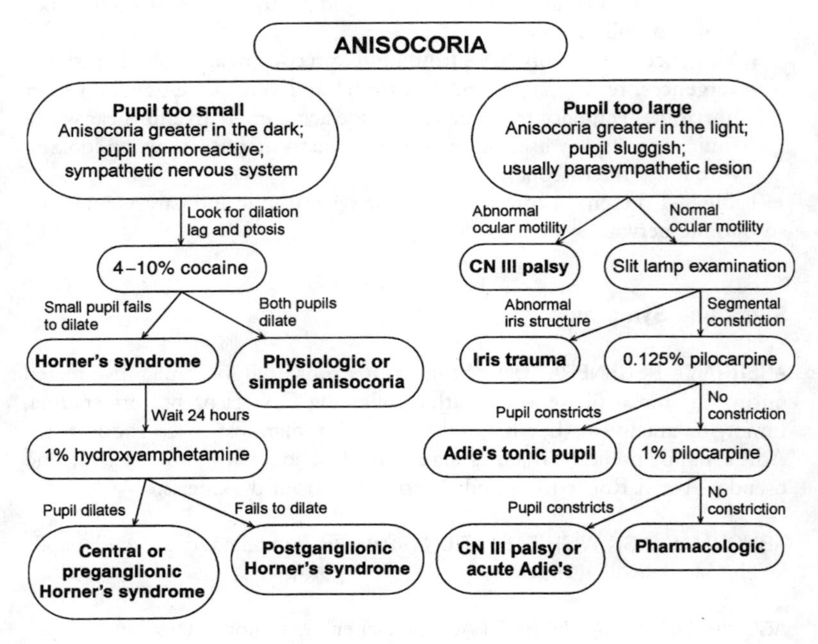

Figure 8–6 Anisocoria flowchart for diagnosis.

  - Fixed dilated pupil: symptomatic of pharmacologic reactions (ask about "red cap" drops, look for a scopolamine patch for motion sickness, consider functional diagnosis), Adie's pupil, CN III lesion (uncal herniation obvious; otherwise, rare; check angiogram), and migraine.
- Anisocoria greater in dark (smaller than normal pupil): suggests sympathetic lesion such as that seen in Horner's syndrome, cluster headache, or pharmocologic reaction. May also be from hyperactive parasympathetic system such as cyclic oculomotor paresis (miosis during the spastic phase).
  - Horner's syndrome: ptosis (and reverse ptosis), miosis, anhydrosis, enophthalmos, decreased tearing, and heterochromia if congenital. Cocaine blocks norepinephrine reuptake and causes normal pupil dilation if the sympathetic chain is intact; however, in Horner's syndrome, no norepinephrine is present in the nerve endings, and thus dilation does not occur. If cocaine test is positive, may perform Paredrine (hydroxyamphetamine) test at least a day later to localize the Horner's syndrome to a first or second order neuron pathway versus a third order. Paredrine stimulates release of norepinephrine and thus causes pupil dilation if third order neuron is intact. More dilation than normally seen with aproclonidine may also suggest alpha-1 hypersensitivity.
    - First order neuron: usually obvious neurologic cause from brainstem disease.
    - Second order neuron: usually C-spine trauma or tumor, or apical lung tumor (Pancoast's tumor).
    - Third order neuron: carotid artery dissection or neck surgery, cavernous sinus lesion, nasopharyngeal CA, migraine, orbital disease or Raeder's trigeminal neuralgia.
- Other causes of anisocoria or pupil abnormalities:
  - Argyll Robertson pupil: miotic and irregular pupil associated with light-near dissociation, tertiary syphilis.
  - Behr's pupil: larger pupil seen on side of hemianopia.
  - Cheyne-Stokes pupil: associated with terminal respiratory pattern.
  - Hutchinson's pupil: seen in comatose patients.
  - Traumatic: sphincter tear causing mydriasis.
  - Wernicke's pupil: associated with optic tract disease.
- Testing for anisocoria: see Table 8–2 for pharmacologic testing for anisocoria.

COMPRESSIVE OPTIC NEUROPATHY Usually from tumor (especially glioma or meningioma), orbital mass, or myopathy. Often presents with progressive loss of vision, and usually disk pallor or atrophy, but can present with unilateral edema.

TABLE 8–2
Pharmacologic Testing for Anisocoria

Pupil Disorder	Drug Challenge	Normal Pupil	Abnormal Pupil
Adie's tonic pupil	Pilocarpine 0.05–0.1%	No reaction	Constricts
Pharmacologic	Pilocarpine 1%	Constricts	Fails to constrict
Horner's syndrome	Cocaine 4–10%	Dilates	Fails to dilate
Preganglionic	Paredrine 1%	Dilates	Dilates
Postganglionic	Paredrine 1%	Dilates	Fails to dilate

CONGENITAL DISK ELEVATION Hemangioma or congenital anomalous optic disk.

CONSTRICTED VISUAL FIELD Bilateral occipital lobe infarcts with macular sparing, RP, glaucoma, chronic papilledema, or functional.

DIPLOPIA, BINOCULAR Strabismus, prism in glasses.

DIPLOPIA, MONOCULAR Dry eye, astigmatism or refractive error, cataract, corneal scarring, blepharitis, polycoria, CME/ICSR/ERM, ARC following strabismus surgery (rare), palinopsia, cerebral polyopia (ischemic occipital lobe), psychogenic.

DISEASES INVOLVING THE ON DUSN, ARN, GCA, VKH, sarcoidosis, toxoplasmosis, CMV, syphilis, sympathetic ophthalmia, Wegener's granulomatosis, toxocariasis, papillophlebitis, AMPPE, Leber's neuroretinitis, scleritis, Behçet's syndrome, SLE, CRAO, papillitis, CRVO, and ischemic optic neuritis.

DYSKINESIS Congenitally misdirected nerve axons, as in Duane's syndrome and Marcus Gunn jaw winking. Differentiate from aberrant regeneration.

HEADACHE DIFFERENTIAL DIAGNOSIS

- Hypertension: usually seen in patients ages 40 to 50.
- Encephalgia: migraine usually with positive family history, seen in patients ages 20 to 30; may be classic "sick headaches" with aura, visual phenomenon, and nausea, or complicated with other neurologic signs, or may be acephalgic.
- Arteritis: GCA
- Definite headache syndromes: trigeminal neuralgia with sharp unilateral pain affecting CN $V_3 > $ CN $V_2 > $ CN V_1, lasting seconds, usually seen in older F > M patients; Gradenigo's syndrome with CN

V or CN VI pain from ear infection; postherpetic neuralgia; temporomandibular joint disease.

- Ocular etiology: asthenopia, uveitis, dry eye, optic neuritis, vascular
- Cervical spine: suboccipital headache
- "Head bone": intracranial tumors, subdural hematoma (SDH), aneurysm, hydrocephalus. Other intracranial causes of headache that should not be missed include:
    - Intracranial hemorrhage: severe headache, focal neurologic defect
    - Pituitary apoplexy, Sheehan's syndrome: postpartum pituitary infarction, hypocalcemia, acromegaly
    - Subarachnoid hemorrhage: worst headache patient has had, stiff neck, usually from trauma or aneurysm
    - Carotid artery dissection: may have Horner's syndrome plus ipsilateral headache; check MRA.
    - Meningitis: nucal rigidity, Lhermitte's sign, photophobia
- Ear, nose, and throat (ENT) causes: ear infection, frontal sinusitis (often has pain in the morning), maxillary sinusitis (often has pain in the evening)
- Psychogenic: consider last because it is a rule-out diagnosis; history of stress.

HETEROCHROMIC IRIDES Fuchs' HIC, long-standing uveitis, congenital Horner's syndrome (involved side is hypochromic) or neuroblastoma causing Horner's, leukemia, chronic IOFB, JXG, prostaglandin analogue drops, HZV, Waardenburg's syndrome, idiopathic.

LESION LOCALIZATION Ocular signs and symptoms from CNS lesions (stroke, tumor, trauma):

- Frontal lobe lesions: tonic eye deviation from involvement of frontal eye fields (controls saccades). Patient looks toward destructive lesions and away from an irritative (seizure) focus. Doll's eyes remain intact.
- Occipital lobe disease (i.e., posterior cerebral artery infarction): may manifest as quadrantic homonymous hemianopsia, macular sparing (if posterior pole of the occipital lobe is spared; usually has normal VA), monocular temporal crescent (if anterior pole is spared), checkerboard field, ipsilateral facial pain (V_1), or loss of high spatial frequency or contrast sensitivity; vision may be blurred despite 20/20, micropsia, macropsia, metamorphopsia, or unformed visual hallucinations. Cortical blindness after cardiac arrest is most often from watershed infarct of the occipital lobe tips.
- Occipitotemporal lesion, medial, bilateral: prosopagnosia (difficulty recognizing familiar faces)
- Parietal, dominant lobe (visual association areas, Brodmann's areas 18, 19; i.e., from left posterior cerebral artery infarction): alexia without

agraphia (reads but cannot write), visual agnosia (sees the image but without meaning), optic agnosia (cannot say name of identified object)
  - Gerstmann's syndrome: left-right confusion, finger agnosia, dysgraphia, dyscalculia.
- Parietal, nondominant lobe (visual association areas; i.e., from right posterior cerebral artery infarction): prosopagnosia, visual hemifield agnosia, hemineglect
- Parietal, bilateral (visual association areas; i.e., from left and right posterior cerebral artery infarction): cortical blindness, usually not simultaneous; pupil reflex is still present. Patients may also have achromatopsia, loss of stereopsis, and stepwise return of vision (motion perception returns first, then LP, color, central vision, then last visual association). Riddoch's phenomenon observed if patients are blind but able to perceive objects in motion.
  - Anton's syndrome: patients deny being blind.
  - Balint's syndrome: bilateral posterior parietal stroke causing pychic paralysis of gaze (ocular apraxia, unable to make voluntary eye movements but spontaneous movements intact), simultanagnosis (difficulty processing more than one thing), and optic ataxia (difficulty looking at more than one thing).
- Temporal lobe disease: formed visual hallucinations

LIGHT-NEAR DISSOCIATION Wernicke's syndrome, Argyll Robertson pupil, Parinaud's dorsal midbrain syndrome/posterior communicating artery (PCA) infarct pinealoma, and diabetes. Also caused by aberrant regeneration of CN III, Adie's tonic pupil, amyloidosis, Charcot-Marie-Tooth syndrome.

MACRODISKS (area $>$ 4.09 mm) Physiologic, congenital ON pit, morning glory anomaly, congenital glaucoma, high myopia

MICRODISKS (area $<$ 1.29 mm) Pseudopapilledema, ON drusen, nonarteritic AION, ON hypoplasia, high hyperopia

OPTIC DISK ATROPHY Trauma, compressive (mass, chronic hydrocephalus), advanced retinal diseases (e.g., RP, CRAO), postpapilledema, pseudotumor cerebri, genetic.

- Schnable's optic atrophy: optic nerve cupping with atrophy; pathology shows cavernous spaces in the anterior nerve, possibly containing vitreous or MPS; not caused by glaucoma. A description, not a functional term; makes good histopathology photos for examinations.

OPTIC DISK EDEMA Determine if the edema is papilledema (almost always bilateral), a unilateral swollen disk, or pseudopapilledema.

- Papilledema: passive optic disk swelling secondary to increased intracranial pressure (ICP); bilateral but may be asymmetric (and an atrophic nerve cannot swell). The first sign is loss of spontaneous venous pulsations (SVPs), along with swelling of the nasal disk, then "doughnut ring" disk swelling with preservation of the physiologic cup (unlike pseudopapilledema) and increased capillarity. MRI is 90% sensitive for the diagnosis. Visual field first shows increased blind spot, then nasal field defect (usually inferior), progressing to arcuate scotoma, then constricted fields and potentially NLP vision. Usually from trauma, idiopathic intracranial hypertension, mass effect (tumor, etc.), or meningitis. See also VINDICTIVES etiologies below.
    - Acute: flame hemorrhages, CWS, "pink" disk, dilated and tortuous vessels
    - Subacute: early disk paleness, resolving hemorrhages
    - Chronic: mildly elevated, pale, "champagne cork" appearance with Paton's lines ("high water" marks), poor vision, and tunnel visual field
- Pseudopapilledema: no CWS or hemorrhage, unlike papilledema, and disk has loss of physiologic cup with scalloped disk borders. Often used synonymously with ON drusen, but may also be associated with hyperopia, myelinated NFL, or tilted disk.
- Swollen disc: unilateral disk edema with or without vision loss; usually with enlarged blind spot secondary to elevated retina (hyperopic shift). Often from anterior optic neuritis, nonarteritic anterior ischemic optic neuropathy (NAION) or arteritic ION, papillophlebitis, compressive optic neuropathy, infiltrative, malignant hypertension, toxic reaction (oral contraceptives, vitamin A, ethambutol, etc.). Mnemonic describes other etiologies: VINDICTIVES: **v**ascular (CHF, dural sinus thrombosis), **i**diopathic/**i**atrogenic (radical neck dissection), **n**eoplasm (carcinomatous meningitis, leukemia), **d**rugs, **i**mmune response, **c**ongenital, **t**rauma, **i**nfection, **v**ascular, **e**ndocrine (eclampsia), **s**ystemic.

OPTIC DISK PALLOR Ischemic optic neuropathy after the acute phase, prior optic neuritis, infiltrative, compressive (TRIO, mengioma, etc.), carcinomatous, toxic response, nutritional, hereditary, radiation

ON ABNORMALITIES WITH SEROUS RD ON coloboma, morning glory anomaly, juxtapapillary staphyloma, ON pit

ON INFECTIONS Syphilis, *Bartonella*, tuberculosis, Lyme disease (papillitis occurs late in the course of the disease, with photophobia, pain)

ON INFILTRATIVE LESIONS Lymphoma, leukemia, malignant histiocytosis, plasmacytoma, sarcoidosis

OPTOCILIARY SHUNT VESSELS Meningioma, glioma, CRVO, ON drusen, fibrous dysplasia, glaucoma (leading cause), arachnoid cyst, idiopathic

PAINFUL HORNER'S SYNDROME Carotid artery dissection

PARADOXICAL PUPILS Congenital stationary night blindness (CSNB), achromatopsia, ON hypoplasia, Leber's congenital amaurosis, Best's disease, albinism, RP. Defined as immediate constriction within 20 seconds after room lights are turned off followed by slow dilation after 1 minute.

PULSATILE TINNITUS Arteriovenous malformation (AVM), aneurysm, pseudotumor cerebri (PTC).

SENSORY NYSTAGMUS WITH "NORMAL EXAM" CSNB, Leber's congenital amaurosis, achromatopsia

TEMPORALIZATION OF DISK VESSELS Situs inversus, albinism

VISION LOSS FROM ON DISEASE Pain is suggestive of inflammatory (intense pain) or compressive (dull pain) etiologies.

- Lasting only a few seconds: transient visual obscurations (TVO)
- Few minutes: amarousis fugax
- Fifteen to 45 minutes: migraine
- Sudden onset (seconds to minutes): occlusive vascular disease (embolic, thrombotic, or arteritic), vascular spastic (migraine)
- Insidious onset (hours to days): inflammatory (multiple sclerosis [MS])
- Gradual onset (weeks to years): compressive (neoplastic, aneurysm, structural)

Exam and Imaging

CALORIC VESTIBULAR TESTING Cold water causes nystagmus beating to the opposite side, and warm water causes ipsilateral beating nystagmus. Indicates the direction of the fast phase of nystagmus in an awake patient with an intact vestibular system. If abnormal, indicates a supranuclear lesion or that a comatose patient with tonic deviation usually has no nystagmus. Bilateral cold water gives fast-phase upward nystagmus.

COLOR VISION TESTING In general, patients with ON disease tend to have decreased red-green color vision (similar to protans and deutans), whereas patients with retinal disease (including the ganglion-cell dysfunction seen with glaucoma) tend to have blue-yellow color deficits (resembles tritans).

- Pseudoisochromatic plates (PIPs): different tests by various manufacturers; frequently used for quick color vision screening, but were designed for diagnosis of congenital defects (patients with acquired defects may not correctly identify the figures).
- Farnsworth-Munsell tests: use color chips mounted in caps. Patients with mildly defective color vision (anomalous trichromats) can pass.
  - D-15: patients asked to order the color hue caps beginning at the fixed blue reference cap.
    - Trichromats: patients arrange caps appropriately from 1 to 15.
    - Deutans: patients arrange colors as follows: 1, 15, 2, 3, 14, 13, 4, 12, 5, 11, 6, 7, 10, 9, and 8. Plotted on the score sheet, the axis of confusion for the deutan is shown to run parallel to the color wheel axis that runs through green and red-purple.
    - Protans: patients arrange hues in order as follows: 15, 1, 14, 2, 13, 12, 3, 4, 11, 10, 5, 9, 6, 8, and 7. On the score sheet, the protan's axis of confusion runs parallel to the red and blue-green axis.
  - FM-100: actually only 85 color chips in four boxes that if arranged in a circle would make a color wheel. Can classify patients with normal color vision as having superior (total error score 0–16, 16% of the population), average (error score 20–100, 68% incidence), or low (score >100, 16% of the population) color discrimination. In addition, it is probably the best test to measure the zones of color confusion for patients with either acquired or congenital color vision deficits.

NEUROLOGIC EXAM Full eye exam, with particular attention to:

- Visual function: BCVA distance and near, color plates, and VF (confrontation, perimetry)
  - May also test stereo vision, brightness, Amsler's grid (tests the central 20 degrees of the visual field), and Pulfrich's phenomen.
  - Photostress test: determine how long it takes the patient to read his or her best line of VA after 30 seconds of bright light exposure. Normal is <60 seconds even with ON disease. However, often >2 minutes is needed to recover with macular disease.
- Pupils
- Motility
- CN V and VII function
- Exophthalmometry
- External, anterior segment, and fundus

NEUROLOGIC HISTORY AND ASSESSMENT Neuro-ophthalmic disease evaluation can often be confusing and daunting; thus, be precise in your thinking, but be flexible. Try to identify one unifying diagnosis if there are several symptoms or signs. Look for patterns. If disease is nonorganic, attempt to prove that the patient has normal vision.

- Elicit chief complaint: a brief sentence summarizing the main problem, such as loss of vision or double vision (monocular or binocular).
- Determine past medical, surgical, ophthalmic, and neurologic histories (headache, migraines, stroke, etc.).
- Take social, family, medication, and allergy histories.
- Review tests: MRI, CT (with or without contrast), lumbar puncture, VEP, EEG.
- Review of systems (especially neurologic symptoms).
- Review the chief complaint, and elicit the history of the present illness, with a chronological history of the chief complaint and a history of any interventions.
- Localization: determine where the lesion is (afferent vs. efferent system) and its etiology.
    - Afferent system: retina, optic disk, optic nerve, chiasm, optic tracts, LGN, optic radiations, occipital lobe, visual association areas, and other supranuclear pathways
    - Efferent system: EOM (intrinsic or extrinsic), neuromuscular junction, cranial nerve, nerve fasicle, cranial nerve nucleus, and supranuclear pathways
- Pathophysiology: organize by diagnosis, then by therapeutics.

OPTIC NERVE EVALUATION Look at the color, contour, capillarity, complement of NFL and the size of the disk. On direct ophthalmoscopy, the smallest aperture in sharp focus is approximately the size of the normal adult ON.

OPTOKINETIC NYSTAGMUS (OKN) Requires at least 20/200 VA and tests pursuits and saccades. Abnormal if asymmetric response, usually from parietal lesions, nonorganic blindness, or homonymous hemianopsia. Reversal of OKN seen with congenital motor nystagmus.

VISUAL EVOKED RESPONSE (VER) Pattern VER can assess VA in preverbal children. False readings from accomodation.

VISUAL FIELD (VF) TESTING (Fig. 8–7) See also Chapter 4 for description of glaucomatous visual field defects.

- Cecocentral scotomas, nasal > temporal defects, and altitudinal defects: localize to the optic nerve.
- Temporal field defect attached to the blind spot: often ON hypoplasia, tilted disk (often superotemporal), or retinal vascular event.
- Monocular VF defects: prechiasmal lesions only, with the exception of an anterior occipital lobe infarct causing a monocular temporal crescent defect.

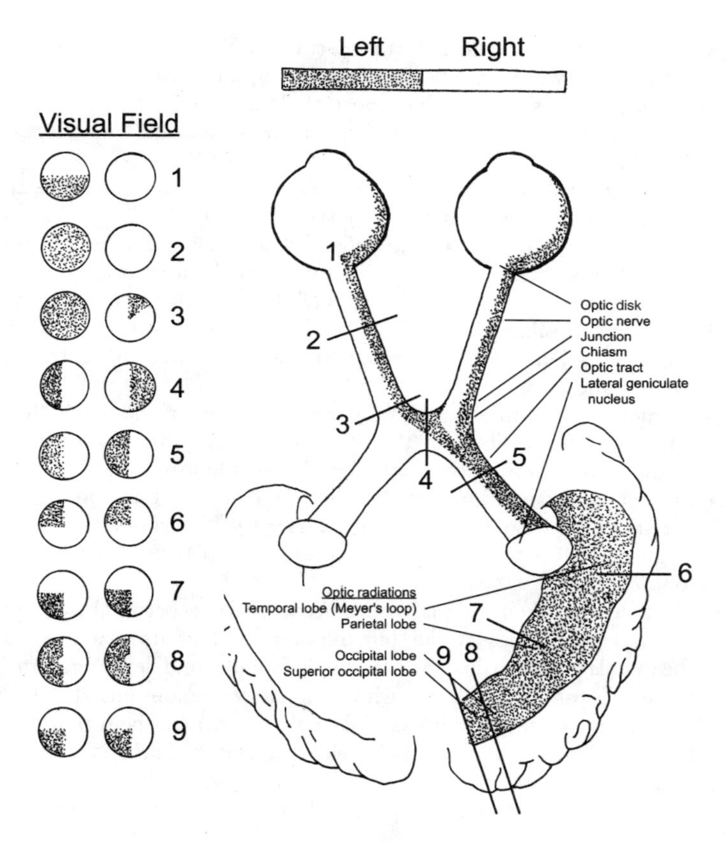

Figure 8–7 Schema, superior view, localizing visual field defects from lesions in the left anterior and right posterior visual pathways. 1, optic disk (e.g., AION); 2, optic nerve; 3, anterior chiasm (junctional scotoma); 4, chiasm; 5, optic tract; 6, temporal lobe optic radiations; 7, parietal lobe optic radiations; 8, occipital lobe; 9, superior posterior occipital lobe.

- Junctional scotoma (a central scotoma in one eye and a contralateral superotemporal VF defect): lesion in the anterior chiasm or optic nerve lesion just anterior to the chiasm involves one entire nerve plus the infranasal fibers (known as Wilbrand's "knee") from the opposite ON that briefly enter that nerve (many experts believe this is no longer anatomically accurate).
- Binasal defects: bilateral retinal or optic nerve lesions, or rarely from lateral compression of the chiasm.
- Bitemporal hemianopia: localizes to the optic chiasm (affects the crossing nasal fibers), usually from pituitary adenoma, meningioma, craniopharyngioma, aneurysm, trauma, or empty sella syndrome.

- Homonymous VF defects that respect the midline: lesions posterior to the chiasm. VF defects become more congruous with more posterior lesions; patients typically have normal VA.
  - Ninety percent of isolated homonymous hemianopias are caused by stroke.
  - Cogan's dictum (especially relevant prior to CT scanning): evaluate a homonymous hemianopsia with the OKN drum. If normal response, then visual field defect is likely from an occipital stroke; if OKN is abnormal, then be concerned about an occipital tumor (pressure forward on the parietal lobe causing the inaiblity to pursue ipsilaterally).
- Incongrous homonymous hemianopia with or without central scotoma: optic tract
- Homonymous superior quandrantanopia ("pie in the sky"): lesion affecting inferior fibers of the optic radiations in the temporal lobe as they sweep around the ventricles (Meyer's loop).
- Homonymous inferior quandrantanopia ("pie on the floor"): optic radiations in the parietal lobe (often have OKN asymmetry).
- Highly congruous homonymous quadrantanopia: posterior occipital lobe.
- Homonymous hemianopia with macular sparing: occipital lobe (posterior cerebral artery stroke, but the occipital lobe tip that represents the macula receives a dual vascular supply from the middle cerebral artery). Other VF patterns associated with occipital lobe lesions include bilateral homonymous altitudinal defects, bilateral homonymous hemianopia with bilateral macular sparing (keyhole field), checkerboard field, and temporal crescent.
- Monocular contralateral temporal defect: anterior occipital lobe

Congenital and Genetic Disease

BERGMEISTER'S PAPILLA Fibrous remnant of hyaloid system arising from the optic disk; may have patent blood vessel.

CHRONIC PROGRESSIVE EXTERNAL OPHTHALMOPLEGIA (CPEO) Generalized ophthalmoplegia and ptosis with no pupil abnormalities. See Chapter 2.

- Myotonic dystrophy: autosomal dominant disorder characterized by abnormal systemic muscle function, including CPEO; also associated with polychromatic lenticular deposits and frontal balding.
- Oculopharyngeal dystrophy: CPEO plus difficulty swallowing, usually seen in French-Canadians.
- Kearns-Sayre syndrome: CPEO with cardiac conduction defects, pigmentary retinopathy. Mitochondrial DNA defect with "ragged red fibers" seen on pathology.

MEGALOPAPILLA Disc size >2.1 mm; bilateral with increased cup:disk ratio, increased blind spot with normal VA.

MORNING GLORY ANOMALY Unilateral, sporadic, large excavated disk (central "coloboma") with a central core of glial tissue; retinal vessels exit from the borders of the defect, and disk is pigmented inferiorly. Defects involve the disk and retina, thus, may have retinal folds, and 30% of patients have RD. Associated with transphenoidal basal encephalocele (look at the hard palate).

MYELINATED NFL Ganglion cell axon myelination from oligodendrites proceeds from the LGN toward the disk; usually stops at the lamina cribosa, but may extend onto the retina as white, feathery radiating fibers. Usually asymptomatic, but if large, may cause VF defect and in the macula may cause decreased VA.

ON ATROPHY Often acquired but may be genetic; also, may be either primary or secondary (genetic causes: Kjer's, Behr's, and Leber's atrophies). Primary or secondary genetic ON atrophy causes usually present with bilateral ON pallor with arteriolar attenuation; most have normal ERG (exception is recessive optic atrophy with cone dystrophy).

- Kjer's dominant optic atrophy, juvenile optic atrophy: insidious onset of moderately decreased VA (20/20–200) seen in preschool children. Typically has temporal disk pallor, temporal peripheral retinal changes (may have a pseudobitemporal hemianopsia), acquired tritan anomaly (blue-yellow color defects as with glaucoma), and no nystagmus. VF shows a cecocentral scotoma or enlarged blind spot. Examine the patient's parents. Atrophy is autosomal dominant with high penetrance and variable expressivity disorder of the ganglion cell. Usually from chromosome 3 defect in the OPA1 gene that interacts with mitochondrial DNA (possibly similar mechanism to Leber's atrophy).
- Behr's recessive congential optic atrophy: rare autosomal recessive disorder with severe vision loss and normal ERG. Technically, only called Behr's if optic atrophy is associated with mental retardation, cerebella ataxia, hypertonia, and spasticity.
- Leber's optic atrophy: progressive optic atrophy seen in young males with decreased VA, often to 20/200 (but patient will usually not go blind). The fellow eye is involved within 3 months. Exam shows triad of circumpapillary telangiectasias, pseudopapilledema (disk edema), with absence of fluorescein disk staining. The acute phase is characterized by the hyperemic disk with tortuous telangiectatic vessels that do not leak on FA; rapidly progresses to late phase with a pale disk. VF shows central or cecocentral scotoma. Typically, only mild APD is present (pupillovisual dissociation with selective sparing of pupillary control axons, and vision loss is often symmetric).

- Maternal mitochondrial DNA (mDNA) inheritance: all children carry the gene, but not all have the disease; males are far more commonly affected than females. Most common defect is the Wallace 11778 gene that codes for subunit 4 of NADH dehydrogenase. Also 14484 gene defect is found in 11% of cases, which carries a better visual prognosis.
- Diagnose by finding mDNA defect in leukocytes. Usually MRI is normal OU. May be associated with heart conduction abnormalities and skeletal muscle disease (findings similar to CPEO).
- No proven treatment. Genetic counseling is important; encourage patients if appropriate to stop smoking and drinking alcohol (which may cause "mitochondrial strain" and increase penetrance).

- Secondary optic atrophy in childhood: metabolic diseases, compressive lesions (bony lesions, craniopharyngioma, ON glioma, hydrocephalus), advanced retinal disease (e.g., RP), and neonatal anoxia
  - Metabolic diseases: gangliosidoses, MPS, adrenoleukodystrophy (pigmentary retinopathy), spinocerebellar ataxia, Friedreich's ataxia, and the following:
    - Wolfram syndrome: DIDMOAD (**di**abetes **i**nsipitus, **d**iabetes **m**ellitus, **o**ptic **a**trophy, **d**eafness); autosomal recessive disorder. Ask about bedwetting from diabetes insipitus; ocular findings and deafness occur in childhood after diabetes diagnosis.
    - Charcot-Marie-Tooth atrophy: sensorineural polyneuropathy that may be autosomal dominant or recessive with late childhood peroneal muscle atrophy, slowly progressive motor neuropathy of legs hands, with deafness and optic atrophy.
  - Bone disease with ON compression: Albright's syndrome, osteopetrosis (anemia, calcium imbalance; patients usually need bone marrow transplant), and the craniosynostoses (Cruzon's, Apert's, Carpenter's).

ON COLOBOMA Failure of fetal fissure and stalk closure with disk excavation, usually inferonasal with no central glial tuft (unlike morning glory anomaly). Usually sporadic inheritance; may be unilateral or bilateral; may have other colobomas that can involve the macula with poor VA or have associated RD.

- Aicardi's syndrome: X-linked dominant (lethal in males) disorder with coloboma of the optic nerve and optic atrophy, peripapillary chorioretinal lacunae; associated with corpus callosum agenesis, infantile spasms, and mental retardation.
- CHARGE association: **c**olobomas, **h**eart defect, **a**tresia choanae, **r**etarded growth, **g**enital anomalies, **e**ar anomalies and deafness
- Systemic associations: Warburg's syndrome, Gorlin-Goltz focal dermal hypoplasia (clefts, syndactyl, coloboma, pigmented linear skin

streaks, X-linked), Meckel-Gruber syndrome, Lenz microphthalmia syndrome (X-linked), renal-coloboma syndrome (autosomal dominant PAX 2 mutation).

ON DRUSEN Calcific deposits within the optic nerve, most commonly seen in the inferior disk. Usually asymptomatic and benign, but 75% of patients with visible drusen have a VF defect. May cause pseudopapilledema, optociliary shunt vessels, AION, and TVO. Clinical diagnosis; may confirm with ultrasound, autofluorescence, or CT. Two percent incidence, often familial, autosomal dominant variable penetrance, usually seen in Caucasian patients. Associated with history of migraine headaches.

OPTIC NERVE HYPOPLASIA (ONH) Small 0.3–0.5 mm disk, with anomalous vessel pattern and double-ring sign (see the round edge of the disk and also the scleral ring, which it does not quite fill). May have profound vision loss, amblyopia, nystagmus, and APD. Is the most common congenital disk anomaly with sporadic inheritance; may be unilateral or bilateral. Thirteen percent of patients have anterior pituitary and CNS developmental anomalies.

- Associated with maternal diabetes (classically superior sectoral ONH) or ingestion of phenytoin/LSD/alcohol/quinine. Also aniridia (may have ON or foveal hypoplasia) or CHARGE association.
- De Morsier's syndrome (septo-optic dysplasia): ONH, midline CNS anomalies (pituitary dysfunction), absence of septum pellucidum. Often presents with growth retardation.

ON PIT Unilateral, inferotemporal small disk excavation that is round or oval, white or yellow. May be considered a minimal coloboma. Forty-five percent of patients have macular serous RD usually in second or third decade (probably has a CSF-vitreous connection). If acquired, associated with NTG.

TILTED DISK Bilateral, nonhereditary, long-axis oblique insertion of the ON showing an optic disk that does not look round. May have VF defect or Fuchs' coloboma (inferior crescent, may have bitemporal visual field defects that do not respect midline, myopic astigmatism with plus axis parallel to the axis of ectasia).

Infectious Disease

BARTONELLA HENSELAE, CAT-SCRATCH DISEASE Causes a neuroretinitis (papillitis plus a macular star); typically has good recovery, but often neuropathy or macular RPE changes persist. May not have known cat bite or scratch. *Bartonella* infection may also cause Parinaud's oculoglandular syndrome, uveitis, branch retinal artery occlusion (BRAO), CRVO, or focal retinochoroiditis. Confirm diagnosis with serum indirect fluorescence Ab. Consider treatment with oral ciprofloxacin, rifampin (89% success), or Septra (58% success) for 6 weeks.

Neoplastic Disease

CARCINOMATOUS OPTIC NEUROPATHY Acute devastating decreased VA from infiltrative malignancy (usually lymphoma or leukemia), often with normal fundus and imaging. Diagnose with lumbar puncture.

CNS ASTROCYTOMA Classified as grade I, II, III (anaplastic astrocytomas), or IV (glioblastoma multiforme characterized by necrosis and very poor life prognosis). Rarely may arise from the optic nerve astrocytes; more commonly, CNS tumor causes mass effect that may cause papilledema. Patients may need palliative ON sheath decompression to preserve visual function.

CRANIOPHARYNGIOMA (SUPRASELLAR) Arises from remnants of Rathke's pouch near the pituitary and often compresses the chiasm, causing a bitemporal hemianopsia; often calcified; almost always occurs in childhood.

FOSTER KENNEDY SYNDROME Frontal lobe tumor causes one pale disk (direct pressure on optic nerve) and one swollen disk (increased ICP). Clinical appearance may be similar to bilateral nonsimultaneous AION.

MELANOCYTOMA Darkly pigmented magnocellular nevus that is benign. See Chapter 7.

NEUROFIBROMA Endoneural fibroma that arises from nerve fibers.

ON GLIOMA Occurence in childhood has a good prognosis and is considered a hamartoma; 50% of patients with ON gliomas have NF1 (15% of NF1 patients have ON glioma). Arising in adulthood, it has a poor prognosis and usually is glioblastoma multiforme. See Chapter 2.

ON SHEATH MENINGIOMA Tumor that arises from the ON meningeal sheath, causing progressive optic atrophy and loss of vision with optociliary shunt vessels. Good prognosis in adults, poor prognosis in children. "Railroad track" sign on CT. Pathology shows proliferation of benign meningiothelial cells in whorls with calcified psammoma bodies. Treatment is controversial. See Chapter 2.

SCHWANNOMA Neurilemmal (nerve sheath) tumor arising in cranial peripheral nerve (usually superior location in the orbit).

Metabolic and Degenerative Disease

ALZHEIMER'S DISEASE Better VA is associated with decreased hallucinations, and visual function is strongly related to cognitive function. Thus, give patients a good refraction, and do cataract surgery if appropriate.

- Visual variant of Alzheimer's disease (VVAD): slowly progressive reading difficulty with a Balint-like picture.

NUTRITIONAL, TOBACCO, OR ALCOHOL OPTIC NEUROPATHY Optic nerve degeneration may be seen with alcohol, drug or tobacco abuse, poor nutrition, or malabsorption syndrome. VF shows bilateral cecocentral scotomas or "biscuit cut" VF. Also check for pernicious anemia.

- Coffee and doughnut maculopathy: inner retinal layer defect with ring scotoma, good VA. Variant of macular neuroretinopathy.

Systemic and Vascular Disease

ARTERITIC ISCHEMIC OPTIC NEUROPATHY, GIANT CELL OR TEMPORAL ARTERITIS Inflammatory infiltration of medium-size arteries by lymphocytes, monocytes, or giant cells, causing closure of the artery and resulting in ischemic optic neuropathy or retinal infarction and potentially blindness. If arteritis causes AION, patients may present with a swollen disk with focal arteriolar narrowing at the rim and altitudinal VF loss. Also consider the diagnosis in patients with PION, CRAO, choroidal infarction (FA shows a vertical watershed zone through the disk, delineating choroidal vasculature), ocular ischemic syndrome, cranial nerve ischemia, or muscle ischemia causing diplopia.

- Clinical diagnosis; thus, treat patients if there is a high index of suspicion. Consider the diagnosis in anyone with transient visual loss over age 55, catastrophic vision loss especially if patients have constitutional symptoms such as polymyalgia rheumatica (PMR), jaw claudication (pain with chewing; do not confuse with temporomandibular joint pain, which is worse at rest and usually seen in younger females with bruxism and stress), fever, or unexplained weight loss.
- Diagnostic tests: usually increased Westergren sedimentation rate (usually > 50) and C-reactive protein (higher sensitivity than ESR) and often positive TAB, which may be positive even on steroids up to 6 months.

- Normal sedimentation rate for men is less than their age divided by 2; for women, their age plus 10 divided by 2.
- Temporal artery biopsy is 100% specific, 85 to 91% sensitive. If the first temporal artery biopsy is negative, then only 3 to 5% will be positive with second biopsy. One clinical scoring method recommends doing a temporal artery biopsy if 6 points are present: 2 points for age >65, headache, ION, jaw claudication, scalp tenderness, or diabetes; and 1 point for fever, weight loss, or muscle weakness.

- Treat with prompt intravenous steroids for 5 days with 10-day taper, then long-term oral steroids to keep ESR <20. Fellow eye becomes involved in one third of cases (75% if untreated).

CAROTID ARTERY DISSECTION Fifty-two percent of cases have eye findings, usually painful Horner's syndrome (44%) or transient visual loss (28%); needs prompt investigation.

CEREBROVASCULAR ACCIDENT (CVA) Thrombotic (far more common) or embolic vascular disease that leads to ischemic (far more common) or hemorrhagic stroke. See Lesion Localization under Signs and Symptoms.

DURAL SINUS THROMBOSIS Decreased CNS venous outflow causes increased intracranial pressure and possibly papilledema that mimics pseudotumor cerebri (PTC). Diagnose with MRI (delta sign from enhanced sinus wall) plus magnetic resonance venography (MRV) (54% have normal CT). Treat with steroids, and rule out hypercoagulable state.

MALIGNANT HYPERTENSION May cause bilateral ON swelling and exudatve RD. See Chapter 7.

MIGRAINE HEADACHE Classic if it has preceding aura, often with scintillating scotoma associated with throbbing headache. Complex migraine if accompanied by neurologic deficits or TIA. Purely ocular variant has scotomata without headache. All cases carry a 3.5 times increased risk of ischemic stroke (same incidence whether simple or classic migraine). Twenty-eight percent of NTG patients have migraines, possible common vascular etiology.

NONARTERITIC ANTERIOR ISCHEMIC OPTIC NEUROPATHY (NAION) Unilateral, painless, swollen disk with VA ranging from 20/20 to NLP, altitudinal VF loss, and presence of APD; on exam, disk shows sectoral edema ("proud flesh" appearance) and focal arteriolar narrowing at the rim. Usually from atherosclerotic plaque occlusion of a posterior ciliary artery; often occurs upon awakening in the morning. Age >50 years old; occurs in the fellow eye in 15 to 40% of cases. Normal VEP and MRI, and FA shows delayed disk filling. May have pseudo–Foster Kennedy syndrome, with one pale disk from old AION and the other disk swollen with acute AION.

- Risk factors: hypertension, hyperlipidemia, disk at risk (small C:D, tighter aperture for vessels to traverse), nocturnal hypotension (also is risk for NTG and POAG). Also consider hypercoagulable state if no vasculopathic history, and rule out hyperhomocystinemia or antiphospholipid Ab (lupus anticoagulant, anticardiolipin Ab).
- Rule out arteritic causes/GCA as appropriate for the patient. Treat with aspirin (protective). NAION is not predictive of coronary artery or carotid disease, stroke, or myocardial infarction. Vision may improve up to 2 years or remain unchanged. L-dopa is not effective.
  - Ischemic Optic Neuropathy Decompression Trial (IONDT): a multicenter, randomized controlled trial (1992–1994), which showed that optic nerve sheath decompression (ONSD) is not effective for NAION. Patients stratified into observation versus surgical groups. Forty percent of observation patients improved versus one third of surgery patients; thus, study terminated early. ONSD patients had higher risk of losing three or more lines of VA (24% surgery vs. 12% of patients that were observed).

PAPILLOPHLEBITIS Unilateral ON swelling with good VA. May be early CRVO, usually in young patients; typically resolves.

POSTERIOR ISCHEMIC OPTIC NEUROPATHY (PION) Similar to AION, but because it occurs more posteriorly in the nerve, no disk swelling or other nerve abnormalities are seen. Work-up similar to AION.

VERTEBRAL BASILAR INSUFFICIENCY (VBI) Basilar artery disease causes brainstem ischemia and may manifest with imbalance, emesis, ataxia, and skew deviation. Check brainstem magnetic resonance angiography (MRA).

Physical Disease

RADIATION OPTIC NEUROPATHY Causes necrosis of the ON and chiasm, usually within 9 to 12 months of treatment (but may be up to 20 years).

TOXIC OPTIC NEURITIS OR NEUROPATHY Usually central scotoma because central small ON fibers from the macula depend on central retinal artery for their blood supply, in contrast to the larger peripheral nerve fibers, which rely more on diffusion from the CSF. Thus, small ON fibers benefit from the blood–brain barrier and are spared until later from toxic/metabolic stress.

- Ethambutol: dose related and reversible. Diagnose by VER; related to zinc chelation.

- Methanol: contaminant of ethanol and its breakdown product, formic acid, is toxic to retinal ganglion cells and the NFL. Usually causes blurred or decreased VA within 18 hours of ingestion with systemic acidosis, early ON hyperemia and retinal edema, and late optic atrophy. VA either recovers within 6 days or is usually lost permanently. Treat with ethyl alcohol and hemodialysis.
- Amiodarone: associated with ischemic optic neuropathy (chemical structure is similar to chloroquine).

TRAUMATIC OPTIC NEUROPATHY (TON) Always consider as cause of vision loss in head trauma patients until proven otherwise. Patients usually have no ophthalmoscopic signs, but have immediate decreased VA with positive APD and dyschromatopsia.

- Mechanism: usually trauma causes indirect injury to the posterior nerve.
  - Direct: rare; from impact of penetrating orbital object compression from ON sheath hemorrhage with CRAO or CRVO, impingement by foreign body, or shearing of nerve fibers.
  - Indirect, anterior: rare; usually from sudden traumatic rotation of the globe (may have CRAO or avulsion of ON head).
  - Indirect, posterior: most common mechanism; typically caused by a blow to the forehead or midface, with force trasmitted posterior along the ON, where it is tethered at the orbital apex and in the optic canal, causing contusion of nerve or shearing of short penetrating blood vessels from deceleration forces. In children, the leading cause is bike accidents (often from not wearing a helmet; most have no loss of consciousness).
- Clinical diagnosis when other causes of vision loss have been ruled out. CT is usually unremarkable, but rule out optic canal fracture with 1 mm cuts through the canal (canal fracture is not prognostic and may be protective by decompressing closed space).
- Treatment: controversial whether to treat or not. Fifteen to 33% of patients improve spontaneously with observation alone; however, steroids may help as an antioxidant effect and to maintain perfusion. Steroids usually given 30 mg/kg load, then 5.4 mg/kg/hour IV infusion for 24 hours or 15 mg/kg every 6 hours for 72 hours. Rarely canal decompression is needed.
  - International Optic Neuropathy Trauma Study (multicenter, nonrandomized comparative interventional study with concurrent treatment groups) concluded that there is no standard of care and that patients should be treated on an individual basis. Study patients were stratified to receive megadose steroids or steroids plus optic canal decompression. The trial was stopped due to small numbers and turned into a case series. Of the 127 patients with TON, 9 received no treatment, 85 received steroids, and 33 had surgery. Trends showed that the timing of treatment made no

difference in outcomes (1 month was similar to 3 months) and that steroid dose made no difference. The VA increased by three lines in one third of surgery patients, half of steroid-treated patients, and half of untreated patients.
  - National Acute Spinal Cord Injury Study (NASCIS), a double-blind randomized clinical trial, found that early high-dose steroids may be neuroprotective for spinal cord lesions. Whether this data apply to optic nerve trauma is unknown, but many clinicians treat TON with high-dose steroids if VA is LP or worse.

TRAUMATIC OPTIC NERVE EVULSION OR TRANSECTION Usually from countrecoup injury; even with apparently minor trauma, the nerve is easy to tear, as CNS tissue has the consistency of warm butter. Characterized by immediate NLP with variable hemorrhage over disk and CRAO-like presentation. May not see avulsion on CT with an intact ON sheath. If not directly transected by trauma, evulsion may be aided by increased IOP that "pushes" ON out of scleral canal or increased intraorbital pressure pushes globe anteriorly, stretching the nerve. If transected posterior in the orbit, the patient may have intact retinal circulation.

Inflammatory and Immune Disease

ANTERIOR OPTIC NEURITIS Monocular vision loss of insidious onset (nadir 7 to 10 days) with gradual recovery in 80% of cases. Typically, patients have pain with eye movement (90% of subjects in Optic Neuritis Treatment Trial [ONTT]—see below; caused by the dural attachment of the SR and MR to the ON sheath), decreased VA (especially contrast and color vision from the PMB fibers), and APD, with or without disk edema (30% of ONTT subjects). Symptoms may increase with increased body temperature or exercise (Uhthoff's sign). Usual age is <50 years old; in adults, is often from multiple sclerosis (60% of optic neuritis progesses to MS), and in children, is usually postviral. FA is normal, and periventricular plaques may be seen on MRI if patient has MS.

- Atypical presentation: painless or sign or symptoms of systemic disease or inflammation such as vitritis, then consider sarcoidosis, syphilis, Lyme disease, bartonellosis, vasculitis, or toxoplasmosis. If patient is not getting better, suspect compressive lesion (e.g., ON sheath meningioma), Leber's optic atrophy, or ischemic etiology.
- Treatment: for acute disease, based on the ONTT, consider treatment with IV methylprednisolone 1000 mg qd (250 mg every 6 hours) for 3 days followed by oral prednisone taper 1 mg/kg for 11 days. (Because oral prednisone is 85% absorbed, the oral equivalent for initial treatment is 1200 mg divided qid.) In children, dose 2 mg/kg IV with slow taper.

- Optic Neuritis Treatment Trial (ONTT) and Longitudinal Optic Neuritis Study (LONS): multicenter study with three treatment groups (intravenous methylprednisolone 250 mg every 6 hours for 3 days, followed by oral prednisone for 11 days, oral prednisone 1 mg/kg/day for 14 days, or oral placebo for 14 days) for acute unilateral optic neuritis presumably secondary to demyelinating disease (seen mostly in young female patients without a diagnosis of MS).
    - Visual recovery begins within 2 weeks in most optic neuritis patients without any treatment, and improvement continues for up to 1 year. Although most patients recover to 20/20 VA, many still have symptomatic deficits in vision.
    - Oral prednisone was ineffective in speeding recovery or in improving the visual outcome after optic neuritis, and actually increased a patient's risk for future attacks in either the affected or fellow eye (27% vs. 15% for placebo patients).
    - Treatment with high-dose, intravenous corticosteroids followed by oral corticosteroids accelerated visual recovery but provided no long-term benefit to vision. The IV steroids also provided a short-term reduction in the rate of development of MS, particularly in patients with brain MRI changes consistent with demyelination. By 3 years of follow-up, however, this treatment effect had subsided.
    - Brain MRI is a powerful predictor of the early risk of MS after optic neuritis (especially if it shows >2 demyelinating lesions).
    - In optic neuritis patients with no brain MRI lesions, the following features of the optic neuritis are associated with a low 5-year risk of MS: lack of pain, optic disk edema (particularly if severe), peripapillary hemorrhage, retinal exudates, and mild visual loss.
    - The probability of a recurrence of optic neuritis in either eye within 5 years is 28%.
- Controlled High-Risk Avonex Multiple Sclerosis Prevention Study (CHAMPS): INF-beta-1-alpha (Avonex) is protective for MS and decreases MS severity with a rapid sustained effect if two or more T2-weighted MRI lesions >3 mm are present. Thus, image patients after their first episode of optic neuritis to rule out MS.

EATON-LAMBERT SYNDROME Autoimmune disease of the neuromuscular junction similar to myasthenia gravis, with muscle weakness and fatigue; less likely to be ocular than MG.

GUILLAIN-BARRÉ SYNDROME Ascending paralysis of the peripheral nervous system, often with antecedent viral illness. Patients may need ventilator support for several months until it resolves.

- Miller Fisher syndrome: bulbar variant. "Guillain-Barré of the head and neck," with ophthalmoplegia and descending paralysis; also has CSF dissociation.
- Acute ophthalmoparesis (AO): forme fruste of Guillain-Barré, affecting only the EOM; positive anti-GQ1B Ab against peripheral nerves.

MULTIPLE SCLEROSIS (MS), CLINICALLY DEFINITE MULTIPLE SCLEROSIS (CDMS) Autoimmune demyelinating disease that presents with optic neuritis in 18%, intranuclear ophthalmoplegia (INO) and horizontal diplopia, nystagmus (oscillopia), and atypical VF (inferior altitudinal, arcuate, cecocentral, or basically any VF defect). Also ask about fatigue, paresthesias, paresis, incontinence, and electric sensation down neck/arms with neck flexion (Lhermitte's sign). Uncommon presentations include chiasmal neuritis with bitemporal hemianopsia (aggressive chiasmitis), CN III, IV, and VI nuclear dysfunction, skew deviation (supranuclear vertical gaze dysfunction), and intermediate uveitis. See Anterior Optic Neuritis above for evaluation and management.

- Immunologic disease: chronic inflammatory demyelinating. Characterized by T-cell activation from myelin breakdown (possible viral beginning). T-cells are then exposed to an antigen that seems "foreign" or through molecular mimicry learns to attack the myelin sheath and migrate into the CNS. As T cells attack the myelinated axons, other antigens are uncovered (epitope spread). At some point, suppressor T cells take over, and the acute episode remits.
- Risks for developing MS: genetic history, young, female, northern latitude (Caucasian, Scandinavian), and increased socioeconomic status
- Two courses and etiologies: primary progressive (15%) and relapsing–remitting (85%), which may progress to secondary or chronic progressive (after 10 years, 40–45% are secondary-progressive). Treatment is aimed to decrease the rate that patients go on to secondary or chronic disease. The progressive form represents actual axonal loss, whereas the relapsing–remitting form is demyelinating attacks.
- Causes of decreased VA that are more prevalent in MS patients: optic neuritis, intermediate uveitis with CME, chiasmitis (transverse myelitis, also known as Devic's syndrome), optic tract plaques, and iritis.
- Diagnosis with clinical findings plus lumbar puncture (increased IgG/oligoclonal Ab) and MRI. MRI often shows white matter demyelinating plaques (especially periventricular, also known as Dawson's fingers) that reach maximum size at 4 weeks after relapse; enhancing lesion in the corpus callosum is pathognomonic.
- Treatment for relapsing–remitting disease: "ABC" drugs reduce the number of attacks, and many clinicians suggest that all three drugs work well as first-line therapy.
  - **A**vonex (interferon beta-1-alpha): per CHAMPS study, was effective in delaying the onset of the next attack.

  - **B**etaserone (interferon beta-1-beta)
  - **C**opaxone (copolymer glatiramer acetate): improves disability and cognition.
- Treatment for progressive MS: treat early to decrease disability and long-term axonal injury sequelae.
  - Mitoxantrone: myelin basic protein that is a chemotherapy drug, like Adriamycin, that may cause a dose-dependent vacuolar cardiomyopathy. Two-year maximum use recommended, or use occasionally as a rescue drug; turns patient blue after injection. MIMS (Mitoxantrone in Multiple Sclerosis) study showed that it increased T-suppressor cells.
  - May also try IV steroids and adrenocorticotropic hormone (ACTH).

MYASTHENIA GRAVIS (MG) Chronic autoimmune neuromuscular junction disorder with weakness and fatigability. Characterized by variable weakness of voluntary muscles, often EOM and limb muscles, which is made worse by use and improves with rest. Eighty to 90% of patients present with ocular findings: primary sign is ptosis (present in 75% of patients with ocular involvement) that may be unilateral or bilateral and worsens with fatigue. Ptotic lid may twitch when patient looks from down to up (Cogan's lid twitch), or the opposite lid droops when the ptotic lid is raised (Schatz lid sign; like Herring's effect). The second most common is strabismus (although diplopia is the main reported symptom), affecting MR > IR > SO; may have paresis of upgaze and an apparent INO. Eye movements are characterized by hypometric (lazy) large saccades and hypermetric small saccades (supernormal saccadic velocities). Also fatigable ophthalmoplegia, uncommonly nystagmus (weak muscles not central origin), orbicularis weakness, peak sign (lids do not close completely). Pupillary and accommodation problems reported but uncommon (for examinations, the pupils are not involved); also, risk of thymic hyperplasia or thymoma.

- Pathogenesis: acquired "autoimmune" antibodies to motor end plates (thus decreased available acetylcholine receptors) and impaired synaptic transmission. Considered neuromuscular junction pathology, not cranial nerve palsy. Acetylcholine receptor usually regenerates every 7 to 10 days, but in MG is 1 day. Similar to Eaton-Lambert syndrome. Patients have increased risk of other autoimmune diseases, such as SLE, RA, and hyperthyroidism.
- May be infantile, juvenile, or adult onset. F:M = 3:2. Average female age of onset is 28 years old; average male onset is 43 years old. Fifty percent of patients have purely ocular MG, and 10% of cases remit spontaneously, usually after 1 year. Of the 40% that remain an ocular disease, 50% will develop generalized symptoms usually within 2 years. If a patient has purely ocular MG >2 years, there is <20% chance of

systemic involvement. Ocular variant has decreased Ab titers and decreased thymoma incidence compared with systemic MG.

- Diagnosis: clinical presentation, proving fatigability and the fleeting, varied, and recurrent presentation.
  - Tensilon (edrophonium chloride) testing: must have objective measure (e.g., millimeters of ptosis) to compare before and after the IV injection of Tensilon. Drug inhibits acetylcholinesterase, thus prolonging the effect of acetylcholine at the synaptic cleft. It has an onset within 60 seconds and lasts about 10 minutes. In children, use neostigmine IM (30 minute duration). Consider monitoring cardiac function during testing; because the drug stimulates muscarinic and nicotinic receptors, it may cause a cholinergic crisis (sweating, nausea, vomiting, salivation, fever). Have atropine available to reverse its effects.
  - Also may use ice testing on the ptotic lid for 2 minutes, which suggests the diagnosis of MG if at least 2 mm of lid improvement is seen (may also be false-positive as a result of the lid resting).
  - Check acetylcholine Ab, which is present in 60% of MG patients, and schedule thyroid function tests, as dysthyroidism is more common. Obtain a chest CT to rule out thymoma (potentially fatal). Also, single-fiber electromyography of the orbicularis muscle may be used for diagnosis.
- Treatment: usually treated by neurologist, using pyridostigmine bromide (Mestinon) or neostigmine (Prostigmin) or chronic immunosuppression. Too much Mestinon floods receptors and may potentiate MG. Ninety-six percent of cases improve with cyclosporine. Consider thymectomy.

PERINEURITIS Disk edema from inflammation of the nerve sheath, with normal imaging and lumbar puncture; usually from sarcoidosis, syphilis, or *Bartonella henselae*.

PSEUDOTUMOR CEREBRI (PTC), IDIOPATHIC INTRACRANIAL HYPERTENSION Usually seen in young, 20- to 40-year-old, obese females who present with headache and papilledema. Vision disturbances include TVO, VF defects, postural bilateral amaurosis fugax, and horizontal diplopia (CN VI palsy). Also, most patients complain of tinnitus.

- Diagnosis of exclusion: must do neuroimaging that shows no mass or dural sinus thrombosis. MRI is 90% predictive of PTC (however, up to 20% have "empty sella," 80% have flattening of the posterior sclera). Lumbar puncture shows increased opening pressure (>20 cm H_20) but otherwise normal CSF studies.
- Fifty percent are idiopathic and 50% are associated with known causes. Pathogenesis is likely hormonal imbalance, as PTC is associated with females, obesity, and exacerbated by pregnancy. May be precipitated by

steroids, vitamin A, tetracycline, nalidixic acid (including ciprofloxacin), venous sinus thrombosis, endocrine abnormalities, Lyme disease, and SLE.

- Treatment: 73% improve with Diamox or other carbonic anhydrase inhibitors and at least a 7% or greater decrease in body weight. Lumboperitoneal shunt may be offered if headache is most prominent symptom; also treats the papilledema in both eyes but has a high failure rate. ONSD may be offered if progressive vision loss is present; ONSD stabilizes or improves VA in 94% of patients, but because it is a unilateral surgery, it does not often help the other eye and will not help headache symptoms. Lasix and steroids are less effective.

Selected Cranial Nerve Abnormalities

CN III PALSY Presents with ptosis, limitation of EOM (SR, MR, IR, IO), with a down and out globe position; may have contralateral lid retraction from overstimulation in trying to lift the ptotic ipsilateral lid, and may have mydriasis. First part of clinical evaluation is to determine if the pupil is involved. The parasympathetic pupillomotor fibers are on the outside of CN III and are thus the first to be injured with compressive lesions (e.g., aneurysm). However, nerve ischemia is by far the most common cause (usually in diabetic patients; 50% have pain), and the central fibers are preferentially affected; thus, <20% of cases involve the pupil.

- Aberrant regeneration: usually occurs after compression (trauma/tumor) as axons are misdirected during repair phase, seen as lid retraction in downgaze (pseudo-Graefe's sign) or abnormal pupillary constriction with adduction (Czarnecki's pupil).
- Work-up: if isolated pupil sparing is observed and patient is >40 years old or there is a history of diabetes, hypertension, or migraine, then can observe patient. If the pupil does not become involved and no other neurologic signs and symptoms develop, then no work-up is necessary and recovery can be expected in about 3 months in most cases. Otherwise, image and consider angiogram.
- Etiology by age: child (trauma, tumor), young adult (aneurysm, demyelinating disease), older adult (ischemia, tumor). Myasthenia may mimic CN III palsy.
- Etiology by location:
  - Nucleus: rare lesions of nucleus, but may be caused by stroke, demyelinating disease, or tumor.
    - Cyclic oculomotor palsy: underlying CN III palsy with intermittent return of function about every 24 hours.
    - Ophthalmoplegic migraine: eye pain, nausea, vomiting, and syncope preceding ophthalmoplegia; usually seen in children with a family history of migraines. Controversial whether it needs angiography.

- Fasciculus syndromes: usually vascular cause.
  - Benedikt's syndrome: ipsilateral III palsy with contralateral decreased sensation and arm tremor or weakness (red nucleus involvement; "nervous traitor").
  - Weber's syndrome: ipsilateral III palsy with contralateral spastic arm and leg hemiparesis (ipsilateral superior cerebellar peduncle involvement).
  - Nothnagel's syndrome: lesions involve the brachyconjunctivum and superior cerebellar peduncle, causing CN III palsy with ipsilateral cerebellar ataxia.
  - Claude's syndrome: Nothnagel's plus Benedikt's syndromes.
- Subarachnoid space: aneurysm, uncal herniation (Hutchinson's pupil is an early sign), tumor, or trauma.
  - Posterior communicating artery (PCA) aneurysm: CN III lies between the posterior cerebral and the superior cerebellar arteries and lateral to the PCA. Aneurysm in this area often causes pain and a pupil-involved CN III palsy. Obtain MRI/MRA and probably angiogram.
- Cavernous sinus: tumor, vascular (small vessel disease, carotid-cavernous sinus fistula), ICA aneurysm, infection (HSV, tuberculosis, fungal), granulomatous disease (Tolosa-Hunt syndrome, sarcoidosis, HZV), or ischemic (may be painful or not; pupil is usually spared, and often complete palsy with all end organs affected).
- Orbital space through the SOF: superior division (innervates SR and levator muscles), inferior division (supplies IR, IO, MR, pupil, and ciliary body). Often divisional palsy, usually from ischemia, trauma, virus (HZV), or tumor.

- Treatment: treat as per etiology. If isolated and ischemic, provide supportive care; may patch eye or use Fresnel prism for the nondominant eye.

CN IV PALSY CN with the longest intracranial course and the most commonly injured CN with head trauma (also known as the "trauma nerve"). Nucleus is contralateral to the nerve, which exits dorsally and then decussates. An ipsilateral SO palsy often has a contralateral head tilt to keep the vertical raphae perpendicular with the horizon. In congenital palsy, vertical fusional amplitudes may be 10–25 pD (normally 3–5 pD); look for head tilt in childhood photos. Forty percent of CN IV palsy is from trauma, 30% miscellaneous causes, 20% ischemia, and 10% tumor related.

CN VI PALSY Most commonly injured by increased intracranial pressure or hydrocephalus (also known as the "tumor nerve"). Unilateral palsy causes an incomitant ET, head turn toward the affected LR, divergence insufficiency (angle less at near than at distance). Incomitance may worsen temporarily (from LR weakness), then range of motion increases, and often becomes comitant (consider an old CN VI paresis in the differential diagnosis of acquired comitant ET). Ninety-four percent of idiopathic cases resolve within 6 months. If condition persists, consider compressive lesion.

- Bilateral CN VI differential diagnosis: ET, thyroid disease, bilateral Duane's syndrome, trauma, convergence spasm, diabetic patient with bilateral ischemia, skull base tumors
- Etiology by age: child (tumor, or more likely postviral; ask about recent upper respiratory infection) or older patients (usually ischemic).
- Etiology by location:
  - Nucleus lesion: causes ipsilateral horizontal gaze palsy because it also involves fibers to the MLF; often associated with ipsilateral CN VII palsy. Usually from pontine infarction or glioma, also Wernicke-Korsakoff syndrome.
    - Möbius' syndrome: congenital CN VI, CN VII palsy.
    - Duane's syndrome: CN VI nucleus hypoplasia causing the LR to be innervated by CN III. Usually sporadic; 5 to 10% of cases are autosomal dominant, associated with spinal or ear anomalies.
  - Fasciculus syndromes:
    - Foville's syndrome: dorsal pons (back of brainstem) with ipsilateral abduction palsy (CN VI), ipsilateral facial weakness (CN VII), deafness (CN VIII), and Horner's syndrome.
    - Millard-Gubler syndrome: ventral pons (closer to fasciculus exit) with abduction palsy, contralateral hemiplegia (pyramids affected), and CN VII palsy.
    - Raymond's syndrome: Millard-Gubler without CN VII involvement.
  - Travels through subarachnoid space, up the clivus (chordoma) and through Dorello's canal (increased intracranial pressure), and across the cistern space. May have bilateral CN VI palsy from cerebropontine angle (CPA) tumors (CN VI exits at the CPA with CN VII; thus, consider the diagnosis of a tumor in a child with Bell's palsy).
  - Petrous space: trauma with fracture of temporal bone or basilar skull fracture. Associated with Gradenigo's syndrome (infection in the mastoid space).
  - Cavernous sinus and orbital space: floating in lumen of the sinus and joined briefly by sympathetics. Palsy often caused by ischemia, vascular lesions, neoplasm, infection, or inflammation.
- Treatment: as per etiology. Consider base out (BO) prism.

CN VII PALSY Nucleus lays inferolateral to and the genu courses around the CN VI nucleus, passing through the pontine cistern with CN VIII. Central nuclear lesions spare the forehead muscles, but peripheral lesions do not. CN VII may be involved in CPA tumors, geniculate ganglion pathology, subarachnoid space lesions, Bell's palsy, facial diplegia, crocodile tears, and Möbius' syndrome, among many others.

- Bell's palsy: idiopathic acute facial nerve palsy with loss of facial muscle tone; patient may be unable to close eyelids. Probably viral or postviral inflammatory etiology. Maximum nerve degeneration by day 2; most patients recover by 3 weeks, and 80% are better within 3 months.
  - Differential diagnosis: a facial nerve palsy is not Bell's palsy until secondary causes are ruled out. Other causes of peripheral CN VII palsy include acoustic neuroma, tumors of the CPA or temporal bone or parotid gland, HZV (Ramsay Hunt syndrome with pain around the ear), HIV (4% incidence; do neuroimage and lumbar puncture), Lyme disease, chronic otitis media, other bacterial or fungal infections, sarcoidosis (affects 22–50% of sarcoid patients due to inflamed parotid gland), trauma, and stroke (only lower face affected). Be especially suspicious of other causes if CN VII palsy is recurrent, bilateral, or does not show improvement after 6 months.
  - Treatment: patients may need frequent ocular lubrication and pressure patch or eyelid taping at night if lagophthalmos is present. May consider upper eyelid gold weight, tarsorrhaphy, Botox injection of the levator muscle, LTS, and punctal plugs or cautery.
- Dystonias: involuntary abnormal muscle movement, often worsened with fatigue or stress, and improves with sleep, relaxation, or massage. May be focal, as in torticollis, blepharospasm, oromandibular, and spastic dysphonia. May be segmental if two or more contiguous areas are involved, as in Meige's syndrome. May be idiopathic or familial, as in blepharospasm, torticollis, and oromandibular dystonia. Also may be secondary, as in Wilson's disease, Hartnup disease, Huntington's disease, tumors, cerebral injury, muscle lesions, L-dopa use, reaction to toxins (manganese, cobalt), Parkinson's disease, tics, Tourette's syndrome, and seizures.
  - Essential blepharospasm: accounts for 62% of dystonias; causes bilateral orbicularis spasms (range from frequent involuntary blinking to complete eyelid closure) that resolve in sleep. Pathology is from a primary basal ganglia/substantia nigra neurotransmitter deficit, but rule out secondary causes such as blepharitis, conjunctivitis, dry eye, keratitis, and iritis. Females are affected 3:1 more than males, with an average age of 63 years (male average age 50 years old). Neuroimage if atypical presentation.
    - No definitive treatment; treat blepharitis and dry eye. Botox injections are 90% effective. May try selective CN VII avulsion or myectomy (Anderson procedure with excision of protractors).

    - Most patients have psychiatric overlay and may improve with psychotherapy, hypnosis, and biofeedback. No improvement proven with anticholinergics, baclofen, Librium, or lithium (one third of patients obtain some relief with placebo).
  - Meige's syndrome: accounts for 12% of dystonias; characterized by blepharospasm plus lower face involvement (oromandibular dystonia). May also have torticollis or upper arm involvement. Related to essential blepharospasm.
  - Hemifacial spasm: accounts for 26% of dystonias; unilateral, involving an entire side of the face. Usually presents in a middle-aged patient; females affected 2:1. Persists in sleep, and 95% are caused by a vascular tortuosity compression of CN VII at the brainstem. Compression of facial nerve axons (usually from the anterior and posterior inferior cerebellar arteries) causes ephaptic transmission (a "hotwire" false synapse between adjacent axons). Symptoms begin with twitches follwed by sustained spasm, and all branches of CN VII are involved. If new onset, rule out tumor (5% incidence, usually brainstem glioma). Treat with Botox injections or neurosurgery (Jannetta procedure to decompress the nerve root at the CPA; 84–97% successful).

Gaze Abnormalities

HORIZONAL GAZE ABNORMALITIES Brainstem or supranuclear disorders that cause gaze deficiency. See also Chapter 9.

- Congenital ocular motor apraxia: deficient voluntary horizontal eye movements in infancy, causing the child to thrust the head toward the desired direction of gaze; improves with age and is usually benign. If acquired (Balint's syndrome), is often from bilateral cerebral disease with deficient saccades and pursuits.
- Internuclear ophthalmoplegia (INO): the ipsilateral eye shows abnormal adduction with contralateral nystagmus in the abducting eye. Caused by lesion in the MLF interfering with interneurons that normally connect the ipsilateral CN III (adduction deficit) to the contralateral PPRF/CN VI nucleus (abducting nystagmus). Usually from MS; in older patients is usually of vascular origin.
  - Wall-eyed bilateral INO (WEBINO): lesions in both MLF tracts, causing a bilateral INO and thus bilateral adduction deficits; pathognomonic for demyelinating disease (MS).
  - "One-and-a-half" syndrome or paralytic pontine exotropia: caused by an ipsilateral gaze palsy and a contralateral INO, allowing the unopposed contralateral PPRF to drive one eye away from the midline.
- Pontine conjugate gaze palsy: ipsilateral gaze palsy from PPRF or CN VI nucleus damage.

- Ocular neuromyotonia: unilateral spasm of a single EOM (usually CN III excitability), causing transient diplopia, especially with sustained eccentric gaze. Rare, associated with previous radiation therapy; may treat with Tegretol 200 mg bid–tid.
- Spasticity of conjugate gaze: lesion of the temporal or parietal lobes, causing gaze up and away from the lesion (Cogan's sign).

VERTICAL GAZE ABNORMALITIES Upgaze palsies are usually from more dorsal lesions (Parkinson's disease, Parinaud's syndrome, etc.), and downgaze palsies are usually from midbrain lesions (e.g., progressive supranuclear palsy). See also Chapter 9.

- Ocular tilt reaction: sustained or paroxysmal cyclovertical deviation with head tilt, often associated with skew deviation. Pathologic head tilt has a contralateral hypertropia (HT) and torsion toward the tilt (normally would be away from the tilt). Caused by an imbalance in otolithic inputs (sustained movement or tonic stimulus).
- Oculogyric crisis: tonic vertical supranuclear deviation; caused by postencephalitis, Parkinson's disease, or phenothiazines (mnemonic: "the three *P*'s").
- Parinaud's dorsal midbrain syndrome: a lesion in the posterior commissure (mnemonic "CLUES"): **c**onvergence-retraction nystagmus (accentuated by a downgoing OKN drum), **l**ight-near dissociation, **u**pgaze paralysis, **e**yelid retraction (Collier's sign), and **s**kew deviation. Etiology by age: hydrocephalus from aqueductal stenosis is the leading cause in children, but also consider pinealomas; trauma, or AVM in young adults, stroke in older patients.
- Progressive supranuclear palsy (PSP), Steele-Richardson-Olszewski syndrome: unrelenting neurodegenerative disease characterized by midbrain and basal ganglia gliosis. Patients are unable to look up ("dirty tie" syndrome) and have progressive dementia and a poor life prognosis. May be a primary disorder or associated with
  - Whipple's disease with vitritis and malabsorption; treat with tetracycline.
  - Neimann Pick variant in teenagers characterized by downgaze deficit, ataxia, and foam cells.
- Skew deviation: cyclovertical deviation that does not isolate to a single muscle. Arises from vertical misalignment of visual axis by disturbance of prenuclear inputs. Usually from brainstem pathology (e.g., trauma, stroke, MS). Often associated with peripheral vestibulopathy and vestibular midbrain lesions (may also have INO), and often has other signs of neurologic dysfunction (e.g., nystagmus).
  - Diagnose with the "four-step test" : the standard three-step test looking at the deviation in primary gaze, side gaze, and with head tilt, plus checking for torsion (e.g., double Maddox rod or look at the fundus).

- The hypertropic eye is intorted, unlike CN IV palsy, in which the HT eye either has no torsional component or up to 7 pD of excyclotorsion. The lower eye is usually on the side of the brainstem lesion, and the head tilt is usually toward the lesion (ipsilateral).
- Wallenberg's syndrome, lateral medullary infarction: skew deviation with lateropulsion of saccades associated with ipsilateral decreased facial pain and temperature sensation, ipsilateral Horner's sydrome, ipsilateral limb ataxia (descending corticospinal tracts affected), and contralateral decreased trunk pain and temperature sensation. Usually from ipsilateral vertebral artery infarction or dissection.

- Treat with prisms, patching, and waiting.

Nystagmus

GENERAL

The word *nystagmus* derives from the Greek *nystagmos*, meaning "drowsiness," to describe head bobbing in drunken sailors. It indicates an involuntary rhythmic beating of the eyes. If acquired, the patient may complain of oscillopsia; otherwise, the nystagmus may just cause decreased VA. It is usually most prominent in primary gaze. Alexander's law states that nystagmus worsens when looking toward the fast phase. May exhibit a glissade, or a residual drift to focus.

- Evaluation: note if it is jerk or pendular nystagmus (if jerk, then note the direction of fast beating); note whether it is horizontal, vertical, circular, elliptical, or torsional; and note if it is conjugate or disconjugate. May help to draw a nine-square noting the presence and direction of nystagmus in each field of gaze (the length of arrow indicates its amplitude: fine, medium, or coarse).
- Etiology: many causes (see below), but the leading cause overall is drug side effect.
    - Unipolar causes of nystagmus (horizontal in any plane): congenital nystagmus, periodic alternating nystagmus (PAN), and peripheral vestibular nystagmus.

AFFERENT OR SENSORY NYSTAGMUS Pendular nystagmus that develops at least 10 weeks after birth when VA is worse than 20/200. Caused by (mnemonic: "seven *A*'s"): **a**lbinism, **a**niridia, **a**chromatopsia, **a**trophic optic neuropathy if it occurs within 3 months, **a**nterior segment disease (cornea, cataract, coloboma), **a**maurosis of Leber's, and **a**ll others (cone dystrophy, CSNB, Chédiak-Higashi syndrome, juvenile X-linked retinoschisis).

CEREBELLAR-OCULAR DYSMETRIA Characterized by ocular flutter, opsoclonus, skew deviation, gaze-evoked nystagmus, and oculopalatal myoclonus.

CONVERGENCE–RETRACTION NYSTAGMUS An attempt to quickly look up (as when viewing a downgoing OKN drum) that causes retraction convergence and horizontal muscle retraction; often associated with Parinaud's dorsal midbrain syndrome with light-near dissociation and deficit of upgaze and convergence.

- Differential diagnosis by age: congenital causes are usually from aqueductal stenosis or hydrocephalus. Patients' age: 10 years old—consider pinealoma; 20 years—most likely trauma; 30 years—often postencephalitis; 40 years—most likely MS; 50 years old or older—often from basilar artery aneurysm or tumors.

DISSOCIATED NYSTAGMUS Asymmetric nystagmus indicating posterior fossa disease, such as abducting nystagmus, as in INO.

DOWNBEAT NYSTAGMUS Downgoing jerk nystagmus in primary gaze that becomes worse with lateral gaze (does not follow Alexander's law). From cervicomedullary junction lesions. (Mnemonic: DoWNBEAT): **d**egeneration, demyelinating, or drugs (lithium); **W**ernicke's encephalopathy; **n**eoplasm or paraneoplastic cerebellar degeneration (especially gynecologic and small-cell lung cancers); **b**rainstem disease (e.g., syringomyelia); **e**ncephalitis; **A**rnold-Chiari malformation; **t**rauma or toxins. Treat with baclofen or Neurontin 1200–2400 mg/day.

DRUGS Leading cause of nystagmus; often from tranquilizers, anticonvulsants, or alcohol abuse, plus others.

EFFERENT OR CONGENITAL MOTOR NYSTAGMUS Jerk or pendular horizontal nystagmus to one side of gaze; onset is within first 3 months, and nystagmus is usually benign. Dampens with eye closure, convergence (thus ET often develops), and head turn to a "null" zone, and disappears with sleep. Head turn and accommodation may cause nystagmus blockage. Patients do not have oscillopsia but often have LN. OKN shows reversal, and EOG demonstrates "sea waves" waveform. VA is relatively good, usually 20/20–70. May treat with contact lenses to decrease astigmatism, prisms to move null point straight ahead, baclofen medication, or Kestenbaum procedure. Better prognosis if OKN is responsive.

GAZE-EVOKED NYSTAGMUS The most common form of pathologic nystagmus, seen when the eye attempts to maintain an eccentric position, with the fast phase in the direction of gaze. Associated with sedatives and anticonvulsant medication and brainstem disease.

LATENT NYSTAGMUS Jerk nystagmus that is brought on by monocular occlusion, when the fixating eye drifts to midline, then jerks to abduction and away from the occluded eye. Associated with congenital ET and dissociated vertical deviation (DVD), with onset >1 year old. EOG waveform shows a convex upstroke with straight downstroke. Patients have better VA with both eyes open, and condition rarely needs to be treated.

OCULOPALATAL NYSTAGMUS Pendular vertical nystagmus with synchronous contraction of the palate and pharynx.

OPSOCLONUS Saccadomania (eye movements all over the place), usually from hydrocephalus in children or postviral encephalitis in adults. Always consider metastatic neuroblastoma with myoclonus and cerebellar ataxia. Also known as "dancing eyes and dancing feet."

PERIODIC ALTERNATING NYSTAGMUS (PAN) Horizontal nystagmus that alternates directions, with a brief null point. If congenital, it is usually from cervicomedullary junction pathology (Arnold-Chiari malformation); it may also be associated with posterior fossa tumors, trauma, MS, stroke, syphilis, and spinocerebellar degeneration.

PHYSIOLOGIC NYSTAGMUS Normal nystagmus at the end point of gaze (usually >30 degrees); fatigues.

SEESAW Dissociated pendular vertical nystagmus with conjugate torsional oscillation (twists in same direction). One eye deviates up, the other down; "roll down the plank" appearance. May be congenital (septo-optic dysplasia, etc.) or from craniopharyngioma (rostral midbrain/third ventricle locations, frequently with temporal hemianopia) or trauma (lesions in the "myoclonic triangle" involving the red nucleus or inferior olive, with delay of nystagmus onset after injury from inferior olive pseudohypertrophy).

SPASMUS NUTANS Triad of monocular or dissociated shimmering, asymmetric, small-amplitude nystagmus, head bobbing, and torticollis or head tilt. Onset at age 4 to 18 months. Usually benign and disappears within 2 years of onset, but rule out chiasmatic gliomas and subacute necrotizing encephalomyopathy (optic atrophy, irritability, vomiting, and increased intracranial pressure).

VESTIBULAR NYSTAGMUS Horizontal rotary jerk nystagmus; if peripheral, is associated with definite torsional component and vertigo or tinnitus. A common cause of acquired horizontal jerk nystagmus (Table 8–3).

UPBEAT NYSTAGMUS Upgoing jerk movements in primary gaze. From lesions in the midline cerebellum or anterior vermis (medulloblastoma,

TABLE 8–3

Distinguishing Characteristics of Peripheral versus Central Causes of Nystagmus

Characteristic	Peripheral Nystagmus	Central Nystagmus
Nystagmus Character	Usually horizontal-rotatory (never purely vertical)	Any direction, may be purely vertical; usually jerk nystagmus
Torsion	Present	Absent
Direction of fast phase	Away from the side with lesion	Toward the side with lesion (may change with direction of gaze)
Vestibular symptoms	Vertigo, tinnitus, nausea; may have hearing loss	Unlikely
Romberg's sign	Falls toward slow side, changes with head turn	Does not change with head position
Visual fixation	Suppresses nystagmus	No effect
Lesion	Unilateral, usually labyrinth or CN VIII	Unilateral or bilateral, usually brainstem or cerebellum
Onset and course	Acute, finite	Slow-growing lesion, persists

alcoholic degeneration, etc.), posterior fossa, or intrinsic lower brainstem disease (rarely drugs). Treat with baclofen or Neurontin 1200–2400 mg/day.

VOLUNTARY NYSTAGMUS Unable to sustain frequency; associated with blinking.

Psychiatric Diseases

FUNCTIONAL PATIENTS Usually present with constricted VF or decreased VA, unilateral or bilateral. Try to elicit better VA by response to OKN drum (at least 20/200 VA), shifting mirrors, stereopsis, and prism shift test. Tangent screen or HVF may show fields that tunnel, spiral, or have isopters that cross or are too close. Pattern-evoked VEP may be used to evaluate ON function.

- Hysterics: lack insight into their disease; demonstrate belle indifference. Treat the primary psychiatric disorder.
- Malingerers: have a secondary gain, and often have an "attitude" about their condition. Document well, and give them a way out when discussing their condition.

CHAPTER 9

Pediatrics and Strabismus

Anatomy and Physiology

EMBRYOLOGY All muscles arise from mesoderm, and connective tissue from neural crest origin. Primordial muscles appear at the second month, and the sclera condenses at the third month. Histologically, the developing eye shows long cylindrical ciliary processes and peripheral retinal folds (Lange's folds, probably a pathology artifact).

EYE AT BIRTH Axial length 16–17 mm; horizontal palpebral fissure is nearly adult size, but the vertical fissure is 50% of the adult; corneal diameter 10 mm; relative miosis from immaturity of pupillary dilator muscle; lens is disproportionately large compared with globe size. By age 3 years, the anterior–posterior diameter is 90% of adult size.

MUSCLES All EOM originate at the anulus of Zinn, except the IO (which originates from the maxillary bone at the base of the anterior lacrimal crest), the SO (which originates from the sphenoid bone), and, some would say, the levator muscle. Both obliques travel beneath their corresponding rectus muscles.

- All muscle bellies are 37–40 mm long except the SO, which is 32 mm. Rectus muscle tendon widths are about 10 mm, and tendon length is about 7 mm, except the MR tendon, which is 4.5 mm long. Arc of contact for all EOM is about 7 mm, except the LR, which is 12 mm.
    - SO tendon length is 30 mm, with a diaphanous, broad, variable insertion under the SR (thus, hook SO from the temporal side). The anterior portion of the SO tendon is responsible for incyclotorsion.
    - The IO has little or no tendon with two to six heads. The IO inserts near the macula.
- Spiral of Tillaux (Fig. 9–1) describes the distances of the rectus muscle insertions from the limbus (superotemporal is most posterior): roughly, the MR is 5.5 mm, the IR is 6.5 mm, the LR is 7.0 mm, and the SR is 7.5 mm.
- EOM are striated muscles that have a higher nerve to muscle ratio than skeletal muscle and smaller nerve terminals than other skeletal

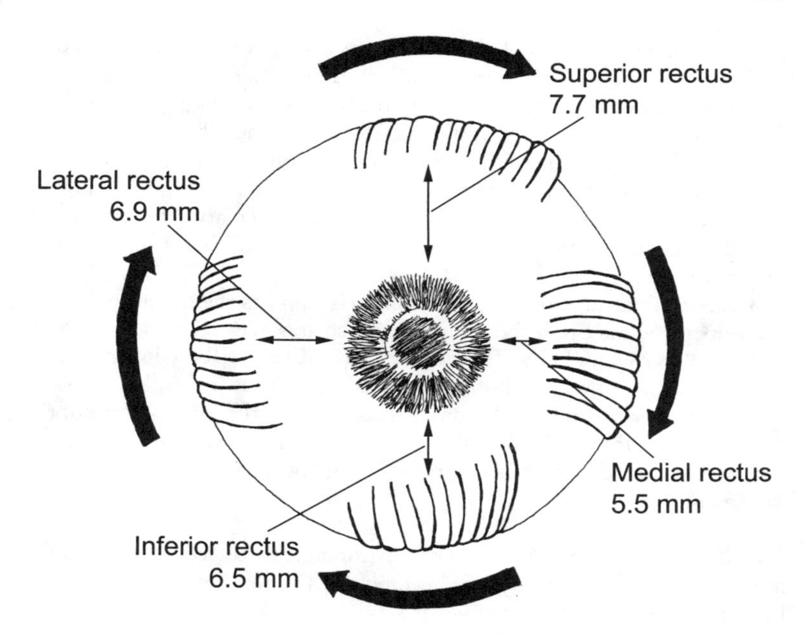

Figure 9–1 Right globe, anterior view, showing the distance of the rectus muscle insertions from the limbus. The increasing distance from the tendon to the limbus beginning at the medial rectus muscle and progressing clockwise is known as the spiral of Tillaux.

muscle, and thus finer control. Two distinguishable types of EOM muscle fibers on histologic evaluation:

- ○ Fibrillenstruktur: larger glycolytic fast-twitch fibers with en plaque (single) nerve endings; preserved in myasthenia, thus patients can fast saccade.
- ○ Felderstruktur: smaller aerobic tonic/slow fibers, similar to "dark meat" skeletal muscle, with en grappe (multiple, small, grapelike) nerve endings that respond to acetylcholine; preserved in cranial nerve palsy, they thus have "molasses-like" eye movements.

- Action: superior muscles (SR, SO) intort and inferior muscles (IR, IO) extort. Vertical rectus muscles adduct (synergy with MR) and obliques abduct (synergy with LR). Vertical rectus muscles work best in abduction (23 degrees), and obliques work maximally in adduction (51 degrees). Horizontal rectus muscles are weak elevators in upgaze and weak depressors in downgaze.
- Blood supply: anterior ciliary artery gives two branches to each muscle except the LR, which receives one branch (usually from the lacrimal

artery). The IR has a plethora of vessels and appears to have more than two branches. Muscular branches continue anteriorly onto the sclera and dive deep about 3.5 mm from the limbus, terminating in the major arterial circle of the iris. With age, anterior segment blood supply from the long posterior ciliary artery is compromised; thus, there is an increased risk for anterior segment ischemia following muscle surgery. Prior to muscle surgery, look for the anterior ciliary arteries beneath the conjunctiva to evaluate blood flow; may check iris FA if ischemia is a concern.

- Innervation: superior division of CN III supplies the levator palpebrae superioris and SR; inferior division innervates MR, IR, and IO; CN IV supplies SO; and CN VI innervates LR. SO and SR are innervated by contralateral nuclei, all others are ipsilateral; thus, no unilateral ptosis is found with a nuclear lesion. Nerves enter on the inner surface of the muscle at the junction of the posterior third and anterior two thirds, except the IO, which is innervated on its outer surface at the halfway point.

CONNECTIVE TISSUE For surgery, cut through three layers to get to the muscles: conjunctiva (inserts at the limbus), Tenon's layer (inserts 1 mm from the limbus), and intermuscular septum.

- Tenon's layer extends from the limbus to the ON and separates the moving surface of globe, muscles, and tendons from the orbital fat. The rectus muscles posterior to the equator and oblique muscle anterior to the equator penetrate Tenon's layer. Anterior to the rectus muscles, Tenon's is thicker than it is posterior to rectus muscle penetration, where Tenon's is thinner and in direct contract with the scleral surface.
- Intermuscular septum extends from the border of the muscle capsule to the nearest adjacent muscle, located within sub-Tenon's space, and fuses with anterior Tenon's into a single fascial plane 3 mm from the limbus. It joins the conjunctiva 1 mm from the limbus.
- Muscle capsule surrounds the muscle and tendon.
- Check ligaments forming a single sheet across the width of vertical rectus muscles and two or three radial folds on the horizontal rectus muscles. Lockwood's suspensory ligament in the lower eyelid is fused muscle capsules of the IO and IR. Lower eyelid retractors are cordlike attachments from the inferior border of the tarsal plate, conjunctival fornix, and skin, and pass through sub-Tenon's space, penetrate Tenon's layer, and attach to the external surface of the IR. The SO tendon passes beneath the SR, and the intermuscular septum of both are attached and prevent the SR from slipping posteriorly.
- Orbital fat: intraconal fat is separated from the sclera by posterior Tenon's layer with sparse septae. Extraconal fat is separated by anterior Tenon's layer and begins about 10 mm from the limbus. If fat is

allowed into the sub-Tenon's space, it incites a fibrofatty proliferative response.

- Sclera is thickest at the ON (1 mm), then limbus (0.8 mm), and thinnest under muscle insertions (0.3 mm).

VORTEX VEINS Usually four veins that drain the choroid, exiting 6 mm behind the equator. Inferotemporal vortex vein is 8 mm posterior to the IR insertion along its temporal border. The superotemporal vortex vein exits at the tip of the SO tendon insertion under the SR muscle. Vortex vein disruption induces choroidal effusion.

MOVEMENT OF THE EYE Six cardinal positions are the diagnostic positions in which each of the six EOM have maximal effect (Table 9–1); eye moves about 50 degrees each direction. Arc of contact is the "grip" of the muscle, and changed by Faden procedure. The eye looks about 15 degrees before the head turns.

- Axes of Fick: central anteroposterior axis (y-axis) allows incyclotorsion and excyclotorsion. X-axis runs from ear to ear → elevation and depression. Z-axis runs from head to toe → abduction and adduction.
- Listing's plane: coronal section along the x-axis or through the y-axis.
- Sherrington's law of reciprocal innervation: simultaneous and equal contraction and relaxation of antagonistic muscle in one eye (mnemonic: "share in one"); involves ductions.
- Herring's law: bilateral stimulation of yolk muscles; involves versions.

NORMAL BINOCULAR VISION Based on corresponding retinal points receiving input via nodal point from the horopter (concave line of focus in space). The eye permits a limited amount of image disparity where it can still fuse the images; this is represented by Panum's spatial area (a second convex line distal to the horopter makes Panum's space look like a minus lens and shows less Panum's area centrally. Thus, less macular disparity is tolerated, and there is greater area peripherally).

TABLE 9–1

Eye Movement and Responsible Extraocular Muscles

Cardinal Position of Gaze	Primary Eye Muscle	Yoke Muscle
Up and right	Right SR	Left IO
Up and left	Left SR	Right IO
Right	Right LR	Left MR
Left	Left LR	Right MR
Down and right	Right IR	Left SO
Down and left	Left IR	Right SO

TABLE 9–2
Average Normal Fusional Amplitudes (in prism diopters)

Fusion	**Distance**	**Near**
Convergence	18 pD	36 pD
Divergence	6 pD	12 pD
Vertical	3 pD	6 pD

- Fusion occurs for images within Panum's area and is an automatic sensorimotor reflex (motor arc is lost with brain disease or anomalous retinal correspondence [ARC]). Perceptions of images outside Panum's area causes physiologic diplopia, which may be consciously ignored (physiologic suppression); images are subconsciously perceived as being nearer if heteronymous (image on bitemporal retinas) or farther away if homonymous (binasal retinas).
  - Sensory fusion: excitation of corresponding retinal elements receiving equal images; retinal rivalry develops when sensory fusion is not permitted.
  - Motor fusion: retinal disparity causes vergence movements in order to maintain sensory fusion.
  - Fusion amplitudes: Table 9–2 presents the average normal fusion amplitudes.
- Stereopsis is depth perception by fusing horizontally disparate images from Panum's area. Excellent stereo from the fovea, up to 14 seconds of arc; poor stereo from peripheral retina, usually 200 arc seconds. Retinal cells project to special cortical cells responsible for stereoperception.
- Symmetric motor processing: nasal bias that normalizes by 5 months; Panum's area is "close enough."
- Abnormal binocular vision characterized by abnormal motion processing (e.g., infantile ET) and abnormal stereopsis; patient uses monocular clues.

ADAPTATION TO DIPLOPIA, CONFUSION, OR STRABISMUS Macula ceases to function with disparate images; diplopia and visual confusion cause an instant and simultaneous extramacular retinal suppression and ARC. Both develop quickly and easily within the first decade. Diagnose with Worth four-dot test (W4D) or Bagolini glasses for ET or base-in prism test for XT. Treat with occlusion, alignment (plus lenses, surgery, prisms), but not orthoptics; ARC will gradually disappear when aligned (may have postoperative diplopia; do not patch, as this delays normal retinal correspondence [NRC]).

- Supression: the brain suppresses area of conscious regard in the deviating eye, creating an absolute scotoma that changes location as fast as alignment changes; transfers to the other eye if fixation changes; can be mapped with binocular perimetry. Treat with proper refraction, occlusion (i.e., for CN VI palsy), alignment of the visual axis (i.e., for intermittent XT), or orthoptics.
  - ET scotoma is a 5 degree horizontal oval (corresponds to the macular projection of the fixating eye) that is nasal to the hemiretinal vertical line through the macula.
  - XT scotoma is larger half-moon shape up to the hemiretinal line temporal out to image; facultative (can come and go as in intermittent XT).
- Anomalous retinal correspondence (ARC): deals with the rest of the extramacular retina outside the area of conscious regard around the suppression scotoma. It represents the hardwiring of the brain to accept a different "macula" in order to eliminate diplopia; an attempt at crude binocularity. ARC persists despite switching fixation and spontaneously reverts to NRC if alignment is corrected to within 8 pD. Patients have no true fusion and no binocularity (if monocular, they have eccentric fixation). Diagnose with Bagolini or afterimage tests; diagnose eccentric fixation with Visuscope. Treat like suppression. (See Table 9–3 for the dual pathways of binocular vision.)
- Amblyopia (from the Greek *amblys*, meaning "dull," and *opia*, meaning "vision"), which affects 2 to 4% of children in the United States, represents cortically decreased VA from disparate retinal images (binocular suppression of amblyopic eye). Development of the visual brain requires well-focused retinal images with high spatial frequencies and high contrast that occurs prior to the age of visual maturity (<age 10 years). The immature visual system is much more sensitive to unilateral than bilateral abnormalities because of the natural competition between the right and left eyes.
  - Clinical features: decreased VA, typically two lines or greater; abnormal contour interaction and abnormally large receptive fields cause crowding (amblyopic eye sees individual letters much better than lines of letters). Persistently dark-adapted, decreased contrast sensitivity; at low illumination, VA is often equal to the fellow eye (compare with organic macular disease, which has a dramatic loss of vision with decreased illumination). May have eccentric fixation, spatial jitter (vertical line appears bent), and increased reaction times, and rarely will have an afferent pupil defect.
    - Amblyopia masquerades: subtle nystagmus, subclinical retinal abnormalities, and undiagnosed lesions (tumors, masses, CNS disease)
    - Neonatal amblyopia: often associated with LN, DVD, and nasotemporal asymmetries.

TABLE 9–3

Comparison of the Dual Pathways for Binocular Vision

	Macular Retina	Extramacular Retina
Image projects onto retina from	Central Panum's area; "area of conscious regard"	Peripheral Panum's area; "outside conscious regard"
Ganglion cell type	Parvoganglion (P cells)	Magnoganglion (M cells)
Contribution to LGN	90% of LGN; areas 3, 4, 5, and 6	10% of LGN; areas 1 and 2
Enters occipital cortex	Layer IV-C	Layer IV-B
Projects to	Occipitotemporal cortex	Occipitoparietal cortex
Characteristics	"What" information; slow processing; color; requires attention to process; sees stationary objects in fine detail	"Where" information; fast processing; no color; subconscious; sees moving objects at a glance
Stereoacuity	Fine; maximal; low threshold (20 minutes of arc)	Coarse; high threshold (240 minutes or 4 degrees of arc)
Fusional vergence amplitudes	Minimal (only fine tuning); check with amblyoscope	Maximal; keeps eyes straight
Images beyond threshold	Monofixation plus contralateral macular scotoma	Simultaneous perception
Reaction to diplopia or visual confusion	None, ceases to function; misalignment tolerance is 20 minutes of arc (two thirds of pD)	1. Suppression of part of VF by brain to eliminate diplopia within the area of conscious regard 2. ARC by brain rearranging retinal inputs to permit fusion of disparate images outside area of conscious regard
Haploscopic presentation of dissimilar images	Retinal rivalry	Fuse but with diplopia
Adaptation to dissimilar images or strabismus	No visual confusion (instant macular scotoma in the nonfixating eye)	1. Diplopia (same image on dissimilar retinal areas) 2. Visual confusion (dissimilar images on similar retinas)
Reinforcement needs	Requires constant use or vanishes after 3 months	Continues to function (no critical period)

        - Bilateral amblyopia: isoametropic amblyopia, symmetrical hyperopia; not typically seen with high myopia. Treat with glasses; do not patch. Response is slow.
    - Deprivation amblyopia: lack of patterned input stimulation causing M cell maldevelopment; most severe form of amblyopia. A 20/40 corneal opacity may result in 20/200 vision from amblyopia. Often does not respond well to therapy; accounts for <3% of all amblyopia.
    - Anisometropic amblyopia: more likely from hyperopic anisometropia (can be present with 2 D or less of anisometropia); only the amount of accommodation necessary to focus the image in the less hyperopic eye is utilized. Amblyopia in myopes is unusual unless the difference between the two eyes is greater than 5 or 6 D. Anisometropic amblyopia is the least profound; high spatial frequencies (P cells) are mainly affected; limited effect on low spatial frequencies (M cells). Better outcomes than with pattern deprivation → more than half have final acuities of 20/120 or better.
    - Strabismic amblyopia: abnormal binocular input in the form of diplopia and confusion leads to suppression and M cell maldevelopment. More likely to develop in ET, which frequently has a fixation preference, versus XT, which frequently has a freely alternating fixation pattern. The severity of the amblyopia is not correlated with the angle of strabismus.
    - Treatment: first treat the underlying cause, then correct dominance; always treat amblyopia before surgery (mnemonic: *A* precedes *S*). In general, patching may be stopped around age 9. Surgery is appropriate when no further improvement is seen from patching.
        - High-grade occlusion of the better eye up to 90% of waking hours (out of patch 1 hour after awakening and 1 hour before bed). Disrupts binocular interaction, may cause occlusion amblyopia. Follow-up full-time patching 1 week per year of life; do not use high-grade occlusion in infants.
        - Low-grade occlusion 10 to 50% of waking hours allows binocular interaction, less risk of causing occlusion amblyopia, less effective for reversing severe amblyopia, excellent for maintenance patching.
        - Atopine penalization is best for mild to moderate amblyopia and may be the most effective.
    - Complications: reverse amblyopia, noncompliance, unresponsive (reassess diagnosis), recurrence (reinstitute patching)
- Monofixation syndrome diagnostic criteria: (1) Patients have straight or nearly straight eyes (<8 pD of deviation), (2) central scotoma with extramacular NRC, and (3) normal fusional amplitudes. May or

may not have good stereopsis (usually not unless straightened by age 2 years) but have absence of binocular vision (lost after 3 months). Often have large latent phoria; may have amblyopia.

- Etiology: end result of strabismus surgery (74%), anisometropia (6%), macular lesion (1%), primary genetic inability to bifixate (1% of population; 14% of first-degree relatives of ET patients).
- Thirty-seven percent of patients are orthophoric, 63% have microstrabismus as determined by cover test (mostly postoperative strabismus patients). Patients have a 3-degree macular scotoma (not suppression) in the nonfixating eye, diagnosed by 4 pD base-out test.
- Treat amblyopia and anisometropia; alignment is already stabilized by extramacular NRC. Monofixation is best result after infantile ET correction and is a good predictor of long-term alignment.

Signs and Symptoms

CARTILAGE IN EYE Patau's syndrome (trisomy 13), PHPV, teratoma

DECREASED VA (ACQUIRED, NEW ONSET) Myopia (usually develops between age 6 to late teens, compared with hyperopia, which typically increases up to age 6, then plateaus), hydrocephalus, tumor, neurodegenerative disease, infection/inflammation, toxins, and previously undiscovered decreased VA

DECREASED VA (CONGENITAL) WITH A "NORMAL" FUNDUS Achromatopsia, CSNB, and Leber's congenital amaurosis (all may have paradoxical pupils)

EYE DISEASE WITH DEAFNESS Usher's syndrome (RP), Wolfram syndrome (optic atrophy).

EYE-POPPING REFLEX Pronounced widening of the PF after abrupt decrease in ambient light or after loud noises. Present in 75% of infants within 3 weeks of birth.

FACE TURN Nystagmus null point, nerve palsy, and astigmatism

FORCED DUCTIONS POSITIVE Brown's syndrome, congenital fibrosis, blowout fracture, thyroid eye disease, and fat adherence syndrome

FOVEAL HYPOPLASIA Albinism, aniridia, and PHPV

HETEROCHROMIA IN CHILDREN Congenital Horner's syndrome, JXG, and Waardenburg's syndrome (autosomal dominant [AD], eyelid abnormalities, white forelock, sensorineural hearing loss)

INCREASED FUSIONAL AMPLITUDES Intermittent strabismus and congenital CN IV palsy

LEUKOCORIA Larval eosinophilic granuloma (*Toxocara*), embryonal meduloepithelioma, uveitis, Coats' disease, organizing hemorrhage, cataract or PHPV (leading cause at birth), ON coloboma, retinoblastoma (average age 18 months) and retinopathy of prematurity (stage 5), idiopathic, and assorted other causes (congenital retinal folds, hamartoma, hemangioma, Norrie's disease, FEVR).

MITOCHONDRIAL DNA INHERITANCE Leber's optic atrophy, exercise-induced myopathy, Leigh's syndrome, Kearns-Sayre syndrome, NARP (neurogenic muscle weakness, ataxia, and RP), and infantile lactic acidosis

NYSTAGMUS AND DECREASED VA CSNB, albinism, Leber's amaurosis, and achromatopsia.

STRABISMUS, THREE PRIMARY ETIOLOGIES:

- Childhood: brainstem, central, vestibular (signal problem)
- Restrictive: myopathic, compressive, thyroid (muscle problem, tendon spared), orbital pseudotumor
- Paralytic: neuropathic (peripheral/central), cranial nerve, neuromuscular junction, myasthenia

VIOLATES HERRING'S LAW DVD, aberrant regeneration, Duane's syndrome

VIOLATES SHERRINGTON'S LAW Duane's syndrome

X-LINKED DISORDERS Adrenoleukodystrophy (optic atrophy), Aicardi's dominant optic neuropathy (XLD), Alport's syndrome (85% X-linked), choroideremia (XLR), Hunter's (XLR), incontinentia pigmenti (XLD), Lenz microphthalmia syndrome, Lowe's syndrome (XLR), megalocornea (XLR), Norrie's disease, ocular albinism (Nettleship-Falls syndrome), Fabry's disease (XLR), X-linked CSNB, X-linked retinoschisis (XLR), X-linked RP

Exam and Imaging

EVALUATION, STRABISMUS Consider family history of strabismus or amblyopia, birth and developmental history, red reflex history, age of onset, abnormal head position, and constant or intermittent strabismus. Check stereopsis prior to VA or cover testing; do W4D; look at facial structure, angle kappa, EOM, A or V pattern, and oblique dysfunction; and measure alignment in primary and secondary positions.

STEREOACUITY In order not to disrupt fusion, check stereopsis first, then check VA and alignment. The Titmus test stereo fly plate tests about 3000 seconds of arc at 40 cm; lateralization clues can give false-positive results. Randot circles range from 400 to 20 seconds of arc at 40 cm.

VISUAL ACUITY (VA) TESTING May test F/F (patient able to fix and follow) or preferential looking (Teller cards) in infants; then central, steady, and maintained VA (CSM; fixation maintained after cover is removed from the opposite eye), tumbling E, Landolt C, Allen figures, Snellen's chart, etc.

CYCLOPLEGIC REFRACTION 1 drop anesthetic (removes stinging and disrupts epithelium to improve absorption), 1% Cyclogyl (2 doses, or 3 doses for dark irides), with 2.5% phenylephrine; wait 30 to 40 minutes. Cycloplegics are parasympatholytic; thus, there may be anticholingergic side effects (fever, flushing, delirium, etc.). Use with caution, especially with Down syndrome. Phenylephrine is an alpha-stimulating sympathomimetic; thus, it may raise blood pressure and decrease pulse rate. Retinoscopy exam improved by occluding the opposite eye.

ALIGNMENT Place plastic prisms in the frontal plane; place glass prisms in plane perpendicular to deviation.

- Hirschberg: corneal light reflection; 1 mm deviation = 7 degrees = 15 pD.
- Krimskey: prism placed over the fixating eye until deviation is neutralized; modified-Krimskey if prism is held over the nonfixating eye.
- Bruckner: pupillary light reflection brighter in strabismic eye (do not confuse with leukocoria).
- Angle kappa: misalignment of visual and anatomic axis, is not strabismus. If positive angle kappa, the patient looks like XT; light deviates nasally from slight temporal rotation of the globe from temporally displaced fovea relative to optical axis. If negative angle kappa, the patient looks like ET (Hirschberg deviates temporally).

COVER TESTING Two diagnostic tests (CT, alternate cover test [ACT]), two quantitative tests (simultaneous prism cover test [SPCT], prism and cover). If alternating tropia, there is less concern for amblyopia.

- Cover test (CT): reveals tropia.
- Alternating cover test (ACT): shows phoria and tropia by dissociating the eyes. If there is no movement, consider orthophoria.

- Simultaneous prism cover test (SPCT): simultaneously place a prism for the amount of tropia on one eye, and cover over the other eye; test reveals tropia without phoria. Useful in discerning small tropias with large phorias.
- Prism and cover: uncovers tropia and phoria.

ACCOMMODATIVE CONVERGENCE/ACCOMMODATION (AC/A) RATIO Normally about 5 pD convergence per D of accommodation. Child can neutralize high AC/A by fusional divergence. Can roughly determine that a high AC/A ratio exists if the measured ET' (near) is ≥ 10 pD more than measured ET (distance).

- Heterophoric method (clinical use; test distance varies; uses prisms): pupillary distance (cm) + [(pD near − pD distance) ÷ (D near − D distance or D of accommodation)]. Usually larger than gradient method.
- Gradient method (research use; test distance remains constant; uses lenses): (pD with lens − pD without lens) ÷ D of lens. AC/A is due to proximal convergence.

MOTILITY Ductions deal with monocular movements; versions deal with binocular conjugate or disconjugate movements. May describe normal motility as full ductions and conjugate versions, or draw cardinal fields of gaze and note underaction or overaction from −3 to +3. Urest measurements are more objective and noted as the distance from the corneal light reflection in primary gaze when looking up, down, left, and right (stated in degrees if light reflection is on the cornea or millimeters if past the cornea).

- A pattern: more XT in downgaze and reading position or more ET in upgaze, as in bilateral superior oblique overaction (SOO). A and V patterns are defined as >15 pD difference from up- to downgaze.
- V pattern: opposite from above, usually inferior oblique overaction (IOO; hyperdeviation is greater in its field of action)

MADDOX ROD Place over one eye, and have patient view a point source of light. Align the rod bars vertically so that the patient sees a horizontal line. If the patient sees a red and white line that is vertically separated, neutralize the vertical deviation with a prism to obtain the hypertropic amount. The test vertically dissociates the patient and is inaccurate for horizontal deviation because horizontal amplitudes are so large.

DOUBLE MADDOX ROD Use two Maddox rods (preferably one white and one red), placing one over each eye, and ask patient to make the lines parallel. Test measures ocular torsion, and the degrees of torsion are obtained from the angle between the Maddox rods' axes. (Torsion may also be seen with the indirect ophthalmoscope. The fovea should be level with the upper third of the optic disk. If it is higher, then excyclotorsion is present; if it is lower, then incyclotorsion is most likely present.)

SENSORY TESTS XT gives crossed diplopia in all tests except afterimage. Tests for diplopia: Maddox rod, red glass, Bagolini lenses, and W4D. Haploscopic tests: major amblyoscope, Lancaster red-green, and afterimage. Tests for suppression: W4D, Bagolini lenses and 4D base-out prism.

- Afterimage: most dissociative; uniocular test for ARC. Do not perform with eccentric fixation. Flashes each fovea separately; flash the suppressed eye in the vertical plane (tends to be a horizontal macular scotoma), and flash fellow eye horizontally. Interpretation is opposite of Bagolini: ET + ARC = crossed, XT + ARC = uncrossed.
- Bagolini striated lenses: least dissociative test; best for ARC with ET. Patients recognize and report their scotoma while viewing a light 15 inches away through striated lenses (can smear ocular lubricant on glasses): streak OS at 45 degrees (up and left), streak OD at 135 degrees (up and right). This produces a line of light perpendicular to the striations, and the normal eye sees an *X*. Examiner can simultaneously evaluate the ocular alignment.
    - If the strabismic patient sees an *X*, then ARC is present. If ARC is not present, then the ET patient sees an uncrossed image, like a *V* with the bottom cut off, and the XT patient sees a crossed image, like an *X* crossed high.
    - Suppression causes a break in the streak or no streak. Most patients with the monofixation syndrome (if they are directed to it) see their macular scotoma as a gap in the nonfixating eye's light streak.
- Base-in prism test for XT: increasing base-in prism before nonfixating eye moves the object of regard across the hemiretinal line onto the nasal retina out of the large scotoma and causes sudden recognition of diplopia. If ARC is present, images appear apart; for NRC, images are "kissing."
- Euthyscope: a retinoscope with an aperture that tests fusional vergence amplitudes. Macular testing: photostressing the retina with macular area shielded bleaches out the peripheral retina and relies only on macular area to fuse (weak fusion capability). Photostressing retina with extramacular area shielded bleaches out the macula and relies only on the peripheral retina to fuse (strong fusional capability).
- 4D base-out prism: test for microstrabismus or monofixation syndrome; the normal response is movement of the contralateral eye away from the prism followed by a refixation movement. With the prism OD: no movement = suppression OD; OS moves but no refixation = suppression OS; OS moves and refixates = normal.
- Major amblyoscope: best ARC test; if the objective angle = subjective angle, then NRC is present. If subjective angle = 0, then harmonious ARC (compensated) is present; if subjective angle is not 0, then patient has unharmonious ARC.

- Red glass test: dissociative test for suppression versus ARC. With red lens placed over right eye, patient fixates on point source of light. If the eyes are straight, patient should have retinal rivalry and see red or white alternately. ET patients have uncrossed diplopia, and XT shows crossed diplopia.
- Worth four-dot test (W4D): dissociative test for testing suppression, monofixation, or ARC with ET. With glasses with red lens on right eye and green lens on left eye, patient views a flashlight that has two red, two green, and one white point sources of light. Light is viewed at a distance (subtends 0.125 second of arc on the macula) and then nearby (subtends 6 seconds of arc, an extramacular test). If the patient sees two red lights = suppressing OS; if three green = suppressing OD; four lights = normal or if strabismic, then ARC is present; five lights = diplopia; >5 lights = functional issues. If distance is normal, then near test is not needed. In ET, the suppression scotoma is small (5 degrees); thus, patient should suppress W4D at a distance but have a fusion response in near test because extramacular has adapted with ARC.

VISUAL EVOKED POTENTIALS (VEPs) Can document 20/20 VA by age 6 to 8 months.

DEVELOPMENTAL AND VISUAL ACCOMPLISHMENTS See Table 9–4

TABLE 9–4
Developmental and Visual Accomplishments

Age	Developmental Milestones	Measured Visual Acuity
<3 months	Blink to light; fixates and follows a 2 inch object; wandering eye movements	20/200
3 months	Fixates and follows a 1-inch object; blinks to threat; rolls from prone to supine	20/50
6 months	Reaches for nearby objects; sits alone	
8 months	Crawls	
1 year	Looks for toys; walks	
3 years	Subjective VA testing (e.g., HOTV); knows colors, copies circle	20/30
4 years	Copies a cross, draws a man	
6 years	Snellen VA possible	20/20

Congenital and Genetic Disease

ALBINISM Reduction or absence of pigmentation from defective production of melanin. There are many variations, depending on the pathway defect, as melanin is produced from tyrosine. Incidence 1:17,000; all types of albinism are autosomal recessive, except X-linked ocular and autosomal dominant albinoidism. May be total versus partial absence of pigmentation, and ocular alone versus oculocutaneous. Patients have decreased VA from foveal hypoplasia, absent stereovision from abnormal chiasmal decussation (75% cross vs. 53% normally; CNS pigment guides neural development), ON hypoplasia, photophobia, sensory nystagmus, decreased uveal and RPE pigmentation, iris TID. Also have increased incidence of strabismus, high refractive error, and cataract. VEP shows asymmetry (larger response of contralateral eye), normal ERG.

- Albinoidism: autosomal dominant; decreased pigment without ocular abnormalities.
- Oculocutaneous albinism (OCA): reduced melanin but normal number of melanosomes.
  - Type I, tyrosinase negative: OCA1A most common; autosomal recessive. Seen with Caucasian patients (no pigment) with VA 20/200 or worse. Tyrosinase, a chromosome 11 gene product, converts tyrosine to dihydroxyphenylalanine (DOPA). OCA1B "yellow" variant has some retained tyrosinase function.
  - Type II, tyrosinase positive: P gene on chromosome 15 codes for normal tyrosinase enzyme but has transport abnormalities and is autosomal recessive; patient has some pigmentation with VA 20/200 or better. Two potentially lethal forms:
    - Chédiak-Higashi syndrome: autosomal recessive (chromosome 1q43) disorder of microtubule formation with abnormal leukocytes that cannot release enzymes from lysosomes, causing reticuloendothelial incompetence, with recurrent sinopulmonary pyogenic infections, and increased risk of lymphoreticular malignancies. Patients also have neutropenia, lymphocytosis, anemia, thrombocytopenia, and impaired chemotaxis of PMNs. Histologic examination shows giant perioxidase-positive granules in leukocytes.
    - Hermansky-Pudlak syndrome: autosomal recessive (chromosome 10q23) disorder of platelets that leads to easy bruising and potentially lethal bleeding diathesis; usually seen in patients of Puerto Rican descent.
  - Type III: OCA3, gene map locus 9p23, tyrosinase-positive; patients have some pigmentation.
  - Type IV: OCA4, "brown" OCA, chromosome 9p.
- Ocular albinism (OA): skin is normal, but eye tissues are hypopigmented.

- OA1 (Nettleship-Falls albinism): X-linked defect at Xp22 with giant pigment granules (macromelanosomes in retina and skin). Only males have full syndrome; females may have mosaicism (look for subtle iris TID).
- OA2: autosomal recessive.

ANIRIDIA Ocular developmental disorder, especially involving failure of the iris to develop (although usually stump of iris is present). Also has anterior polar cataract, ectopia lentis, corneal pannus (epitheliopathy) from hypoplasia of limbal stem cells, foveal (enlarged FAZ on FA) and ON hypoplasia, nystagmus, and often glaucoma (50–75% angle-closure glaucoma, as iris stump may obstruct TM).

- Two thirds of cases are familial: autosomal dominant; no Wilms' tumor risk.
- One third of cases are sporadic: 98% bilateral; 7q mutation at PAX6 gene, which is adjacent to Wilms' tumor suppressor gene (like RB, need homozygous deletion to form tumor). Thus, a large PAX6 deletion is seen in 20% of patients, who will also get Wilms' tumor (nephroblastoma).
  - Nephroblastoma has 90% mortality if untreated or 10% mortality if treated with chemotherapy and radiation.
  - WAGR syndrome: Wilms' tumor, aniridia, genitourinary abnormalities, and retardation. Also known as 11p- or Miller's syndrome.

CHARGE ASSOCIATION Acronym for the major features of this association: **c**oloboma of the eye, congenital **h**eart disease, choanal **a**tresia, mental **r**etardation, **g**enital and **e**ar anomalies. Need three major signs to make diagnosis. Eye is involved in 80% of cases, with uni- or bilateral coloboma of the iris, retina, choroid, and ON. Rarely may also see micro- or anophthalmos or cataract. Also associated with uni- or bilateral facial palsy, renal anomalies, tracheoesophageal fistula, micrognathia, cleft lip, cleft palate, and omphalocele.

CHROMOSOMAL ABNORMALITIES May involve whole genome (triploidy, tetraploidy, polyploidy) and be numerical (monosomies, trisomies) or structural (translocations, insertions, deletions, or duplications). Unlike genetic mutations involving a single gene, chromosomal changes are larger and involve multiple genes.

- Trisomy 13 (Patau's syndrome): most common chromosomal abnormality associated with congenital ocular malformations. Incidence 1:20,000; associated with advanced maternal age; M = F. Usually involves severe mental retardation, seizures, and holoprosencephaly, and is lethal. May have microphthalmia, anophthalmia, colobomas, cartilage in the CB, PHPV (may be bilateral), and retinal dysplasia.

- 18q-deletion (de Grouchy syndrome): severe mental and motor retardation, short stature, abnormal external ears, microcephaly, nystagmus, and optic atrophy.
- Trisomy 18 (Edwards' syndrome): second most common autosomal trisomy overall (1:6000); F:M = 3:1; associated with advanced maternal age. Every organ system is affected, and condition is lethal; patients tend to die from apnea. May have microphthalmia, anophthalmia, hypoplastic orbits, ptosis, lid phimosis, strabismus, coloboma, congenital glaucoma, and abnormally long eyelashes.
- Trisomy 21 (Down syndrome): many abnormalities seen, including mental retardation, hypoplastic midface, short, protruding tongue, and congenital heart disease (50%). Increased incidence of Alzheimer's disease seen in patients >35 years old, along with retinoblastoma and leukemia. A 1:800 incidence is found after the 75% that are spontaneously aborted. Associated with advanced maternal age; risk for affected subsequent child 1%. Thirty-year survival rate is 71%.
  - Ophthalmic findings: upward slanting palpebral fissures and epicanthal folds, NLDO (33%), syringomas, strabismus (33–50%), astigmatism (20%), keratoconus (15%), cataract incidence (300x), Brushfield's spots in one third of cases, especially light irides (called Wolfring's spots if in non-Down patients), and "spoke wheel" appearance to the vessels as they emerge from the optic disk. Patients have better vision than hearing.
  - Ninety-five percent of cases are from meiotic nondisjunction (trisomy) of chromosome 21, 4% are Robertsonian translocations (heritable), and 1% are mosaic.
- XXY (Klinefelter's syndrome): primary hypogonadism with delay of secondary sex characteristics in males; also developmental delay. Eye findings uncommon.
- XO (Turner's syndrome): females with sexual ambiguity; may have ptosis, cataract, blue sclera, and nystagmus.

CONGENITAL INFECTIONS Maternal infections that particularly cause fetal morbidity; maternal IgM does not cross the blood–placental barrier (mnemonic: TORCH)

- Congenital **t**oxoplasmosis
- **O**ther: HIV/AIDS and syphilis. Fetal syphilitic infection is from maternal *Treponema pallidum* spirochetemia. If mother has primary- or secondary-stage syphilis, then approximately one half of fetuses will be infected. If mother has untreated tertiary syphilis, then about 30% of infants will be infected. Patients may have saddle nose, peg teeth, hearing loss, IK, and salt and pepper fundus appearance.
- **R**ubella: salt and pepper fundus, heart defects, growth retardation, mental retardation, cataract (if early in pregnancy), or glaucoma (if later in pregnancy).

- Cytomegalovirus (CMV) most common congenital infection; 95% are subclinical and have chorioretinitis, optic atrophy, and CNS calcifications. Pathology shows basophilic cytoplasmic inclusions.
- Herpes simplex virus (HSV): 70% are type 2; 60% mortality.

FETAL ALCOHOL SYNDROME (FAS) Multiple systemic and ocular abnormalities, including epicanthal folds, strabismus, blepharophimosis, long eyelashes, microphthalmia, telecanthus, anterior segment dysgenesis, and persistent hyaloid vessel in up to 30% of infants born to mothers who abuse alcohol. May consider disulfiram (Antabuse) treatment.

GOLDENHAR'S SYNDROME, OCULO-AURICULAR-CERVICAL DYSPLASIA Characterized by preauricular skin tags, cervical spine dysplasia, mandibular hypoplasia, hemifacial microsomia, and cardiac defects. May have multiple choristomas (especially limbal dermoids), dislocated lens, Duane's syndrome, and upper lid colobomas.

MUCOPOLYSACCHARIDOSES See Table 9–5 for ophthalmic presentations of mucopolysaccharidoses.

PEROXISOMAL DISORDERS Intracellular organelles that are defected. all disorders are characterized by hypotonia, seizures, and mental retardation.

- Adrenaleukodystrophy: X-linked, incidence 1:15,000. Patients have adrenal insufficiency, spastic paresis, fluctuant vision, and RP.
- Refsum's disease: autosomal recessive disorder of lipid metabolism from decreased phytanic acid alpha-hydroxylase (chromosome 10p) with accumulation of phytanic acid in RPE and serum, causing atypical RP (granular RPE appearance), cerebellar ataxia, peripheral neuropathy, nerve deafness, anosmia, and EKG conduction defects.

TABLE 9–5
Ophthalmic Presentations of the Mucopolysaccharidoses

MPS	Cornea	Glaucoma	RPE	Optic Nerve
Hurler I-H	+++ (6 months)	+	+++	+++
Scheie I-S	+++ (1–2 years old)	+	++ (late)	+
Hunter II	–	+	+/–	++
Sanfilippo III	+ (mild)	–	++	+/–
Morquio IV	+++ (10 years old)	–	–	–
Maroteaux-Lamy VI	+++ (5 years old)	++	–	++
Sly VII	++ or –	–	–	+

Note: All are autosomal recessive, except Hunter's syndrome, which is X-linked recessive.
Spectrum of involvement from (–) not affected up to (+ + +) significant tissue pathology often seen.

Treat with low phytol diet (no dark green vegetables), and maintain body weight.

- Zellweger syndrome, cerebro-hepato-renal disease: cartilage calcification with joint disorder, nonrecordable ERG, and optic atrophy.

SPHINGOLIPIDOSES Cell membrane components are not degraded but instead accumulate in cells.

- Fabry's disease: X-linked deficiency of alpha-galactosidase; 90% have corneal verticillata, tortuous conjunctival and retinal vessels, and posterior spokelike cataract.
- Farber's disease: deficient ceramidase, with cherry red spot.
- Gaucher's disease: deficient glucocerebrosidase, with choroidal and conjunctival macrophage accumulation.
- Krabbe's disease: deficient galactocerebrosidase beta-galactosidase in 50% of patients, with white matter necrosis and cherry red spot.
- Niemann-Pick disease, type B: deficient sphingomyelinase, causing macular halo, hepatosplenomegaly, lung infiltration, bone marrow foam cells, and no mental retardation, unlike the others.
- Sandhoff disease: GM_2 type II gangliosidosis from deficient hexosaminidase alpha, causing a cherry red spot.
- Tay-Sachs disease: GM_2 type I gangliosidosis from defect in hexosaminidase beta, with accumulation in ganglion cells (highest concentration in the macula), causing a cherry red spot, mental retardation, and early death.

WAARDENBURG'S SYNDROME Autosomal dominant developmental anomalies of eyelids, nasal root, and eyebrows, with heterochromia iridis, white forelocks, and sensorineural deafness.

Congenital Disease: Phakomatoses

OVERVIEW The word *phakomatosis* means "lentil, or a spot on the body," because most disorders have skin findings. Most are hamartoma disorders that are autosomal dominant, except the diseases with *W* in their names (Sturge-**W**eber syndrome [SW] and **W**yburn-Mason's syndrome [WM]), which are sporadic, and (ataxia-telangiectasia [AT]), which is autosomal recessive. The diseases with *S* in their names, **S**turge-Weber (SW) and tuberous **s**clerosis (TS) are characterized by seizures.

ATAXIA-TELANGIECTASIA (AT), LOUIS-BAR SYNDROME Autosomal recessive phakomatosis of abnormal DNA repair from chromosome 11q22.3, causing telangiectasias on the face, neck, and conjunctiva; also has cerebellar ataxia, mental retardation, hypoplastic thymus with recurrent sinopulmonary infections; increased lymphoma, leukemia, and insulin resistance; increased glucose; and no CNS abnormalities.

NEUROFIBROMATOSIS I, VON RECKLINGHAUSEN'S DISEASE Classical, peripheral, autosomal dominant phakomatosis with variable penetrance from chromosome 17q-defect (mnemonic: 17 letters in *neurofibromatosis*), characterized by hamartomas of neural crest tissue. Occurs in 1 in 3000 births. Neurofibromas are tumors are from the peripheral nerve sheaths; patients also have CNS tumors such as glioma, meningioma, and increased risk of breast, gastrointestinal, and genitourinary cancers, pheochromocytomas, and cutaneous and uveal melanomas. Diagnosis established by two or more of the following:

- Café au lait spots: six or more >5 mm in children or >15 mm in adults. Pathology shows normal skin except increased pigmentation in the basal layers; present in 99% of NF patients.
- Cutaneous neruofibromas: two or more; can degenerate into fibrosarcomas.
- Plexiform neurofibroma: may cause S-shaped eyelid; 50% of unilateral upper lid plexiform neurofibromas have ipsilateral glaucoma. May cause significant ptosis.
- Axillary or inguinal freckling
- ON glioma: 15% prevalence; fusiform ON enlargement. Glioma is actually a JPA.
- Absence of sphenoid wing: may cause pulsatile proptosis; may have other osseous deformities.
- Lisch nodules: two or more melanocytic hamartomas on the iris; seen in 92% of NF cases. Useful for establishing or excluding the diagnosis because they are not found in normal patients.
- Family history: first-degree relative with NF1.

NEUROFIBROMATOSIS II Central phakomatosis with hamartomas of neural crest tissue, from chromosome 22q defect; characterized by CNS tumors such as acoustic schwannoma. Diagnosis needs one of the following:

- Bilateral acoustic neuroma
- Unilateral acoustic neuroma with first-degree relative affected
- Two of the following: meningioma, glioma (15% prevalence, fusiform and kinked appearance on CT), schwannoma, neurofibroma, presenile PSC cataract
    - Other findings may include pheochromocytoma (15%), Lisch nodules, plexiform neurofibroma, ipsilateral glaucoma with upper lid neurofibroma, prominent corneal nerves, choroidal hamartomas (flat, 51% prevalence), retinal and RPE hamartomas, choroidal melanoma, proptosis from ON glioma, orbital neurofibromas, and sphenoid dysplasia.

ORGANOID NEVUS SYNDROME, NEVUS SEBACEOUS OF JADASSOHN Alopecia anterior to ear and 20% BCC in that area; associated with posterior scleral cartilage, epibulbar complex choristomas, seizures, mental retardation, and cardiovascular, renal, hepatic, skeletal abnormalities.

STURGE-WEBER SYNDROME (SW), ENCEPHALOTRIGEMINAL ANGIOMATOSIS Nonhereditary (sporadic) phakomatosis with unilateral facial cutaneous angioma (nevus flammeus or port-wine stain, usually V_1-V_3 distribution) and choroidal cavernous hemangioma ("tomato catsup" fundus). Thirty-three percent of cases have ipsilateral glaucoma when lid or conjunctiva is involved (60% from congenital trabeculodysgenesis and 40% from late-onset increased EVP). Eighty percent have unilateral meningeal hemangioma with contralateral epileptic attacks, mental retardation, and calcification of gyri ("railroad tracks" on skull films).

- Klippel-Trénaunay-Weber syndrome: bilateral cutaneous hemangioma with extremity hypertrophy and systemic vascular anomalies.

TUBEROUS SCLEROSIS (TS), BOURNEVILLE'S SYNDROME Autosomal dominant (but incomplete penetrance) phakomatosis, from defect on chromosome 16 (50%) and chromosome 9 (50%), with retinal or ON astrocytic hamartomas (50%), seizures (90%), and mental retardation secondary to CNS astrocytic hamartomas ("tubers" or, if calcified, "brain stones"). May also have retinal peripheral depigmentation (ash leaf spot equivalent), fine facial acne (adenoma sebaceum, which is really angiofibromas; seen in 83% of cases), skin ash leaf spots (shagreen patches; pathology shows smaller melanosomes with less pigment; seen in 80% of cases) or café au lait spots, periungual fibromas, renal/pulmonary/bone cysts, and cardiac rhabdomyosarcoma.

VON HIPPEL-LINDAU DISEASE (VHL), ANGIOMATOSIS RETINAE Autosomal dominant phakomatosis, from defect on chromosome 3p- tumor supression gene (controls VEGF production; like RB, patients inherit one hit, then acquire second hit), characterized by capillary hemagioblastomas of the retina fed by dilated tortuous artery drained by engorged vein; may have exudative RD. Up to 60% of cases have a cerebellar hemangioblastoma (vertigo, ataxia), 25% renal cell carcinoma (most common cause of VHL deaths; usually about age 50, with 50% mortality; check urinanalysis for hematuria). May also see renal, pancreatic, or hepatic cysts, meningiomas, and pheochromocytomas; no skin involvement like other phakomatoses. May laser small (<2 DD) retinal lesions or cryotherapy larger ones.

WYBURN-MASON SYNDROME (WM), RACEMOSE HEMANGIOMA Sporadic defect of a single AV communication (no capillary bed; also known as congenital retinal macrovessel) with dilated, tortuous retinal vessels; also found in ipsilateral brain, orbit, and face (reported fatal hemorrhage following dental extraction).

Strabismus: Esotropia

EPIDEMIOLOGY ET comprises 70% of strabismus and may be congenital/infantile or acquired; most are comitant but may be incomitant.

PSEUDOESOTROPIA Wide nasal bridge, prominent epicanthal folds, or negative angle kappa give the appearance of ET, but patient is aligned on cover testing; recheck patient in 3 months.

CONGENITAL OR INFANTILE ESOTROPIA Large-angle (usually >35 pD) constant ET; onset within 6 months. Patients have normal refraction (+1.5 D average) and usually alternate/cross-fixate; thus, amblyopia is sometimes seen. ET is horizontally comitant (pD near = distance) and may have effort nystagmus in abduction. Infantile esotropia is characterized by poor abducting kinetics, usually a positive family history, and is genetic; thus, it is more acurately considered a syndrome. MR may be anteroplaced (i.e., 3.5 mm from limbus). Angle may be variable when associated with cerebral palsy.

- Differential diagnosis: Duane's syndrome type I, nystagmus blockage syndrome, Möbius' syndrome, early-onset accommodative (also known as mixed ET), and congenital CN VI paralysis.
- Associated deviations (in order of prevalence):
  - DVD or combined cyclovertical deviation: seen in 46 to 90% of cases, usually occurs at a later age, seen especially in abduction. Diagnose with remote cover test.
  - IOO: causes V-pattern ET, usually occurs after age 1, and is present in two thirds of patients by age 8.
  - Nystagmus: latent in 50% of cases, which is horizontal jerk when other eye is covered (to get VA, may need to fog with +10 lens and not occlude the other eye). Rotary nystagmus present in 30% of cases; rarely may have manifest nystagmus.
  - Accommodative component: check cycloplegic refraction if the ET "recurs" after initial surgery.
  - Ciancia's syndrome: extreme congenital ET with large angle, LN, restricted movements.
- Treat refractive error first if present (usually not an issue), then treat amblyopia before surgery. Surgical goal is to align within 10 pD of ortho; usually wait until patient is 4 to 6 months old; usually perform bilateral MR recessions or LR resections (Table 9–6). Treat DVD/IOO with anterior transpositions of SO (Harada-Ito procedure). Amblyopia management requires constant surveillance until patient is 7 to 8 years old.
  - Early intervention study: designed to find out if the angle is stable by 4 months. Previously, surgery was usually performed at 18 months.

TABLE 9–6
Surgical Recession and Resection for Esotropia

ET	Recess MR OU	Resect LR OU
15 pD	3.0 mm	4.0 mm
20 pD	3.5 mm	5.0 mm
Increase by 5 pD	Increase by 0.5 mm	Increase by 1.0 mm
50 pD	6.0 mm	10 mm
60 pD	7.0 mm	10 mm

- Surgical goal is monofixation syndrome (horizontal deviation <10 pD, with a scotoma in the nonfixating eye under binocular conditions, with peripheral NRC). Only 39% of patients have stereopsis. No binocular vision if not surgically corrected by age 2 years.

ACCOMMODATIVE ESOTROPIA Cause of 70% of ET and 50% of all strabismus cases; characterized by acquired, comitant, moderate deviation (20–30 pD), with onset at 18 months to 7 years (average age 2.5 years; not surprising, as most neonates are not yet accommodating, and it often takes full accommodation to bring out the ET). Often intermittent and variable, then becomes constant; often hereditary and usually asymptomatic. Patients are either hyperopic or have high AC/A. May be precipitated by trauma, illness, accommodative targets with high spatial frequency, or fatigue at end of the day. Amblyopia is common due to a fixation preference or anisometropia; no motility restriction like acquired CN VI palsy. Have facultative suppression scotoma in the nasal retina (suppression only when eyes are deviated).

- Four subtypes:
  - Nonrefractive (57%): high AC/A (>10 pD near vs. distant shows excessive convergence when patient accommodates); normal refraction. A higher AC/A ratio is predictive of deterioration of PET (Table 9–7).
  - Refractive (43%): hyperope (average + 4.75 D) with normal AC/A and sensitive accommodation
  - Partially accommodative: part congenital ET
  - Decompensated accommodative ET: occurs from delay to spectacles or high AC/A
- Treatment: amblyopia treatment and spectacles, then eventual surgery for residual ET.
  - Spectacles: give full cycloplegic prescription if patient is <6 years old, and give tolerated prescription if patient is >6 years old. Instruct parents to obtain glasses promptly and to use glasses full

TABLE 9–7
Rate of Deterioration of Accommodative Esotropia

AC/A Ratio	Grade	Deterioration
Normal (0–9 pD)	Normal	8%
High (10–19 pD)	I	25%
Moderately high (20–29 pD)	II	44%
Very high (30+ pD)	III	52%

Based on data from Ludwig IH, Parks MM, Getson PR, Kammerman LA. Rate of deterioration in accommodative esotropia correlated to the AC/A relationship. J Pediatr Ophthalmol Strabismus 1988;25:8–12.

time; caution that patient may need to use bifocals and change prescription soon and that glasses are being used to improve alignment, not help the child to see better.

- At follow-up, ask parents if ET is improved and if child is wearing glasses full time; check glasses with lensometer to ensure correct dispensing, and check glasses' fit, patient stereopsis, and fusion and alignment in spectacles. Hold minus lenses in front of prescription; if patient holds fusion, may decrease plus prescription to wean off.
- After visual maturity, can often wean down plus power.

- High AC/A or if ET persists at near with full hyperopic correction. If patient is able to fuse at distance, consider
  - Bifocals: give +3.00 bifocal (write for executive style or large flat-top segment if polycarbonate, which bisects pupil) to decrease near ET.
  - Miotics: parasympathomimetic, long-acting cholinesterase inhibitors facilitate acetylcholine transmission, and augment accommodative response and decrease AC/A ratio (vs. atropine, which increases the AC/A). Echothiophate iodide (PI) 0.125% every AM; at follow-up, look for miosis, ET controlled at distance and near after 3 to 4 weeks, then taper down. Many adverse drug reactions, including ciliary spasm with brow ache, blurred vision, cataract, iris cysts (prevent with concomitant phenylephrine drops), abdominal cramps, nausea, vomiting, diarrhea, salivation, and potentiates depolarizing agents; thus, patient should wear medical alert bracelet.
  - May consider bilateral medial rectus recession (BMRR) with or without Faden procedure.
- Consider surgery if patient has residual >15 pD in glasses. Operate for distance angle plus 1 D or near deviation.
- Prism Adaptation Study: a multicenter, randomized clinical trial (1984–1989) to determine whether preoperative use of prisms

could improve surgical outcome for acquired esotropia. Patients with residual ET > 12 pD after full correction were treated with preoperative use of base-out (BO) Fresnel prism equal to the angle of ET. Responders, defined as simultaneous cover test deviation 0.8 pD or fusion on W4D, had 83% surgical success versus 72% for nonresponders ($p = 0.04$).

CYCLIC ESOTROPIA Comitant, intermittent ET every 48 hours that usually breaks down to constant ET; 1:4000 incidence.

DIVERGENCE INSUFFICIENCY ESOTROPIA ET > at distance; normal neurologic exam. Treat with BO prism.

DIVERGENCE PARALYSIS ESOTROPIA Similar to divergence insufficiency with no fusional vergences; need neurologic work-up to rule out pontine tumors, trauma.

DUANE'S RETRACTION SYNDROME (DRS) Accounts for 1% of all strabismus cases; characterized by horizontal gaze abnormalities (head turn), palpebral fissure narrowing from globe retraction, and up- or downshoot on attempted adduction. Most are sporadic, but some may be familial; usually unilateral, but 20% are bilateral. From congenital agenesis of the abducens nucleus with the LR abnormally innervated by CN III that also supplies the MR. This aberrant innervation violates Sherrington's law. More common in left eye and in females. Associated with cataract, iris abnormalities, Marcus Gunn jaw winking, microphthalmia, crocodile tears, Goldenhar's syndrome, and Klippel-Feil syndrome. Treat amblyopia (present in 10–14% of cases), and consider surgery with MR Faden procedure to reduce the upshoot on adduction (fixate near the equator), or transpose SR and IR over toward the LR. Three types:

- Type I: limitation of abduction (mnemonic: 1 "d" in abduction); most common type. Majority of patients are straight but may have esodeviation. Electromyogram shows no LR electrical activity on abduction with paradoxic activity with adduction.
- Type II: limitation of adduction (mnemonic: 2 "d"s in adduction); majority of patients are straight but may have exodeviation. Electromyogram shows LR active with both adduction and abduction.
- Type III: limitation of abduction and adduction (mnemonic: 3 "d"s in abduction and adduction); least common type. Electromyogram shows both LR and MR active with both adduction and abduction.

INCOMITANT ACQUIRED ESOTROPIA MR or LR restriction or dysfunction as seen with thyroid, postoperative, fracture, myasthenia gravis, and congenital CN VI palsy.

- Beware of late-onset ET: rule out pontine glioma with MRI.
- Abduction deficit of myopia: long axial length with tight MR and abduction deficit.

MIXED CONGENITAL AND ACQUIRED ESOTROPIA Patients born with ET and high hyperopia.

MÖBIUS' SYNDROME Congenital bilateral palsies of CN VI (ET, lateral gaze paralysis), CN VII (flat facies, facial diplegia, weak orbicularis), and CN XII (early suck and feeding problems; atrophy of anterior third of the tongue). No abduction; has adduction with convergence, decreased forced ductions with abduction and adduction. Usually partial and asymmetrical. Also associated with poly-, micro-, macro-, and syndactyly, clubbed feet, and peroneal muscle atrophy (wide-based gait), with or without mental retardation and autism.

NEUROIMPAIRMENT Often seen with cerebral palsy, FAS, meningiomyelocele, and intracranial hypertension. Patients often have hypotonia and strabismus; treat amblyopia, and often delay surgery until other medical issues are resolved.

NYSTAGMUS BLOCKAGE SYNDROME (NBS) Fixating eye adducts and converges to dampen horizontal nystagmus; adduction continues when eye is occluded; head turn toward fixating eye to maintain the adduction; and pupil constricts, indicating accommodative mechanisms. Typically large, variable ET angle as compared with other ETs.

SENSORY ESOTROPIA Poor vision leads to ET and often comitant XT later; often from cataract or media opacities OU, RB (11%), ONH, albinism, aniridia, Leber's amaurosis, and cone or cone-rod dystrophy.

SPASM OF NEAR SYNKINETIC REFLEX Acquired comitant ET, usually in female teenagers with miosis, accommodative spasm, headache, and difficulty reading. Treat with cycloplegia, and give maximum plus in any refraction. Usually benign, but may be associated with posterior fossa tumors.

STRESS-INDUCED ESOTROPIA From illness, trauma, or older age (likely latent accommodative ET).

Strabismus: Exotropia

EPIDEMIOLOGY XT comprises 20% of strabismus cases.

PSEUDOEXOTROPIA Appearance of XT from wide IPD or positive-angle kappa (visual axis falls nasal to the macula), as may be seen in retinopathy of prematurity patients.

EXOPHORIA Latent, manifests with fusion interruption. XT up to 5 pD is normal, and XT of 15 pD is naturally seen in fusion-free states (e.g., sleep).

EXOTROPIA Usually presents at age 1 to 4 years; characterized by squinting in light (patient closes one eye in the sun), tiring with visual tasks, or diplopia, and usually has a normal refraction. May see IOO, DVD, lateral incomitance, A pattern (more XT in downgaze and reading position), V pattern (usually IOO), or X pattern (tight LR). Patient has temporal suppression with ARC and a half-moon-shaped suppression scotoma (compare with ET, which has a tight, small, round scotoma). Typically begins as exophoria, then intermittent XT, then constant XT.

- Intermittent exotropia: fatigue, inattention, or illness brings out XT; caused by "wimpy" convergence. Ninety percent of cases get worse, and some will convert to full-time phoria. Operate at stage II (before constant XT) when the tropia increases and/or there is increased ease of dissociation or poor recovery of fusion (not size of deviation). Exhibits facultative suppression (only when eyes are deviated); thus, during periods of visual concentration, patients often maintain bifoveal fusion and develop excellent stereopsis.
- Constant XT: most are broken down intermittent exotropia; if congenital, look for ocular or systemic problems. Four main types:
  - Basic: distance XT = near XT'
  - Convergence insufficiency: XT < XT' from increased near point of convergence (NPC); comprises 33 to 62% of XT cases. Patients often present with asthenopia and reading complaints. Treat with orthopic exercises with BO prism.
  - Divergence excess: XT > XT'. Differentiate from pseudodivergences excess with 30-minute patch test to dissociate the eyes and reveal the full latent deviation. Then measure with +3.00 add to determine if high AC/A ratio is present; important because these patients are prone to surgical overcorrection (up to 75%). Counsel parents regarding poor surgical alignment prognosis and need for bifocals postop.
  - Pseudodivergence excess: strong convergence and accommodation, causing appearance like XT > XT', but after 30-minute patch test, the XT = XT' (knocks out fusional and accommodative vergence, and NPC is normal).
- Treatment: treat amblyopia, over-minus the hyperope, and give myopes their full prescription; try orthoptics for convergence insufficiency and prisms for small angle deviation. May try 3-month patching

trial of the fixating eye half time or alternate eye patching. If the tropia converts to a phoria, may delay surgery; if not, go to surgery.

- Surgery goal is to preserve good binocular fusion; thus, operate when patient is X(T). If patient has constant XT, operate for diplopia, asthenopia, or cosmesis. R & R the amblyopic eye versus unilateral or bilateral lateral rectus recession (BLRR) if small angle (corrects about 3 pD per millimeter of muscle weakened). Do vertical offset for A or V pattern if there is no oblique overaction.
- A pattern or bilateral SOO: may cut SO to correct 10–15 pD in primary and 40–45 pD in downgaze, but must have >45 pD downgaze deviation, 3–4+ SOO, and no IOO. In patients with high-grade stereopsis, SO tenotomies could cause consecutive SO paresis with intractable torsional diplopia; thus, may want to do vertical offsets or Wright SO silicone expander (controls amount of SO weakening, is reversible, and alleviates the hypertropia in side gaze).
- IOO: surgery if >2+ or 10–15 pD in upgaze, 5 pD in primary (do not have to factor this into the primary measurement).
- Aim for overcorrection in children, often 10–20 ET postoperative, as half will have gradual exodrift (0.5 pD/year). The other half remain stable; 5 to 10% need reoperation.

CONSECUTIVE EXOTROPIA XT following ET; comitant; spontaneous or seen after trauma or surgery.

FAMILIAL CONSTANT EXOTROPIA Large angle in infancy with strong family history; image if no family history elucidated (50% neurologic pathology).

SENSORY EXOTROPIA Monocular decreased VA causing a large-angle, progressive XT. Patients may have difficulty fusing ("horror fusionus") following surgery for long-standing dense cataract that caused them to lose the ability to fuse.

Strabismus: Vertical Deviations

EPIDEMIOLOGY Comprises 4% of strabismus cases. Most are incomitant, but some may be comitant.

PSEUDODEVIATIONS May be caused by vertically displaced macula (positive or negative angle lambda), eccentric fixation, ptosis, orbital asymmetry, or process displacing globe vertically.

BROWN'S SYNDROME SO tendon or trochlea restriction, causing limitation of elevation in adduction; typically unilateral, but may be bilateral in 10% of cases. Patients have overshoot in downgaze with adduction; eye may be hypotropic; may have PF widening. May remember by mnemonic Brown bREAD (**r**estriction of **e**levation in **ad**duction). Also known as "canine tooth syndrome" (dog bite that severs the trochlea). Patients must have positive forced ductions (differentiates Brown's from IO palsy), and usually have head tilt toward the affected side (looks like a big IO underaction without SO overaction).

- Slight predominance in females and right eye. May be congenital or acquired (e.g., collagen-vascular disease).
- Treat for head tilt or diplopia in primary gaze; wait if acquired, as condition may improve spontaneously. Typically treat with SO tendon expander or weakening procedure.

COMITANT HYPERDEVIATION Often seen in older patients with small angle and mild diplopia from muscle contractures. Treat with prism, or recess one vertical muscle if <15 pD or two muscles if >15 pD, but avoid vertical R & R (may cause lid asymmetry).

CONGENITAL FAMILIAL FIBROSIS Rare EOM restriction of unknown etiology causing incomitant strabismus that is uni- or bilateral.

DISSOCIATED VERTICAL DEVIATION (DVD) During periods of visual inattention or under cover, the eye slowly elevates, extorts, and abducts, then drops down when uncovered. No corresponding hypotropia of fellow eye on ACT; thus, because the fixating eye shows no associated movement, DVD does not respect Herring's law. The hypertropia is the same in abduction, adduction, and primary gaze, unlike IOO (hypertropia greatest in field of action). May be torsional or horizontal, and usually latent but may be manifest. Variable; usually OU, but rarely symmetric. Worse DVD eye is usually amblyopic.

- Often seen with LN and 40 to 75% of ET cases (60–80% of congenital or infantile ET). Caused by early disruption of binocular development (seen in flatfish normally).
- Measure out-of-field of action with a base-down prism; Krimsky method, grade 1–4+. Bielschowsky's phenomenon: DVD recenters and fixates as neutral density filters are placed over other eye.
- Treatment: benign neglect, but if there are manifest or functional problems, may do SR recession, IR resection, with or without Faden procedure. Usually do OU symmetric surgeries; if IOO, then do IO transposition and anteriorization (makes it a depressor).

DOUBLE-ELEVATOR PALSY, MONOCULAR ELEVATION DEFICIT (MED) Unilateral limitation of upgaze in all fields (unlike Brown's syndrome), from supranuclear deficit of SR and IO (both eye elevators) with or without IR restriction (rule out blowout fracture). Hypotropia in the involved eye increases with upgaze. Twenty-five percent of cases are associated with Marcus Gunn jaw winking (especially with ptosis). No surgery is recommended unless there is large vertical deviation or diplopia in primary gaze. If forced ductions are positive, then do IR recess; if negative, then do transposition of horizontals toward SR.

ENDOCRINE MYOPATHY Incomitant deviation from TRIO; positive forced ductions; affected muscles IR > MR > SR > LR. Treat with Fresnel prisms; when TRIO and deviation are stable (after orbital decompression and before lid surgery), may operate, but do recessions only.

INFERIOR OBLIQUE OVERACTION (IOO) Elevation in adduction; primary cause unknown, secondary cause is SO palsy (hypertrophy of antagonistic muscle). Incomitant; not variable; usually presents in infancy. Has a V-pattern ET because IO is an abductor, and has hypotropia in the other eye (unlike DVD). Measure in field of action (adduction); determine how many millimeters vertical difference there is between the 6 o'clock limbus light reflections of both eyes (1+ if 1 mm, 2+ if 2mm, etc.). Treat primarily for cosmesis with myectomy, myotomy, or a graded recession (1+ = 6 mm, 2–3+ = 10 mm, 4+ = denervation/extirpation).

INHIBITIONAL PALSY OF THE CONTRALATERAL ANTAGONIST Incomitant "fallen eye" syndrome when fixating with the nonparetic eye. For example, when fixating with a paretic right SR, the left SR overacts and may look like a paretic left IR. From Herring's law, the secondary deviation is > than the primary.

ISOLATED CYCLOVERTICAL PALSY Incomitant deviation, usually from CN paresis; most are SO palsies. Always rule out trauma, myasthenia gravis, and thyroid or neurologic/demyelinating disease. Five steps in the work-up:

- Isolate with three-step test; for example, a right hypertropia that is worse in left gaze and right head tilt = right SO palsy. (See Table 9–8.)
- Compare ductions to versions.
- Measure torsion: synoptophore, double Maddox rod, or pencil test, or look at fundus.
- Look at old photos: "FAT" scan (**f**amily **a**lbum **t**omography) for compensating head position.
- Look for suppression scotoma on W4D.

ISOLATED IO PALSY A pattern (ET in upgaze); etiology unknown. Rule out Brown's syndrome.

TABLE 9–8
Three-Step Test for Vertical Strabismus

Hypertropia	Worse with	Worse with	Affected Muscle
Right hypertropia	Right gaze	Right head tilt	Left IO
		Left head tilt	Right IR
	Left gaze	Right head tilt	Right SO
		Left head tilt	Left SR
Left hypertropia	Right gaze	Right head tilt	Right SR
		Left head tilt	Left SO
	Left gaze	Right head tilt	Left IR
		Left head tilt	Right IO

ISOLATED IR PALSY Local trauma is leading cause (e.g., retrobulbar needle muscle trauma); wait 6 months to ensure stability before surgery. Differential diagnosis: includes blowout fracture or double elevator palsy.

ISOLATED SO PALSY Common cause of hypertropia that increases with ipsilateral head tilt because the two incyclotorters (SO and SR) try to work to counteract the tilt and because the SO is palsied, the SR overacts, thus causing increased elevation and hypertropia.

- Congenital SO palsy: uncertain onset, prominent head tilt, no subjective torsion or diplopia, with large vertical deviation and fusional amplitudes; may have facial asymmetry on the dependent side and ptosis.
  - If fixation preference is present, may have contralateral SR underaction (inhibitional palsy of the contralateral antagonist), or the contralateral IR can undergo contracture (double elevator palsy).
  - Patients usually have a flaccid SO tendon, so tuck until tight, and recess the contralateral IO.
- Acquired SO palsy: acute onset of variable vertical deviation; head tilt not as prominent; positive subjective torsion; good fusion and spread of comitance (trying to fuse). Etiology includes trauma, diabetes, HZV, muscle disease, vascular lesions, or tumor.
  - Unilateral SO palsy: tilt in one direction, small angle, V-pattern ET, <10 degrees excyclotorsion, large hyperdeviation.
  - Bilateral SO palsy: tilt both directions, large V-pattern ET, >10 degrees excyclotortion (double-Maddox rod test), chin down position, no tilt, small hypertropia in primary.
  - Treatment: prisms or surgery for large vertical deviation, diplopia, and abnormal head position. If <15 pD, do one muscle surgery; if >15 pD, do two muscle surgeries. Operate for gaze position with

the most diplopia. For torsion, may do Harada-Ito procedure (split SO, and advance the anterior/torsional half). If deviation is worse up and nasal, then weaken the IO or resect SR. If it is worse down and nasal, then recess IR (if torsion is not a big problem), or tuck the SO (will have iatrogenic Brown's syndrome).

ISOLATED SR PALSY Very rare; usually from orbital disease or superior blowout fracture.

SKEW DEVIATION Acquired, incomitant, supranuclear vertical deviation that is a diagnosis of exclusion. Rule out muscle, cranial nerve palsy, and myasthenia. See Chapter 8.

Surgery

STRABISMUS GENERAL PRINCIPLES Conjunctival incision may be fornix based (better cosmesis, often limited view), limbal (better view), or direct (Swan). Hook the IR from the nasal side, LR superior (don't sweep broadly or may incorporate IO fibers), SR temporal (don't get SO), MR superior and pass muscle hook in a tangential plane. Always clamp before cut, and generally use a spatulated needle with Vicryl suture.

ADJUSTABLE SUTURING Best for re-operations, TRIO, small angle deviations, or diplopic patients.

BOTULINUM TOXIN (BOTOX) Muscle injection to weaken the muscle that is antagonistic to the muscle causing the strabismus. Best for nonrestrictive strabismus, XT or ET < 40 pD; also small-angle strabismus, early postoperative over-/undercorrections, cyclic ET, and acute paralytic strabismus (muscle contraction begins within 6–8 weeks). Botulinum toxin type A binds to acetylcholine receptors on presynaptic motor nerve terminals and interferes with release of acetylcholine into the synaptic cleft.

- Injected IM produces localized chemical denervation muscle paralysis within 2 days, lasting 5 to 8 weeks in EOM and 3 months in the orbicularis.
- Do not exceed 200 units in 1 month. Use 0.1 cc for EOM injection and electromyogram (EMG) lead on the needle to localize the muscle; have the patient sit up afterward.
- Side effects: 17% have ptosis or vertical strabismus complications; also diplopia and spatial disorientation. No systemic toxicity (injected dose is 1/100 of the toxic dose).

HORIZONTAL OFFSETS For hyper- or hypodeviation; 1 pD = 1 mm graded response.

INFERIOR OBLIQUE MUSCLE (IO) SURGERY Weaken with myotomy or recession. Fibers are interspersed with orbital fat; thus, use care when bluntly dissecting (risk of adherence syndrome). Often has multiple insertions; use care to not disinsert the IR, and cut IO under direct visualization. Can cut it free, move IO to the border of IR (small recession), 3 mm posterior to IR (large recession), or anterior transposition.

SUPERIOR OBLIQUE MUSCLE (SO) SURGERY Isolate from the nasal side, but cut laterally (lies 4 mm posterior to SR insertion). Weaken with myotomy, tuck, or expander (may use 6 or 8 mm retinal band). Strengthen with resections (variable techniques) or tuck, which is good after scleral buckle procedure or multiple muscle procedures (does not compromise ciliary arteries) and for congenital palsy (usually has a long, floppy tendon); fold tendon, and place permanent suture.

STRENGTHENING PROCEDURES Resections increase the length-tension curve. Pass double-arm partial thickness suture in a "weaving" fashion through the muscle; two-loop locking pass at each side of muscle. Pull up muscle, cut tendon, measure forward, and reattach anteriorly, or cut section out of muscle and reattach at insertion.

TRANSPOSITIONS Several variations, including Knapp (two muscles, full tendon), Jensen (split muscle and suture together), and Hummelstein (take half of SR/IR and move lateral).

- Harado-Ito procedure: anterior half of SO is torsional, posterior half is vertical, so split the tendon and advance the anterior half to the border of LR to enhance incyclotorsion.
- A or V patterns: horizontal muscle offset changes the vector of forces and can correct up to 30 pD of and A or V pattern without significant IOO. Move MR toward the apex of the A or V, and move the LR the opposite direction a half tendon width to correct up to 15 pD (only if there is no oblique overaction).

WEAKENING PROCEDURES Recessions in effect "lengthen" the muscle, giving it more "play," by moving its insertion more posterior. Pass a double-arm suture partial thickness through the muscle, in a "weaving" fashion, then do two-loop locking pass at each side of muscle. Pull up muscle, cut tendon, measure back, and reattach.

- Marginal myotomy: Z myotomy, not accurate or often used; attenuates the length-tension curve.
- Faden procedure: posterior fixation suture for nystagmus dampening, DVD, etc. The procedure "tacks" the muscle to the globe without moving tendon (changes the arc of contact in field of gaze, but not in primary gaze). Use permanent suture (Mersilene, etc.).

STRABISMUS SURGERY COMPLICATIONS

- Adherence syndrome: occurs if orbital fat is violated; not easily treated.
- Anterior segment ischemia: short posterior ciliary arteries are compromised when muscles are disinserted, and the long posterior ciliary arteries are tasked more to provide blood supply to the anterior segment. Thus, usually do only two muscles at a time, as ischemia is likely to some degree after three-muscle surgery, even in young healthy eyes. May see cornea edema, Descemet's folds, and iritis. Treat as iritis in general.
- Astigmatism: usually with-the-rule and resolves within 6 weeks.
- Conjunctival inclusion cyst: pale, nontender, cystic nodule; if excised, use caution, as cyst may extend deeply. May cause dellen.
- Conjunctival scarring: usually from Tenon's layer that was closed or reapproximated too close to the limbus, or plica semilunaris on the bulbar conjunctiva violated.
- Eyelid changes: widening of palpebral fissure with SR or IR recession or narrowing of PF with SR or IR resection.
- Foreign body granuloma: red, tender nodule from suture reaction.
- Globe perforation: 1:100 incidence with scleral passes. Do a DFE intraoperative if you are suspicious of perforation, then cryotherapy or laser around the needle track. Usually benign unless there is VH, RD, or infection. Dilate all strabismus patients at one of the postoperative visits looking for the "snake eyes" (two holes) appearance of a perforation; if there are RPE changes around the site, then there is a low risk of any future complications and can tell patient it has scarred around the area.
- Infection: preseptal or orbital cellulitis, usually within 72 hours.
- Malignant hyperthermia: rare (incidence 1:6000–30,000) but carries a 10% mortality (historically 70%); triggered by succinylcholine or inhalational anesthetics (not local anesthetics). Ptosis, strabismus, and porphyria patients are at increased risk.
  - Earliest signs are tachycardia and increased end tidal CO_2, then unstable blood pressure, tachypnea, sweating, muscle rigidity, cyanosis, dark urine (increased CPK in 2/3), and a rise in temperature later.
  - Treat with dantrolene 2–3 mg/kg up to 10 mg (muscle relaxant that stabilizes cell membranes and prevents release of calcium from sarcoplasmic reticulum); stop anesthetics, cool, hydrate and hyperventilate the patient with O_2, and treat acidosis.
- Pupil changes: IO surgery may damage parasympathetic fibers to the pupil.
- Slipped muscle: diminished muscle function; can find it in its capsule and can usually reattach the muscle.
  - Lost muscle: can often find it against the orbital wall.

- Unsatisfactory alignment: can reoperate in 6 weeks; most cases of horizontal strabismus have a gradual trend toward exodeviation over many years.

Other

INFANT WITH DECREASED VISION Give a vision estimate (<20/70 normal, >20/200 legally blind), but avoid using the word *blind* with the patient's parents. Check VF when older in order to counsel caretakers about the field of vision. Always give genetic counseling when appropriate (failure to do so is the leading cause of malpractice in pediatric ophthalmology).

- Vision estimate: recognize parents (patient age 2–3 months when the fovea develops), OKN response = at least 20/200, and reactive pupils are good signs. Poor vision signs include nystagmus (usually 20/200 or worse), wandering eye movements, staring at bright lights, oculodigital massage.
- Usually a sensory anomaly, typically accompanied by a horizontal nystagmus and decreased VA. Etiology includes (mnemonic: NOSE):
  - **N**eurologic disease: cerebral palsy, anoxia, seizures, etc.
  - **O**bvious diagnosis on exam: cataract, glaucoma, aniridia, toxoplamosis scar, retinopathy of prematurity, ONH, optic atrophy, etc.
  - **S**ubtle disorder: albinism, etc.
  - **E**RG abnormality: CSNB, achromatopsia, Leber's congenital amaurosis

CHAPTER 10

Medications

General

PHARMACOKINETICS Average drop = 50 μL; however, the tear lake holds only 10 μL. Tear turnover is 16% per minute; thus, approximately 50% remains at 4 minutes. Most drops act by first-order kinetics: a constant fraction is absorbed and eliminated (e.g., 100 → 50 → 25 → 12.5, etc.).

DRUG PERMEABILITY Penetration into the eye is dependent on
- Lipid solubility: characterized by the partition coefficient; a higher coefficient indicates more lipid solubility and thus greater permeability. Partition coefficient = (drug in lipid phase) ÷ (drug in aqueous phase).
- Corneal permeability: cornea structure is soluble to fat (epithelial layer), then water (stroma), then fat (endothelial layer). Thus, the more lipid that is soluble, the greater the permeability, up to a point. Surfactants and increased concentration of the drug (up to the point of increased tearing) increase corneal permeability.
- Ionization status: Henderson-Hasselbach equation demonstrates that a substance with higher pH is more nonionized or uncharged and is more lipid soluble.

Antibacterials: Aminoglycosides

PROPERTIES Bind 30S bacterial ribosomal subunit, irreversible and thus bactericidal. Active against many gram-negative and staphylococcal organisms.

AMIKACIN 20–50 mg/mL fortified topical, 0.4 mg intravitreal.

GENTAMICIN (Garamycin) 1 drop every 4 hours or ½ inch ribbon of ointment bid–tid (solution 0.3%, ointment 0.3%).

NEOMYCIN Significant topical hypersensitivity.

TOBRAMYCIN (Tobrex) 1 drop every 1 to 4 hours or ½ inch ribbon of ointment every 3 to 4 hours or bid–tid (solution 0.3%, ointment 0.3%), or fortified topical 14 mg/mL solution, 0.1–0.2 mg intravitreal. Slightly more active against *Pseudomonas* than gentamicin.

Antibacterials: Cephalosporins and Penicillins

PROPERTIES Beta-lactam antibiotics that inhibit bacterial transpeptization enzymes necessary for cell wall synthesis; bactericidal.

CEFAZOLIN (Ancef) 50 mg/mL fortified topical solution or 100 mg subconjunctival injection. First-generation cephalosporin that is active against most gram-positive cocci.

CEFTAZIDIME 2.25 mg intravitreal. Third-generation cephalosporin with greater activity against gram-negative organisms, including *Pseudomonas.*

PENICILLIN G 200,000 units/mL fortified topical, 1 million units subconjunctival, 2 million to 18 million units intravenous every 4 to 6 hours. Active against most streptococci, gonococci, and anaerobes. Most staphylococci produce beta-lactamase and are resistant. Hypersensitivity in 3 to 10%.

Antibacterials: Fluoroquinolones

PROPERTIES Inhibits bacterial DNA gyrase, thus interfering with DNA replication; bactericidal and inhibitory. Active against most gram-negative organisms, staphylococci, and many streptococci. Avoid fluoroquinolones in children, as they may inhibit cartilage and growth plate development.

CIPROFLOXACIN (Ciloxan) 1 gtt every 1 to 6 hours or ½ inch ribbon ointment bid–tid (solution 0.3%, ointment 0.3%). Second-generation fluoroquinolone.

GATIFLOXACIN (Zymar) 1 gtt every 1 to 6 hours (solution 0.3%). Fourth-generation fluoroquinolone.

LEVOFLOXACIN (Levoquin, Quixin) 1 gtt every 1 to 6 hours (solution 0.5%). Third-generation fluoroquinolone.

MOXIFLOXACIN (Vigamox) 1 gtt every 1 to 6 hours (solution 0.5%). Fourth-generation fluoroquinolone.

NORFLOXACIN (Chibroxin) 1 drop every 2 to 6 hours (solution 0.3%).

OFLOXACIN (Ocuflox) 1 drop every 1 to 6 hours (solution 0.3%).

Antibacterials: Inhibitors of Cell Wall Function

BACITRACIN Ointment every 3 to 4 hours or bid–qid. Polypeptide that inhibits early steps in peptidoglycan synthesis. Treats *Neisseria, H. flu, Actinomyces*, and most gram-positive bacteria.

POLYMYXIN B AND GRAMICIDIN Detergent-like action to increase cytoplasmic membrane permeability. Polymyxin B is mixture of basic peptides that dissolve cell membranes with greatest activity against gram-negative bacteria.

VANCOMYCIN Fortified topical 50 mg/mL, 1 mg in 0.1 mL intravitreal, 2 g every 6 to 12 hours intravenous. Inhibits early steps in peptidoglycan synthesis. High level of activity against most gram-positive cocci and bacilli.

Antibacterials: Inhibitors of Nucleic Acid Synthesis

PYRIMETHAMINE Inhibits conversion of dihydrofolic acid into tetrahydrofolic acid, but also more active against host cell and thus more toxic than trimethoprim; bacteriostatic.

RIFAMPIN Binds to bacterial DNA-dependent RNA polymerase.

SULFACETAMIDE (Sulamyd, Bleph-10, Sulf-10, Isopto Cetamide) 1 drop every 2 to 6 hours (solution 10, 15, 30%) or ½ inch ribbon of ointment every 3 to 8 hours (ointment 10%). Bacteriostatic inhibition of folic acid synthesis by competing with PABA for conversion into dihydrofolic acid. Active against many gram-positive, gram-negative, *Chlamydia, Actinomyes,* and *Nocardia* organisms.

TRIMETHOPRIM Inhibits conversion of dihydrofolic acid into tetrahydrofolic acid; bacteriostatic.

Antibacterials: Inhibitors of Protein Synthesis

CHLORAMPHENICOL (Chloroptic) 1 drop every 4 to 6 hours (solution 0.5%), or small amount of ointment up to every 3 hours (ointment 1%), or make 5 mg/mL fortified topical drops from 100 mg subconjunctival solution. Binds to the 50S ribosomal subunit; bacteriostatic. Active against many gram-positive, gram-negative, and anaerobic organisms. Idiosyncratic fatal aplastic anemia occurs with similar frequency to that of fatal anaphylaxis following penicillin therapy (about 1 in 50,000); also, can cause dose-related bone marrow suppression.

CLINDAMYCIN 50 mg/mL fortified topical. Binds the 50S subunit of bacterial ribosomes.

ERYTHROMYCIN (Ilotycin, AK-Mycin) ½ inch ribbon of ointment every 3 to 4 hours or bid–qid (ointment 0.5%). Binds ribosomal 50S subunit. Similar activity to penicillin against gram-positive bacteria; also active against *Hemophilus, Neisseria,* and *Chlamydia.*

TETRACYCLINE Binds 30S bacterial ribosomal subunit like aminoglycosides but has reversible binding and is thus bacteriostatic. Active against many gram-positive, gram-negative, *Chlamydia, Actinomyes,* and *Mycobacterium* organisms.

Antibacterials: Combinations

NEOSPORIN (neomycin + bacitracin + polymyxin B) 1 drop every 1 to 6 hours for 7 to 10 days or ½ inch ribbon of ointment every 3 to 4 hours for 7 to 10 days.

POLYSPORIN (polymyxin B + bacitracin) ½ inch ribbon of ointment qid or every 3 to 4 hours for 7 to 10 days.

POLYTRIM (polymyxin B + trimethoprim) 1 gtt every 3 to 6 hours for 7 to 10 days, maximum 6 drops/day.

Antibacterial and Corticosteroid Combinations

CORTISPORIN (neomycin + polymyxin + hydrocortisone 1%) 1 drop or ½ inch ribbon of ointment every 3 to 4 hours.

MAXITROL (dexamethasone + neomycin + polymyxin) 1 drop every 1 to 8 hours or ½–1 inch ribbon of ointment qd–qid.

TOBRADEX (tobramycin + dexamethasone) 1 drop every 2 to 6 hours or ½ inch ribbon of ointment bid–qid.

Antifungal Agents

AMPHOTERICIN B (AMB) 0.15% topical every 30 to 60 minutes initially for fungal corneal ulcers (mix AMB powder with sterile water), 5–10 μg intravitreal or 1 mg/kg/day intravenous for fungal endophthalmitis (limited by renal toxicity). Highly effective polyene antibiotic against a broad range of fungi.

IMIDAZOLES Inhibit ergosterol in fungal cell membranes, but activity is limited by metabolism. Clotrimazole, miconazole, econazole, ketoconazole, and thiabendazole all may be made into topical preparations.

NATAMYCIN (Natacyn, Pimaricin) 5% solution every 1 hour (50 mg/mL). Only commercially available topical antifungal. Polyene binds to sterols, damaging cell membranes of filamentous fungi, with activity similar to AMB; especially active against *Fusarium* and *Aspergillus*. Local hypersensitivity reaction is common, but it is the least toxic of the polyenes.

TRIAZOLES Action similar to imidazoles but less vulnerable to host metabolic degradation. Fluconazole (most active against *Candida*) and itraconazole may be made into a topical preparation.

Anti-inflammatory: Allergy

ANTAZOLINE, PHENIRAMINE, PYRILAMINE Traditional antihistamines.

AZELASTINE (Optivar) 1 gtt bid. Dual-mechanism antihistamine and mast cell stabilizer.

COMBINATION ANTIHISTAMINE PLUS OCULAR DECONGESTANT Naphcon-A, AK-Con-A, Opcon-A (pheniramine + naphazoline), Vasocon-A (antazoline + naphazoline).

CROMOLYN SODIUM (Crolom, Opticrom) 1 drop 4 to 6 times per day (solution 4%). Inhibits mast cell degranulation and thus blocks histamine release; used for prevention of allergic effects, not acute treatment.

EMEDASTINE (Emadine) 1 gtt qid (solution 0.05%). Potent, selective H_1-antagonist.

KETOTIFEN (Zaditor) 1 gtt every 8 to 12 hours (solution 0.025%). Mast cell stabilizer.

LEVOCABASTINE (Livostin) 1 gtt qid (suspension 0.05%). Long-acting, highly potent, and selective H_1-antagonist.

LODOXAMIDE (Alomide) 1 drop qid (solution 0.1%). Mechanism similar to cromolyn.

NAPHAZOLINE (Albalon, AK-Con, Vasocon, Naphcon) 1 gtt every 3 to 4 hours prn up to qid (solution 0.012, 0.02, 0.03, 0.1%). Vasoconstrictor that provides symptomatic relief by decreasing conjunctival edema and hyperemia.

OLOPATADINE (Patanol) 1 drop bid (solution 0.1%). Dual action as a mast cell stabilizer and highly selective H_1-antagonist antihistamine.

PEMIROLAST (Alamast) 1 gtt qid (solution 0.1%). Mast cell stabilizer.

Anti-inflammatory: Antifibrotic

5-FLUOROURACIL (5FU): 50 mg/mL, 0.1 mL in 5–10 subconjunctival injections post-trabeculectomy, or 50 mg/mL on sponge for 3 to 5 minutes intraoperative. Pyrimidine analogue, inhibits thymidylate synthesis and DNA synthesis, incorporated during and aborts S phase, inhibits fibroblast proliferation; application effective for about 3 weeks. Epithelial toxic. Also used in breast, gastrointestinal, and skin CA.

MITOMYCIN C (MMC) 0.2–0.5 mg/mL, 2 mL administered intraoperatively. Alkylating agent that cross-links DNA, not cell cycle specific; dose is effective for about 5 hours. Has 100× > potency than 5FU. May cause avascular blebs, wound leak, hypotony, and intraocular toxicity.

Anti-inflammatory: Corticosteroids

PROPERTIES Binds to cytoplasmic glucocorticoid receptor that binds to DNA to increase or decrease gene transcription (over 100 steroid-responsive genes). Clinical effects include decreased capillary permeability, chemotaxis inhibition, and suppression of fibrin deposition.

- Also decreases eicosanoids (lipids derived from arachidonic acid in the cell membrane phospholipids):
  - Inhibits cyclooxygenase-created prostaglandins: vasodilation, increased permeability of blood–ocular barrier, corneal neovascularization, decreased IOP via prostaglandin E2, prostaglandin D2, and prostaglandin F2-alpha.
  - Inhibits lipoxygenase-created leukotrienes: chemotactic for PMNs and eosinophils, conjunctival and uveal edema, immune modulation.
- Also decreases platelet-activating factor, cytokines, tumor necrosis factor, nitrous oxide, and adhesion molecules. Downregulates ICAM-1, which is responsible for white blood cell (WBC) migration, and decreases growth factors and beta-adrenergic receptors.
- May suppress endogenous steroids from adrenal cortex; created from cholesterol into corticosteroids (21 carbons) or androgens (19 carbons).

DEXAMETHASONE (Decadron, Maxidex, AK-Dex) 1 drop every 1 to 8 hours or ½–1 inch ribbon of ointment qd–qid (suspension 0.1%, solution 0.1%, ointment 0.05%). Has >48 hours half-life; 30–40× more potent than hydrocortisone. Alcohol derivative is more effective than dexamethasone sodium phosphate.

FLUOROMETHOLONE (FML, FML Forte, Flarex) 1 drop every 1 to 12 hours or ½ inch ribbon of ointment every 4 to 24 hours (suspension 0.1, 0.25%, solution 0. 1%, ointment 0.1%). Fluorinated structural analogue of progesterone that is less effective than dexamethasone or prednisolone but with a lower potential for elevating IOP. Acetate derivative (Flarex) is more effective than alcohol derivative (FML).

LOTEPREDNOL (Alrex, Lotemax) 1 drop qid (suspension 0.2, 0.5%).

MEDRYSONE (HMS) 1 gtt up to every 6 hours (suspension 1%). Least potent topical steroid.

PREDNISOLONE (AK-Pred, Pred Forte, Pred Mild) 1 gtt every 1 to 12 hours (suspension 0.12, 0.125, 1%, solution 0.125, 1%]. Has 12- to 36-hour half-life and is 4× more potent than hydrocortisone.

RIMEXOLONE (Vexol) 1 drop every 1 to 6 hours (suspension 1%). Synthetic steroid that has same anti-inflammatory efficacy of 1% prednisolone but no greater risk of elevated IOP than fluorometholone.

Anti-inflammatory: Nonsteroidals

PROPERTIES Blocks prostaglandin synthesis by inhibiting cyclooxygenase (and some affect lipoxygenase).

DICLOFENAC (Voltaren) 1 gtt qid (solution 0.1%) or 75 mg PO bid. Inhibition of postsurgical inflammation. Oral preparation has less bleeding than other nonspecific NSAIDs.

FLURBIPROFEN (Ocufen) Used for allergy or inhibition of intraoperative miosis (solution 0.03%).

KETOROLAC (Acular) 1 gtt qid (solution 0.5%). Relief of allergic conjunctivitis itch and inhibition of postsurgical inflammation.

ORAL AGENTS Aspirin, ibuprofen, indomethacin, etc. Celecoxib (Celebrex) and others selectively inhibit COX-2 enzyme and thus have decreased systemic side effects.

SUPROFEN (Profenal) 1 gtt qid (solution 1.0%).

Antiseptics

BENZALKONIUM CHLORIDE (aqueous zephiran)

CHLORHEXIDINE GLUCONATE (Hibiclens) 4% solution

POVIDONE-ETHYL ALCOHOL SOLUTION

POVIDONE-IODINE SOLUTION Lowers conjunctival bacterial counts preoperatively and is effective for ophthalmia neonatorum prophylaxis. Lowest risk of conjunctival and corneal toxicity of all the antiseptics.

SILVER NITRATE 1% solution used for ophthalmia neonatorum prophylaxis (however, it is not active against *Chlamydia*). May cause local argyrosis (black deposits in the conjunctiva).

Antiviral Agents

ACYCLOVIR (Zovirax) For HSV, use 200–400 mg PO 5x/day for 7 to 10 days, or HZV 600–800 mg 5x/day for 10 days; use IV if immunosuppressed. All current antivirals are virostatic.

- Synthetic guanosine analogue that is tri-phosphorylated by thymidine kinase (TK) to acyclovir triphosphate. The triphosphate accumulates in infected cells and competes with doxyguanosine triphosphate for viral DNA polymerase and terminates replication after incorporated into DNA.
- 200× greater affinity for viral thymidine kinase (TK) than mammalian cell TK, thus low toxicity. Activity greatest for HSV-1 > HSV-2 > HZV > EBV > CMV.
- Most viral resistance is from alteration of TK gene.

CIDOFOVIR Nucleotide analogue inhibits viral DNA polymerase, used for CMV infection; does not require viral activation; long intracellular half-life. May cause profound hypotony (CB destruction) and severe uveitis (14% of intravitreal usage).

FAMICICLOVIR (Famvir) 500 mg PO every 8 hours to treat HZV and genital herpes, typically treated for 7 days.

FOMIVIRSEN (Vitravene) Exonuclease used as intravitreal injection for CMV retinitis.

FOSCARNET Inhibits CMV DNA and RNA polymerase, demonstrates improved AIDS survival; use limited by nephrotoxicity.

IDOXURIDINE (IDU) First topical antiviral, pyrimidine nucleoside, similar to thymidine and incorporated into DNA; very toxic.

GANCYCLOVIR May be delivered PO, IV, or intravitreal. Structurally similar to acyclovir, as it is phophorylated to gancyclovir triphosphate; blocks DNA polymerase and is incorporated into DNA instead of doxyguanosine. Is 10–20x more active than acyclovir against CMV, equally active against HSV and EBV, and has 10x greated affinity among virus-infected cells.

PROTEASE INHIBITORS HAART has demonstrated increased CD4 count, decreased HIV load, improves CMV retinitis, and may cause increased CME (overall a good sign, in that the body is responding with inflammation).

TRIFLURIDINE (Viroptic) For HSV, 1 gtt every 2 to 4 hours for 7 to 14 days, maximum 9 drops/day (solution 1%). Structural analogue of thymidine and is thus incorporated into viral DNA; also directly inhibits thymidylate synthase.

VALACYCLOVIR (Valtrex) 1 g PO tid; begin at earliest signs of HZV or genital herpes, typically for 7 days, and adjust dosage for renal insufficiency. Prodrug that is converted to acyclovir in small intestine and liver; increased concentration with concurrent cimetidine; effective for HZV.

VIDARABINE (Vira-A) ½ inch ribbon of ointment bid up to 5 times daily for 5 to 7 days (ointment 3%).

Glaucoma: Beta-Blockers

PROPERTIES Decreases cAMP in ciliary epithelium, which causes decreased active secretion and thus decreased aqueous production. Peak 2 hours, some effect up to 4 weeks; 10 to 20% of patients do not respond. Additive effect to most drops (especially miotics), except epinephrine/dipivefrin. See Table 10–1 for side effects and precautions.

BETAXOLOL (Betoptic, Betopic-S) 1 drop bid (suspension 0.25%, solution 0.5%). Beta-1 cardioselective (safer to use in mild, intermittent asthma, but generally should not be used in CHF). Less IOP control than nonselectives; possibly increased ON blood flow (may be better in NTG); more additive effect with Propine.

TABLE 10–1
Beta-Blocker Precautions

Side Effects		Contraindications
Bronchospasm	Confusion or depression	Asthma
Bradycardia	Impotence	Obstructive pulmonary disease
Arrhythmia	Masked diabetic hypoglycemic symptoms	Heart block
Hypotension		Congestive heart failure
Syncope	Exacerbated myasthenia gravis	Cardiogenic shock
Decreased HDL cholesterol	Punctate keratitis	Hypersensitivity
	Corneal anesthesia	

CARTEOLOL (Ocupress) 1 gtt bid (solution 1%). Nonselective with intrinsic sympathomimetic activity (decreased systemic effects), better lipid profile, less ocular irritation.

LEVOBUNOLOL (Betagan) 1 drop qid–bid (solution 0.25, 0.5%). Nonselective.

METIPRANOLOL (Optipranolol) 1 gtt bid (solution 0.3%). Nonselective; inexpensive. May cause rare granulomatous uveitis.

TIMOLOL (Timoptic, Betimol) 1 gtt bid (solution 0.25, 0.5%). Timoptic XE: 1 gtt qam (solution 0.25, 0.5%). Nonselective; decreases IOP up to 30%. Substantial systemic levels may be obtained with topical usage; thus, decreased effectiveness if on systemic beta-blocker.

Glaucoma: Carbonic Anhydrase Inhibitors

PROPERTIES First discovered in the ciliary epithelium, carbonic anhydrase (CA) is a zinc metalloenzyme that catalyzes the reversible hydration of CO_2 to bicarbonate. Carbonic anhydrase inhibitors have free sulfonamide ($-SO_2\ NH_2$) linked to aromatic ring that competes with bicarbonate binding to CA in its acidic form → decreased bicarbonate synthesis → decreased Na+ and water influx → decreased aqueous production by up to 30%. See Table 10–2 for side effects and precautions.

ACETAZOLAMIDE (Diamox) 250 mg PO up to qid (immediate release) or 500 mg PO up to bid (Diamox Sequels or timed-release) (tablets 125, 250, extended release capsules 500 mg). In addition to lowered IOP, resultant

TABLE 10–2
Carbonic Anhydrase Inhibitor Precautions

Side Effects		Contraindications
Paresthesias	Hemolysis	Sulfa allergy
Dizziness	Aplastic anemia (sulfa)	Kidney or liver disease
Confusion	Gastrointestinal upset	Na^+/K^+ depletion
Tinnitus	Polyuria	Hyper-Cl acidosis
Anorexia	Kidney stones	Chronic obstructive lung disease
Metallic taste	Stevens-Johnson syndrome	

metabolic acidosis may increase ON perfusion and increase visual function. May cause hypokalemia when used with K^+-depleting diuretics such as Lasix and HCTZ. Not metabolized but excreted in urine. Diamox Sequels are better tolerated but have limited immediate effect.

BRINZOLAMIDE (Azopt) 1 gtt tid (suspension 1%). Less acidic, less stinging, but blurs vision more than dorzolamide. Can be dosed bid with a beta-blocker.

DICHLORPHENAMIDE (Daranide) 50 mg PO qd–tid. Many side effects, thus not commonly used in humans (veterinarians often use it).

DORZOLAMIDE (Trusopt) 1 gtt tid (solution 2%). Most common adverse effect is superficial punctate keratitis and local allergy. Can be dosed bid with a beta-blocker.

COSOPT (dorzolamide 2% + timolol 0.5%) 1 gtt bid.

METHAZOLAMIDE (Neptazane) 25–50 mg bid–tid. Has longer half-life than Diamox, is better tolerated and metabolized in the liver, not primarily excreted by the kidneys; thus, there are fewer stones and less metabolic acidosis (also less potent).

Glaucoma: Hyperosmotics

GLYCERIN (Osmoglyn) 1.0–1.5 g/kg PO (50%). Nauseating; give with cracked ice.

ISOSORBIDE (Ismotic) 1.5 g/kg PO (45%). Preferred in diabetic patients, as it is a nonmetabolized sugar.

MANNITOL (Osmitrol) 0.5–2.0 g/kg IV (5–20%). Because solutes are freely filtered by the glomerulus, serum osmolarity is increased and vitreous volume is decreased by 3 to 4%, resulting in decreased IOP. More potent than urea.

UREA (Ureaphil) 0.5–2.0 g/kg IV (30%).

Glaucoma: Miotics/Cholinergic, Direct Acting

PROPERTIES Parasympathetic agents that mimic the effect of acetylcholine on muscarinic nerve endings. Used to lower IOP by stimulation of the longitudinal ciliary muscle to pull open and increase outflow through the TM (also closes intramuscular spaces and thus causes decreased uveoscleral outflow). In addition, may be used in the control of accommodative esotropia. Miotics cause accommodation and miosis and thus may have decreased patient compliance.

ACETYLCHOLINE (Miochol) Up to 3 mL intraocular; short acting.

CARBACHOL (Isopto Carbachol, Miostat intraocular) 1 drop tid (solution 0.75–3%), or intraocular injection 0.5 mL. Dual action as a direct muscarinic cholinergic agonist and also indirect-acting agent. Longer acting than Miochol.

PILOCARPINE (Pilocar, Isopto Carpine, Ocusert P-20 and P-40) 1 drop tid–qid or ½ inch ribbon of gel at bedtime (solution 0.25, 0.5, 1.0, 2.0, 3.0, 4.0, 5.0, 6.0, 8.0, 10%, gel 4.0%). Solution effect peaks in 2 hours, and half-life is 6 hours. Gel decreases IOP for 18 to 24 hours. Ocusert is left in place for 5 to 7 days and releases 20 μg (equivalent to 1% drop qid) or 40 μg (equivalent to 2% qid). Works as a direct muscarinic agonist. Used for glaucoma control, prior to LPI, and 0.125% solution confirms an Adie's tonic pupil from supersensitive denervated smooth muscle. Binds to melanin; thus, increased dose is needed in darker irides.

- Cautions: RD potential from longitudinal ciliary muscle traction on the vitreous base. Young myopes may have increased myopia with miotics from increased convexity of lens and forward lens movement. Miosis causes nyctalopia and is especially troublesome in older patients with cataracts. May increase relative pupillary block; thus, 4% is contraindicated in acute and chronic angle closure, as there is increased anterior movement of the lens–iris diaphragm. Avoid in patients with uveitis who may have increased inflamation and pain; with chamber shallowing, may have posterior synechiae and may progress to pupillary block.

- Pilocarpine used with phospholine iodide (PI) actually causes slight pupillary dilation because acetylcholine (potentiated by PI) binds stronger than pilocarpine, which acts to displace acetylcholine from its receptor.
- Mnemonic: "4-3-2" rule: pilocarpine maximum concentration is 4% and is used qid, carbachol maximum is 3% and is dosed tid, and echothiophate maximum is 0.25% and is used bid.

Glaucoma: Miotics/Cholinergic, Indirect Irreversible

PROPERTIES Acetylcholinesterase is a ubiquitous enzyme in all cell membranes that hydrolyzes acetylcholine to inactive choline + acetic acid. Acetylcholinesterase inhibitors allow individual acetylcholine molecules to repeat their effect at muscarinic receptors (miosis, accommodation, longitudinal ciliary muscle) and with some agents at nicotinic receptors (as with edrophonium). Used in glaucoma to stimulate the longitudinal ciliary muscle that pulls open the TM. See Table 10–3 for side effects and precautions.

DEMECARIUM BROMIDE (Bromide) Indirect-acting cholinesterase inhibitor that irreversibly carbamylates acetylcholinesterase. Most carbamylating agents are shorter acting (physostigmine, enostigmine, pyridostigmine) and not used for glaucoma, except demercarium, which is longer acting.

DIISOPROPYL PHOSPHOROFLUORIDATE (DFP) Similar to phospholine iodide, irreversibly phosphorylates acetylcholinesterase.

TABLE 10–3
Cholinergic Precautions

Side Effects		Contraindications
Salivation	Myopia	Concurrent MAOI use
Lacrimation	Cataract	Anterior uveitis
Urination	Miosis	RRD risks (relative contraindications in young, high myopes)
Diarrhea	AV heart block	
Gastrointestinal upset	Bronchoconstriction	
Excessive sweating	Confusion, ataxia	
Pupil cysts	Hypotension	
Brow ache	Bradycardia	

AV, atrioventricular; MAOI, monoamine oxidase inhibitor.
Mnemonic: SLUDGE describes the common side effects.

ECHOTHIOPHATE IODIDE (phospholine iodide) 1 gtt bid (solution 0.03, 0.06, 0.125, 0.25%). Needs to be fresh and refrigerated. Indirect-acting cholinesterase inhibitor; longer duration and more potent than direct-acting agents. Used to lower IOP and decrease AC/A ratio in accommodative ET; also, is an insecticide that could be used topically for lice infestation of the eyelashes. Use only in pseudophakes or aphakes, as miosis is poorly tolerated in phakic patients.

- Irreversible phosphorylates not only acetylcholinesterase of the synaptic cleft and also pseudocholinesterase in the plasma that may cause prolonged succinylcholine paralysis and potentiate ester-type local anesthetics (like tetracaine, not lidocaine).
- Systemic side effects are uncommon, but there are many local effects: orbicularis or ciliary muscle spasm, intense miosis, cataractogenic (primarily in adults), iris pigment epithelium cysts (usually in children; may be prevented by coadministration with phenylephrine to constrict the dilator muscle), disruption of blood–aqueous barrier, anterior subcapsular cataract, punctal stenosis, and pseudopemphigoid.
- Treat overdose of phosphorylating cholinesterase inhibitors acutely with pralidoxime (2-PAM) that also treats organophosphate poisoning (e.g., insecticides).

Glaucoma: Prostaglandin Analogues

LATANOPROST (Xalatan) 1 gtt qhs (solution 0.005%]. Onset 2 to 3 hours and works by enhancing uveoscleral outflow (thus, theoretically not useful in acute increased IOP or ACG, although it may help). Prodrug that is changed by corneal esterases into acidic form that acts at the ciliary body to mimic prostaglandin F2-alpha (from arachidonic acid). This increases matrix metalloproteinase (MMP) enzyme release, causing degradation of extracellular matrix collagen and thus increased uveoscleral outflow. Up to 25 to 35% decreased IOP (approximately equivalent to timolol bid). May cause a permanent increased brown iris pigmentation or heterochromia, exuberant eyelash growth, and may increase postoperative CME or inflammation. Dose before pilocarpine, as it decreases latanoprost's access to uveosceral outflow.

BIMATOPROST (Lumigan) 1 gtt qhs (solution 0.03%). A prostamide analogue that works like latanoprost, except a higher concentration is needed because the corneal esterases do not cleave it. Causes conjunctival hyperemia.

TRAVAPROST (Travatan) 1 gtt qhs (solution 0.004%). Similar to latanoprost.

UNOPROSTONE (Rescula) 1 gtt bid (solution 0.15%). Prostanoid (docosanoid) with action similar to latanoprost.

Glaucoma: Sympathomimetics

APRACLONIDINE (Iopidine) 1 drop tid (solution 0.5, 1.0%]. Mainly used perioperatively for anterior segment laser treatment.

- Action: relatively selective $alpha_2$-adrenergic agonist that inhibits norepinephrine release from sympathetic nerves that are destined for beta-receptors in the ciliary epithelium (thus, it is an indirect beta-blocker). This leads to decreased aqueous humor formation and may increase uveoscleral outflow.
- Side effects: may cause follicular conjunctivitis and vasovagal response; up to 33% of patients develop tachyphylaxis. Some $alpha_1$ effect seen that causes pupil dilation, lid retraction, and does not cause systemic hypotension like clonidine.

BRIMONIDINE (Alphagan) 1 gtt bid–tid (solution 0.2%) now released as Alphagan P (0.15%) with a different preservative and less side effects.

- Action: highly selective $alpha_2$-adrenergic agonist (same mechanism as Iopidine) that decreases aqueous formation by up to 20%. Also increases uveoscleral outflow, and theoretically may be neuroprotective.
- Side effects: dry mouth, headache, fatigue, conjunctival blanching, lid edema, depression, syncope; in children, has been reported to cause respiratory distress or arrhythmias. Contraindicated with MAOI, use and use caution with concomitant beta-blockers or other antihypertensives, cardiac glycosides, and tricyclic antidepressants.

DIPIVEFRIN (Propine) 1 gtt every 12 hours (solution 0.1%).

- Action: nonselective prodrug of epinephrine that penetrates cornea better because it is more lipophilic. It is transformed by corneal esterases into active epinephrine; thus, it allows a 0.1% strength to be dosed rather than epinephrine (0.5%, 1.0%, 2.0%) and causes fewer systemic side effects than epinephrine.
- Side effects: often causes toxic follicular conjunctivitis or contact dermatitis.

EPINEPHRINE (Epifrin, Glaucon, Epinal, Eppy/N, Epitrate) 1 gtt qd–bid.

- Action: nonselective alpha and beta agonist that decreases aqueous formation acutely (may also have a paradoxical increased IOP) and increases uveoscleral and TM outflow by $beta_2$ stimulation. This leads

TABLE 10–4
Sympathomimetic or Adrenergic Agonist Precautions

Side Effects	Contraindications	
Hypertension	Cardiovascular disease	Narrow angles
Tachycardia	Hypertension	Aphakia
Arrhythmia		

to increased cAMP and decreased outflow resistance and thus decreased IOP by up to 20%.
- Side effects: mydriasis may precipitate ACG in narrow angles, may cause adrenochrome deposits, rebound hyperemia, hypertension, headache, and CME in aphakes and pseudophakes. See Table 10–4 for sympathomimetic precautions.

Immunosuppressives: Antimetabolites

AZATHIOPRINE (Imuran) 1 mg/kg up to 100 mg PO qid for RA, Wegener's granulomatosis, pars planitis, VKH, sympathetic ophthalmia, Behçet's syndrome (2.5 mg/kg), increased corneal graft survival in high-risk eyes, scleritis, and OCP. Purine analogue, active as 6-MP, causes decreased T-cell mediated immunity, slow activity.

METHOTREXATE (Rheumatrex) 5–25 mg every week for RA, scleritis, or chronic uveitis. Folate analogue that inhibits dihydrofolate reductase (DHFR) conversion to tetrahydrofolate → decreased purine nucleotide and thymidylate synthesis → decreased DNA synthesis. Give folinic acid (Leucovorin), a DHFR coenzyme, to protect normal tissues. Inhibits proliferating tissues (malignancy, bone marrow, gastrointestinal); causes decreased B and T lymphocytes. Hepatotoxic, pulmonary fibrosis, and gastrointestinal toxicity adverse reactions.

Immunosuppressives: Alkylating Agents

CHLORAMBUCIL (Leukeran) Like Cytoxan, very slow acting. Causes bone marrow suppression and reproductive organ damage (thus, offer sperm or egg banking prior to use).

CYCLOPHOSPHAMIDE (Cytoxan) 1–2 mg/kg for Wegener's granulomatosis and many other uses. Nitrogen mustard; causes decreased humoral and cellular immunity. May be myelotoxic (leukopenia, macrocytic anemia, thrombocytopenia) and cause nausea, sterility (thus, bank sperm or eggs prior to use), hemorrhagic cystitis, increased risk of infection and malignancy. Has slow onset. Check CBC weekly for first month, then every other week for 2 months, then monthly, and check liver function tests occasionally.

Immunosuppressives: Noncytotoxic

LEFLUNOMIDE (ARAVA) Decreases T cells; used in RA and chronic uveitides.

MYCOPHENALATE MOFETIL (CellCept) Decreases T and B cells.

COLCHICINE Decreased PMN response; inhibits leukocyte migration.

CYCLOSPORINE (Neoral) 2.5–5.0 mg/kg/day in two doses for many diseases, such as uveitis, Wegener's granulomatosis, and corneal melts, to delay rejection in high-risk corneal grafts (91% success if cyclosporine begun 2 days before surgery), severe vernal or ligneous keratoconjunctivitis, and RA. Topical cyclosporine (Restasis) is available for inflammatory dry eye syndrome.

- Action: affects cell-mediated (T-cell) immunosuppression. Binds intracellular receptor (cyclophilin), like FK-506, altering gene regulation and decreasing many modulators, especially interleukin-2. Metabolized by cytochrome P-450.
- Side effects: nephrotoxic; may cause hypertension and infection.

DAPSONE 25 mg bid; adjust to clinical response and to keep the hematocrit about 30%. Used for immune complex disease and diseases mediated by PMN (OCP has a 70% response). May cause hemolytic anemia, especially with G-6-PD deficiency; avoid in patients with sulfa allergy.

ETANERCEPT (Enbrel) Soluble tumor necrosis factor (TNF)-alpha receptor, which decreases the levels of TNF.

FK-506 Like cyclosporine but more potent; inhibits T-cell function. Cytoplasmic receptor inhibits genes for interleukin-2, -3, and -4, interferon gamma, TNF-alpha, granulocyte colony stimulating factor, and c-myc gene that is normally responsible for early T-cell activation.

INFLIXIMAB (Remicade) Decreased TNF (bound by monoclonal AB), may be effective in chronic uveitis.

Miotics: Cholinergic, Indirect Reversible

(See also Glaucoma: Miotics)

EDROPHONIUM (Tensilon) Reversible indirect nicotinic (parasympathomimetic) agonist that competitively inhibits acetylcholinesterase by binding to the active site of ganglia and skeletal muscle. Used in diagnosis of myasthenia gravis with 2 mg IV rapidly injected followed in 1 minute by 8 mg if first dose had no effect. May have muscarinic side effects (cholinergic crisis: sweating, nausea, vomiting, salivation, and fever) unless atropine 0.5 mg is coadministered.

NEOSTIGMINE (Prostigmin) Reversibly carbamylates acetylcholinesterase. Used to treat myasthenia gravis.

PHYSOSTIGMINE (Eserine) Parasympathomimetic indirect-acting cholinesterase inhibitor that reversibly carbamylates acetylcholinesterase. Used to treat atropine overdose 0.25 mg SQ every 15 minutes up to 4 mg. Also is a louse respiratory poison.

Mydriatics and Cycloplegics: Anticholinergic

ATROPINE (Isopto Atropine) 1 drop before procedure or qd, or ointment qd (solution 0.5, 1.0%, ointment 1.0%). Muscarinic antagonist. Used for cycloplegia, lasts 5 to 10 days; mydriasis lasts 7 to 14 days. Also used to treat ciliary block (malignant) glaucoma and to block oculocardiac bradycardia during surgery with 1 gtt of 1% solution = 0.5 mg (same as ACLS for bradycardia). Treat atropine overdose with physostigmine 0.25 mg every 15 minutes until symptoms resolve. See Table 10–5 for anticholinergic precautions.

CYCLOPENTOLATE (AK-Pentolate, Cyclogyl, Pentolair) 1 drop in 1–2 doses before procedure or examination (solution 0.5, 1.0, 2.0%]. Cycloplegia lasts 6 to 24 hours; mydriasis lasts up to 1 day.

TABLE 10–5
Anticholinergic Precautions

Side Effects		Contraindication
Mydriasis	Flushing	Narrow angles (relative)
Blocks accommodation	Fever, tachycardia	
Increased IOP	Delirium	
Lid swelling	Conjunctival hyperemia	

HOMATROPINE (Isopto Homatropine) 1 drop before procedure or bid–tid (solution 2.0, 5.0%). Cycloplegia and mydriasis can persist 1 to 3 days.

TROPICAMIDE (Mydriacyl) 1 drop before procedure (solution 0.5, 1.0%). Cycloplegia and mydriasis effects last up to 6 hours.

Mydriatics: Adrenergic

PHENYLEPHRINE (Neo-Synephrine, Mydfrin, Relief) 1–2 drops before procedure or examination (solution 0.12, 2.5, 10.0%). No cycloplegic effect; mydriasis may last up to 5 hours.

Neurologic Medications

BOTULINUM TOXIN TYPE A (Botox) 2.5–10.0 units/10 mL (100 units/bottle). Lyophilized (freeze dried) with human albumin (may cause antibodies to develop over years of use, causing increased resistance to Botox effects). Unopened preparation is stable for 2 years; keep refrigerated, with no light exposure. Unstable and should be used in about 2 hours once reconstituted with normal saline.

- Action: binds presynaptic nerve terminals to block acetylcholine release. Neurologic toxins A through G serotypes, related to tetanus toxin. Activated by proteolytic cleavage by bacteria in human gut. Heavy chain responsible for cell entry; light chain gives toxicity. Binds preferentially at cholinergic nerve (i.e., striated muscle) membrane, internalizes (heavy chain), then intracellular poisoning by light chain by possible enzyme effect. Irreversible, but symptoms return due to new nerve growth (perhaps small effect from deactivation).

COCAINE Blocks norepinephrine reuptake and causes pupillary dilation normally, but not in Horner's syndrome.

HYDROXYAMPHETAMINE (Paredrine) Stimulates release of norepinephrine and thus causes pupillary dilation to confirm a third-order neuron lesion in Horner's syndrome.

LIDOCAINE Amide-type anesthetic hepatically inactivated, longer duration.

NEUROMUSCULAR BLOCKING AGENTS (NICOTINIC PARASYMPATHETIC ANTAGONISTS) Nondepolarizing (curare-like gallamine and pancuronium) or depolarizing (succinylcholine and decamethonium), which causes initial muscle contraction. Generally avoid depolarizing agents during general anesthesia for open globe repair cases to avoid EOM contraction. Anticholinergic side effects (like mydriatics): flushing, fever, tachycardia, and delirium

PROPARACAINE (Ophthaine, Ophthetic) 1–2 drops before procedure (solution 0.5%). Do not prescribe for unsupervised use, as corneal toxicity may occur with repeated use. Agent of choice for obtaining corneal cultures.

TETRACAINE (Pontocaine) 1–2 drops or ½–1 inch ribbon of ointment before procedure (solution 0.5%, ointment 0.5%]. Opens ion channels to prevent neuroconduction. Ester-type local anesthetic inactivated by serum cholinesterase (increased risk of systemic toxicity with cholinesterase deficiency as with phospholine iodide, pesticide, exposure, and some congenital conditions). Increased hypersensitivity reaction versus amide-type. Do not prescribe for unsupervised use, as corneal toxicity may occur with repeated use. Disrupts intercellular tight junctions with increased epithelium permeability to topical agents.

TEGRETOL 200 mg bid–tid. Used for seizures, also for chronic pain syndromes. May cause drowiness, nausea, vomiting, and aplastic anemia.

Other Agents

ARTIFICIAL TEARS (Tears Naturale, Hypotears, Lacrilube) 1–2 drops tid–qid prn. Lubrication ointment: Refresh PM Paralube.

BENZALKONIUM CHLORIDE Quaternary ammonium preservative in about 60% of ophthalmic solutions. Antimicrobial that also increases drug penetration by causing mild corneal epithelial disruption.

DAPIPRAZOLE (Rev-Eyes) AND THYMOXAMINE Alpha-blockers that compete with norepinephrine at alpha-1 receptors on the iris dilator muscle and thus reverse phenylephrine mydriasis with incomplete effect on cholinergic (tropicamine, etc.) mydriasis. Produces miosis without effect on accomodation or AC depth.

HYPERBARIC OXYGEN Used to treat arterial gas embolism, chronic CME, rhino-cerebro-orbital mucormycosis, radiation optic neuropathy, and potential reoxygenation following CRAO. Side effects include myopic shift, CWS, and cataract.

SERUM-DERIVED TEARS Two drops every 2 hours used for severe ocular surface disease and after limbal stem cell transplant. Prepare from eight vials whole blood, centrifuge, pipet off the top serum that contains growth factors, and put in bottles. Freeze whatever will not be used within the next couple of days.

THIMEROSAL Organic mercurial preservative found in about 15% of ophthalmic solutions. Allergic sensitivity common.

TISSUE PLASMINOGEN ACTIVATOR (TPA) 12.5 μg/0.1 mL, inject 0.05 mL in the AC or vitreous for fibrin dissolution.

Index

Page numbers in italics indicate that the entry on that page is in a figure or a table.